RED BIOTECHNOLOGY

The Editors

Dr Anjani Singh Tomar is Associate Professor of Law at GNLU. She is recipient of 5 Gold medals from Devi Ahilya Vishwavidyalaya, (DAVV) Indore, for holding merit positions in LL.B. (Hons) & LL.M. exams. She is also holder of M.Sc. degree in Clinical Bio-Chemistry from Holkar Science College, DAVV, Indore. She passed her NET (Law) exam in 2008 & received Ph.D. degree in 2010. She has an experience of more than 11 years as a faculty in Law. She has written books on variety of subjects including labor law, information technology, taxation laws, intellectual property laws etc. She is editor of leading journal of the country, The GNLU Law Review. She has published the papers in leading journals of the country as well. She has also worked as faculty of law at Indore Institute of Law, Indore, & University of Petroleum & Energy Studies, Dehradun.

Dr Viralkumar B. Mandaliya is an Assistant Professor – Research at Gujarat National Law University, Gandhinagar. He was awarded with "Bharat Shiksha Ratan" by Global Society for Health and Educational Growth, Delhi, and "Young Scientist" by Venus International Foundation, India. He hold numerous member positions of Scientific and Educational Society and Council. He has pursued several short term courses from WIPO, Geneva; agMOOCs, Ministry of HRD, GOI; EUIPO, Spain. He has numerous publications (national and international), book and book chapters, paper-presentations to his credit.

RED BIOTECHNOLOGY

Dr Anjani Singh Tomar

Dr Viralkumar B. Mandaliya

2019

Daya Publishing House®

A Division of

Astral International Pvt. Ltd.

New Delhi – 110 002

ISBN: 978-93-5124-962-7 (HB)

Published by : **Daya Publishing House®**
A Division of
Astral International Pvt. Ltd.
– ISO 9001:2015 Certified Company –
4736/23, Ansari Road, Darya Ganj
New Delhi-110 002
Ph. 011-43549197, 23278134
E-mail: info@astralint.com
Website: www.astralint.com

Digitally Printed at : Sanat Printers

Acknowledgements

Team members would like to acknowledge the Government of Gujarat for graciously accepting the research project "The Key Development in Biotechnology and its Impact on the Society, and Creation of Techno-legal Awareness towards the Recent Trends in Biotechnology" to be conducted by GNLU. We are equally obliged & thankful to Director, Gujarat National Law University, Prof. (Dr.) Bimal N Patel, Professor of Law, who have posed his confidence & trust in our team and have given us this opportunity to bring our research into success. We are also thankful to Dean, Research division, Prof. (Dr.) Ranita Nagar, who has been a source of encouragement to us. We would like to thank all the members of Research Division, with special reference to Mr. Rahul B. Pandya, who has been instrumental in the completion of the research project and this book. We would also like to acknowledge the administrative support given to us by the Registrar's office, GNLU.

The entire project and the book could not take up the shape without the hard efforts put in by our Project Assistant, Ms. Urvi Vacchheta. She, being the active support to us, has really worked very hard to bring our project into reality. We are very thankful to her whole hearted contribution, in every aspect of our project.

We are most thankful to the contributions made by Dr. Bindu Vijay, Asst. Professor of Science & Tech. at GNLU in completion of this book.

We express our sincere thanks to all the contributing authors for their contributions that resulted in this book. We also express our sincere thanks to Astral Publishers especially Mr. Kanav for his support and suggestion to bring it in a form of book.

We would also like to thank all our friends and family members who have directly and indirectly supported us to bring out this book.

Preface

Biotechnology is a broad area and its development is dependent on relationship with various disciplines of science. The term "Biotechnology" derives from three Greek words: *bios* - life; *techno* – technology and *logos* - thinking. There exist a vast variety of definitions of Biotechnology. Presumably the most general one is given by the United Nations Convention on Biological Diversity, 1992, which states that "Any technological application that uses biological systems, living organisms, or derivatives thereof, to make or modify products or processes for specific use." Biotechnology has diverse applications. From producing food to designing baby, biotech today is considered as million dollar industry. Today industry and researchers use biotechnology as a tool in their process to a greater extent in a diverse manner.

This diversity has, in turn, brought about the need for a system to classify biotechnology uses based on common features or final purpose. As a result, nowadays there exist **five** main groups in biotechnological applications, which have been identified by a color system.

Red Biotechnology brings together all those biotechnology uses connected to medicine which includes producing vaccines and antibiotics, developing new drugs, molecular diagnostics techniques, regenerative therapies and the development of genetic engineering to cure diseases through genetic manipulation. It also includes reproductive technologies.

White Biotechnology comprises all the biotechnology uses related to industrial processes - that is why it is also called "industrial biotechnology". It includes the use of microorganisms in chemicals production, the design and production of new materials for daily use (plastics, textiles, etc.) and the development of new sustainable energy resources such as biofuels.

Green Biotechnology is focused on agriculture as working field. It includes creating hybrid varieties, new plant varieties and transgenic plants of agricultural interest using modern biotechnology, producing biofertilizers and biopesticides etc.

Purple Biotechnology deals with different domains of Intellectual Property such as Patents, Trademarks, Copyrights and Geographical Indications. It is connected with inventions and trade in biotechnology, especially in an economically globalised scenario, where technology transfers by way of intellectual property protection is now part of global trade.

Blue Biotechnology is based on the exploitation of aquatic and marine resources to create products and applications of industrial interest. Sea has covered ¾ of the planet where diversity of sea creatures is enormous. The researcher has explored a huge portion of the ocean and a lot of species, yet many mysteries are waiting to be discovered.

The present book on the topic **"Red Biotechnology"** aimed at finding out the issues and challenges in medical field and how they can be addressed. The contributions were invited from the people involved in medical field as well as people involved in regulatory framework of issues pertaining to medical biotechnology. The articles have covered the substantive matter from India and abroad. We believe that this edited book will be useful not only to scientific community but also to others who are involved in policy making.

Editors

Contents

Chapter 1

Electroactive Biofilms: Application in Microbial Fuel Cell

Ambika Arkatkar[1,2], Preeti Sharma[2], Arvind Kumar Mungray[1]

[1]Department of Chemical Engineering, Sardar Vallabhabhai National Institute of Technology, Surat, India.

[2]Department of Biotechnology, Veer Narmad South Gujarat University, Surat, India.

Email: saregadesh@gmail.com; preetisharma26@yahoo.com; amungray@yahoo.com

Abstract

The presence of biofilm is a very common feature of our day to day life. Biofilm harbors microbes of varied nature and in varied combinations. The use of microbes in the form of biofilms to remove environmental contaminants, like heavy metals, radio nuclides, oil spills, nitrogen compounds and for the purification of waste water is a popular research area. Biofilms which have electroactive properties are finding their application in the form of the possible source for simultaneous energy generation system and also as a waste water treatment agent. Microbial fuel cell (MFC) systems works on the electroactive nature of microbes in a biofilm, which has the capacity to transfer electrons exogenously towards the external electron acceptor (Electrode). This chapter is an effort towards discussing the various factors that affect the formation of electroactive biofilm in MFC, features of biofilm that can affect the functionality of MFC system, microbes reported to be present in the biofilm, mechanism of electron transfer by the microbes and techniques those are used so far for analyzing biofilm growth in MFCs and inferences to be driven from them.

1. Introduction

In natural environment we can broadly differentiate microbial existence in two types- (i) freely existing; planktonic type and (ii) attached to a surface; sessile type. The sessile forms of microbes when densely get attached to any surface, forms a film like colonial structure termed as 'Biofilm'. A biofilm can be defined as *"a sessile microbial community having cells which are attached to a surface (either biological or non-biological), embedded in an exo-polysaccaride matrix that demonstrate an altered phenotype"* (Characklis *et al.*, 1990; O'Toole *et al.*, 2000; Shirtliff *et al.*, 2000; Garret *et al.*, 2008). First documentation of biofilms was done in 1674 by Antonie van Leuwenhoek. He observed the aggregates from human tooth under a microscope and described them as "animalcules" (Costerton *et al.*, 1999; Garret *et al.*, 2008]). Nearly 99% of microbial population in the world is found in the form of a biofilm. These films are as diverse as the microbial population (Dalton & March, 1998). In environmental conditions biofilms may include cells of one or many microbial species (Garret *et al.*, 2008). Generally biofilm is encased in Extracellular Polymeric Substance (EPS) (Read *et al.*, 2010; Schechter *et al.*, 2014; Baranitharan *et al.*, 2015). The number and type of surfaces and environments, both living and nonliving, that have been inhabited by biofilms are almost infinite (Garret *et al.*, 2008).

Formation of biofilm is one of the survival tactics of microbes acquired under adverse environmental conditions (Kokare *et al.*, 2009). Many industries like dairy (Teh *et al.*, 2015), food, oil, paper (Houdt & Michiels, 2010), water systems (Percival *et al.*, 2000), dentistry and hospitals (Sandholm & Wirtanen, 1992) suffer the hazardous effects of biofilm growth. Product spoilage, corrosion, unpleasant odors/mal-odors, unsightliness, infection (hospital related nosocomial infections and/or contamination in dairy, food and slaughter industry), pipe blockages, fouling and equipment failure (Sandholm & Wirtanen, 1992; Kokare *et al.*, 2009) are examples of the negative side effects of biofilms.

Despite of the hazards caused by the formation of biofilm, scientists are exploring the usefulness of biofilms, especially in the field of bioremediation and biodegradation. Though the use of microbes in the form of biofilms to remove contaminants, like heavy metals (Barkay & Schaefer, 2001), oil spills (Radwan *et al.*, 2002), nitrogen compounds (Celmer-Repina, 2010) and for the purification of industrial waste water is well known on laboratory scale, but little success has been achieved in its large scale applications (Garret *et al.*, 2008).

Microbial Fuel Cell (MFC) systems are one of the notified and lab-scale accepted systems, where biofilms are used for simultaneous production of energy and biodegradation of waste water. Microbes involved in the MFC system metabolize the given substrate and transfer the electrons extracellularly to an electrode in an anaerobic environment leading to the conversion of chemical energy to electrical energy (Franks & Nevin, 2010).

The basic idea behind MFC sounds to be simple, but the implementation of biofilms in this electrochemical device creates many complications. The nature, structure and composition of biofilm in MFC have direct effect on its performance. The energy generation efficiency of MFC is low as compare to commercially utilize non-renewable energy generation systems. In MFC power generation is obstructed by many biochemical factors.

Eminent scientists worldwide are working on the structural modification of MFC. Extensive studies have been done on the optimization of design with respect to the use of mediators, electrolyte (Pant *et al.*, 2010), electrode materials (Liu, *et al.*, 2010; Mustakeem, 2015), and chamber configuration (Logan, 2008). As microbes are the main source of electrons and protons that ultimately generate the current in MFC; now from last few years the researchers are focusing on microbial aspects of MFC. So far, few microbes which can degrade the biodegradable waste (substrate) and transfer electrons to the electrodes have been identified (Kumar *et al.*, 2016). The isolated microbes have been genetically explored for their functional capabilities.

Some studies also explain the microbial mechanism behind the electron transfer from microbes to electrode with the support of experimental observations (Qian *et al.*, 2007; Klimes *et al.*, 2010; Carmona-Martínez *et al.*, 2013).

In this chapter we are going to discuss "Biofilms" in MFC systems. As microbes play a key role in the process of energy generation through degradation of substrate in MFC, they are correctly termed as 'Power House of MFC'. The experimental condition which can affect the growth of biofilm and the effects of biofilm growth on the work efficiency of MFCs as recorded by the earlier studies are incorporated in this chapter.

2. Microbial Fuel Cell (MFC)

The basic H-shape double chambered MFC system as shown in Figure 1 consist of two chamber separated by Proton Exchange Membrane (PEM). In this MFC set up, after the degradation of substrate; electrons are transferred from microorganism to an electrode (the anode). This reaction takes place under anaerobic conditions. The electrons are further conducted via external electrical circuit to another electrode (the cathode), which is having aerobic conditions where reduction of oxygen takes place. Many time when oxygen is not supplied, Ferricyanide (Fe (CN) $^{-3}$6) is commonly used as an electron acceptor in cathode chamber (Figure 1). The protons produced during anaerobic degradation are transferred from one electrode chamber (anode chamber) to other electrode chamber (cathode chamber) through PEM (Figure 1). The flow of electrons between anode and cathode, generate current, which can power electronic devices just like commercial chemical batteries (Logan, 2008; Franks & Nevin, 2010; Lovley & Nevin, 2011).

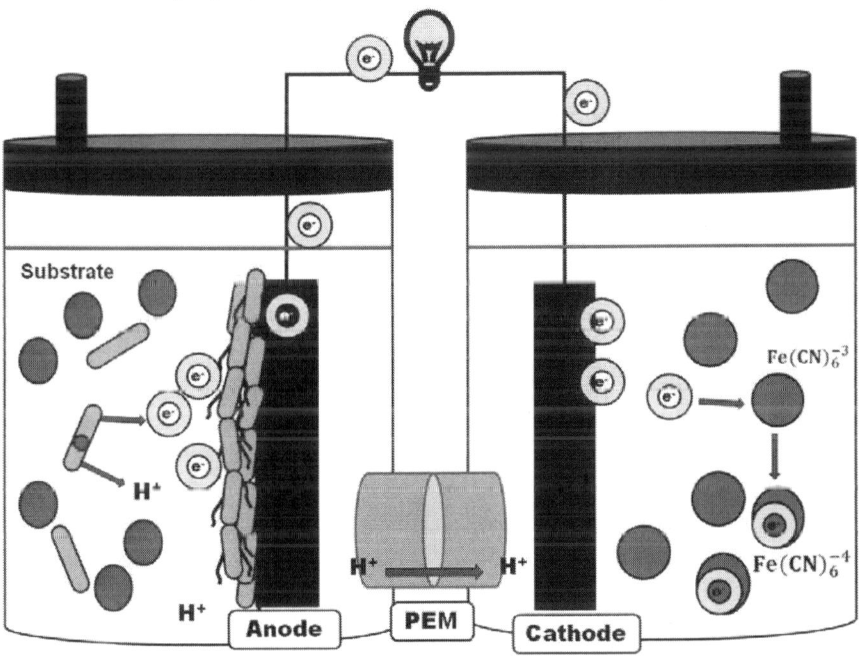

Fig. 1: Basic H- type Microbial fuel cell design

Microorganisms act as a catalyst in MFC. A Catalyst is considered as the one which increases the rate of a reaction. A true catalyst does not receive energy from the reaction they catalyze (Franks & Nevin, 2010). The microbes in a MFC are not considered as true catalysts, because they use the energy from the oxidation of the substrate for their growth. As the microbes in a MFC can obtain all the energy for cellular growth from the oxidation of the substrate present within the system, such MFC technology has been theoretically considered as self-sustaining (Lovley, 2006).

3. Biofilms in MFC

Biofilms are the integral part of any Microbial fuel cell system. The main surface where biofilms are formed in MFC is 'on the electrode'. The stability of MFC system depends on the functional capabilities of the biofilm on the electrode. Biofilms are found to be positively influencing the anode charge transfer and polarization resistance, which affect the MFC operations (Singh *et al.*, 2010). Composition of biofilm in MFC is governed by few factors; whereas there are features of biofilm that ultimately affect the MFC system in terms of performance (Figure 2).

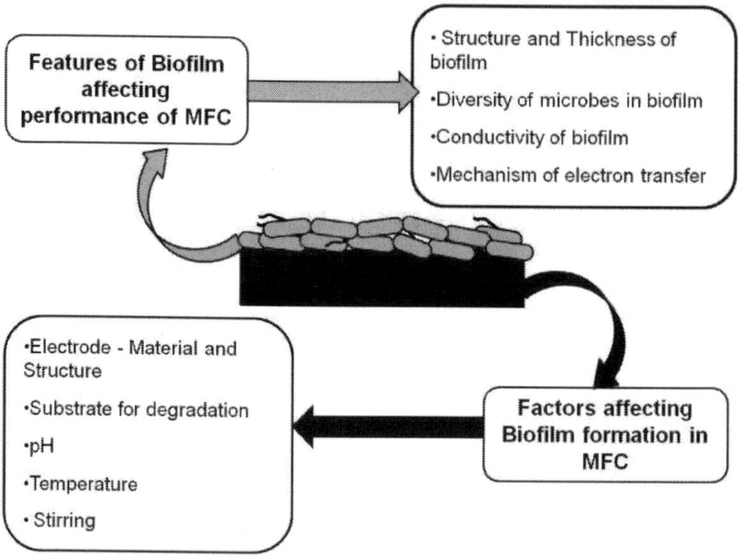

Fig. 2: Conditions affecting biofilm formation in MFC and features of biofilm which can affect the performance of MFC.

4. Process of Biofilm Formation

While studying the factors affecting biofilm formation in mediator less MFC Li *et. al.*, (2010) observed the biofilm formation of *Geobacter metallireducens* systematically. Through SEM and other electrochemical analysis like current generation, substrate consumption and protein estimation on anode surface they quoted that at the beginning of biofilm formation, the interaction among microbes, as well as between microbes and the electrode interface, helped enrich sufficient numbers of *G. metallireducens*, to form biofilm on the electrode surface. During this phase, *G.*

metallireducens multiplied remarkably and secreted extracellular substances. This secretion helped the bacteria to adsorb on the anode surface and also to attach with each other. Simultaneously metabolites started to accumulate in the anode chamber, and the density of suspended cells was increased. A month later, the protein concentration in the anode solution reached to 60 mg L^{-1}. In the anolyte majority of the suspension cells came from the aged and dissociated biofilm. Thus they concluded that the biofilm formed during this study went through the process reported by the different previous studies as follows: reversible adsorption – irreversible adsorption – multiple colony formation and gradual expansion – mature biofilm – aged and dissociated biofilm (Flow chart 1) (Costerton *et al.*, 1995; Costerton, 1999; Dunne, 2002; Hall-Stoodley & Stoodley, 2002; Ghigo, 2003; El Abed *et al.*, 2012). After one month when the solution in the anode was changed, and the metabolites, suspended dead bacteria were removed, it was found that addition of fresh metabolites speeded up *G. metallireducens* metabolism, and increased the traveling rate of electron and proton in the mediatorless MFC (Li *et al.*, 2010).

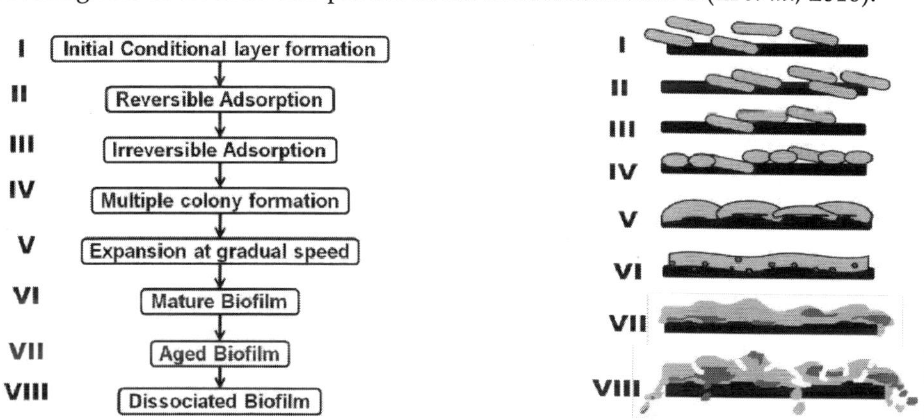

Flow chart 1: Flow chart depicting "The Process of Biofilm Formation"

During their study of enrichment of microbial community in MFC operations, with anaerobic sludge, Kim *et al.*, (2004) reported the formation of biofilm on the electrode surface with electrochemically active bacteria (Kim *et al.*, 2004). It was observed that this enriched biofilm can reduce the charge transfer resistance of the electrode. Ramasamy *et al.*, observed that due to the development of the microbial biofilm on the anode; the anode polarization resistance decreased. The growth of biofilm also facilitated the kinetics of the electrochemical reactions. From the power generation results Ramasamy *et al.* noted that: during the initial biofilm growth period as the growth of biofilm increased the power density produced in MFC increased. These studies confirmed that the microbes growing on the anode surface and the subsequent biofilm formation help in reduction of the anode charge transfer resistance and also decreases the anode polarization, which in turn increases the power generation (Ramasamy *et al.*, 2008; Baranitharan *et al.*, 2015).

The power output of any MFC using pure culture or mixed culture biofilm is very difficult to compare because design (including architecture, electrode type, material, ratio between electrode dimensions and MFC chamber dimensions etc.,), operating conditions, substrates, chemical composition of anolyte and catholyte used in different studies are usually different (Kumar *et al.*, 2016).

5. Properties of Electroactive Biofilm

Biofilm that harbors microorganism which are capable of electron transfer towards solid electron acceptors are called electroactive biofilms (Babauta *et al.*, 2012). Such biofilms are inevitable part of all MFC systems. As depicted in Figure 1, there are two main processes which take place in the anode chamber of MFCs: (a) electron generation by microorganisms during the degradation (oxidation) of the substrate and (b) electron transport from microorganisms to the electrode (Baranitharan *et al.*, 2015). Here, microbes act in a catalytic manner during the process of electron generation and transportation. During the generation of electrons the microorganisms conserve energy to support their growth by oxidizing organic compounds to carbon dioxide. The microorganisms which have capacity to transfer the electron after their metabolism exogenously onto/towards electrode surface are called "Electricigens" or Electrogenic or Exoelectrogens (Lovley, 2006; Franks & Nevin, 2010; Kumar *et al.*, 2016). As depicted in Figure 2 there are different factors that influence the nature of biofilm formed on an electrode and eventually affects the MFC performance.

5.1. Structure and thickness of biofilm

The structure and thickness of biofilm is governed by few factors such as electrode/ substrate properties, microbial growth phase, diversity of microbes in biofilm etc. Studies in the presence mixed bacterial culture and pure bacterial culture added to researchers understanding of different aspects of biofilm structure and behavior.

5.1.1. Electrode/ substrate properties

The microbial growth and attachment is found to be increasing on a rough surface as compare to smooth surface (Characklis *et al.*, 1990). The biofilm thickness has its effect on current density. The microbe which can form thick biofilm has been reported to generate higher current density. *G. sulfurreducens* forms highly structured and thick multilayer biofilms (₹ 50 mm). Though a very thick biofilm formation may limit the electron flow (Kumar *et al.*, 2016). Thus the thickness of biofilm is linearly correlated to current density but up to some thickness limit (Reguera *et al.*, 2006). Depending upon the electrode material, the biofilm in MFC may be in the form of pillar or homogeneous structure. *G. sulfurreducens* has been reported to form a thick homogenous layer of cells with slightly pillar structure on carbon cloth. However, when the same microbe was grown on graphite rod, the biofilm showed heterogeneous pillar structures (Nevin *et al.*, 2008). During another research study with *G. sulfurreducens* DL-1 and KN400 it was observed that the microbial strain DL-1 forms heterogeneous biofilm with pillar structures (Franks *et al.*, 2009) where as KN400 produce thin homogeneous biofilm. *G. sulfurreducens* KN400 was reported to produce more power. So, along with thickness some times the pattern in which cells are arranged in the biofilm is also important (Yi *et al.*, 2009).

5.1.2. Microbial growth phase

The structure and morphology of biofilm also depend on the growth phase of the microbial culture. During the lag phase biofilms of *G. sulfurreducens* had tightly packed single-cell thick clusters and low amount of c-type cytochromes and hence the biofilm generated less current. Whereas, comparatively in exponential phase amount of c-type cytochromes increased by three-to four fold and the biofilms contained two- to three dimension layer of bacterial cells (Lebedev *et al.*, 2014).

The biofilm structure in MFC also varies from Gram-positive to Gram-negative bacteria. During pure culture studies it was also observed that if the MFC is operated as a closed circuit system, the bacterial cell remain more viable and close to anode, but when the system is operated in open circuit mode bacterial cell were more viable on top layer of biofilm that means away from the anode surface (Read *et al.*, 2010).

5.2. Diversity of microbes in MFC biofilm

Biofilm can be formed by mixed bacterial culture comprising of many bacterial species or pure bacterial culture comprising of single bacterial species (Kumar *et al.*, 2016). During MFC studies the biofilms at anode surface are widely studied for their composition, diversity and dominance. As the anode is inoculated with diverse substrate the bacterial population found there is also of diverse nature. The bacterial species belonging to phyla *Proteobacteria, Frimicutes, Bacteroidetes* and *Acidobacteria* exhibit electrogenic activity in MFC (Logan, 2009; Beecroft *et al.*, 2012; Aracic *et al.*, 2014).

Electrogenic bacteria are advantageous for MFC because: 1) After complete oxidation of the organic substrate the microbes transfer the electrons to the electrode resulting in high columbic efficiency as compare to any other non-electrogenic bacteria, 2) long term stability is maintained due to conservation of energy for maintenance and growth on anode with simultaneous electron transfer to the anodes; and 3) direct electron transfer to the anode by the bacteria nullify the need for the addition of any exogenous electron mediators (Lovley, 2008; Franks & Nevin, 2010).

The main electrogenic microorganisms discovered so far in different studies having electroactive property are: *Shewanella putrefaciens, Clostridium butyricum, Desulfuromonas acetoxidans, Geobacter metallireducens, Geobacter sulfurreducens, Rhodoferax ferrireducens, Pseudomonas aeruginosa, Desulfobulbus propionicus, Thermincola sp., Cupriavidus basilensis* and many more (Friman *et al.*, 2013; Schechter *et al.*, 2014).

5.2.1. Mixed bacterial culture

Complex nature of substrate supports the growth of mixed culture from natural inoculum during lab-scale experiments. The synergistic relationship between mixed cultures can always help in biodegradation of complex substrate with simultaneous power generation. As the MFC's are fed by different type of substrate as a fuel component like - acetate (Bond & Lovley, 2003; Logan *et al.*, 2007; Nevin *et al.*, 2008), glucose (Catal *et al.*, 2008), starch (Niessen *et al.*, 2004), cellulose (Ren *et al.*, 2008), wheat straw (Zhang *et al.*, 2009), phenol (Luo *et al.*, 2009), azo dye (Sun *et al.*, 2009) and complex solutions such as domestic waste water (Rodrigo *et al.*, 2007; Lobato *et al.*, 2012), brewery waste (Wang *et al.*, 2008; Wen *et al.*, 2010), land fill leachate (You *et al.*, 2006; Galvez *et al.*, 2009), chocolate industry waste (Patil *et al.*, 2009), mixed fatty acids (Freguia *et al.*, 2009; Teng *et al.*, 2010) and petroleum contaminates (Morris & Jin, 2008; Li *et al.*, 2016; Venkidusamy *et al.*, 2016). Variable biofilm compositions can be observed in different MFC's depending upon the substrate available for utilization (Mathuriya & Sharma, 2009; Franks & Nevin, 2010; Pant *et al.*, 2010). The complex nature of anolyte gives rise to the formation of biofilm containing bacterial mixed culture. As a result, it is inevitable that different bacterial species perform different roles in the anode chamber. While some species are responsible in the fermentation of the complex organic substrate to a simple form; few species may contribute in the oxidation of simple substrates to produce electrons; again few will do the distance electron transport where as few other species lead to the formation of biofilm and direct electron transfer on the electrode surface. So, all the species are important for the biodegradation as well as for the energy generation in a MFC system (Holmes *et al.*, 2006; Jung & Regan, 2007; Lovely, 2008a; Nevin *et al.*, 2008).

It is widely observed and confirmed that when an anolyte harbors mixed culture microbial community, the dominance of microbes on the anode biofilms does not merely dependent on their superior exoelctrogenic capabilities. During the MFC operations also a community shift is documented by many researchers. Kim *et. al.*, (2004) reported a phenomenon of 'community shift' which shows that the initial population in the inoculum could be different from the subsequent microbial population on the electrode biofilm. Such community shift during the operation of the fuel cell indicates that microbial diversity varies significantly. As the biofilm reaches a stable state the change in the diversity would be less (Kim *et al.*, 2004).

5.2.2. Pure bacterial culture

Pure cultures are mainly used in MFC for the genomic studies. Many microorganisms have shown the capability of electron transfer in MFC. *Geobacter spp.*, and *Shewanella spp.*, are extensively studied as model electrogens (Figure 3) because of their occurrence in electrode biofilm, metabolic ability and electron transfer mechanism.

5.2.2.1. *Geobacter species (Deltaproteobacteria)*

The members of Geobacteraceae family of ä- proteobaceria phyla can completely metabolise fermentation products such as acetate, ethanol, propionate, butyrate, and lactate, as well as aromatics such as benzoate, toluene, and phenol (Srikanth *et al.*, 2008). *Goebacter sp* are also used in hydrocarbon bioremediation (Rooney-Varga *et al.*, 1999; Lovley & Anderson, 2000) dechlorination (Sung *et al.*, 2006), and heavy metal bioimmobilization (Anderson *et al.*, 2003; Wilkins *et al.*, 2006).

G. sulfurreducens is one of the most extensively studied microorganisms (Figure 3) capable of high current densities in MFC. *G. sulfurreducens* has become a model microbe for bacterial processes in a MFC due to some of its qualities: (a) it is a commonly isolated and identified bacterial species in the environmental samples used for different MFCS; (b) pure culture studies reported that, *G. sulfurreducens* can produce near or greater than maximum power of mixed species biofilms (Nevin *et al.*, 2008); (c) the full genome sequence is available (Methe *et al.*, 2003) and can be genetically manipulated (Coppi *et al.*, 2001; Bond & Lovley, 2003; Holmes *et al.*, 2004; Franks & Nevin, 2010).

5.2.2.2. *Shewanella species (Gammaproteobacteria)*

Shewanella spp are dissmilatory metal reducing bacteria. They have capacity to use various compounds and metal oxides as terminal acceptors during their anaerobic respiration. It has been proven through many studies that *Shewanella sp.,* has capability to metabolically utilize broad range of carbon substrates like amino acids, lactate, pyruvate etc., and has potential for bioremediation of heavy metals, radionuclides and xenobiotics (Ganesh *et al.,* 1997; Park & Kim, 2001). *Shewanella oneidensis* MR-1 has been used as a model microorganism for the study of electron transfer mechanism. It can gain energy by reducing many electron acceptors including oxygen, fumarate, nitrate, trimethylamine and other metal oxides. It was the first environmental bacteria to have its genome completely sequenced. So far 25 *Shewanella spp.,* (or stains of same speceies), have been sequenced. Comparative genome analysis revealed that *Shewanella* strains can metabolize preferably two and three-carbon carbohydrates. The genomes of these strains lack the key enzymes in glycolysis (e.g., glucokinase). It is well documented that most *Shewanella spp.,* cannot use glucose as a carbon source unless an aerobic adaptation occurs before exposure to glucose (Heidelberg *et al.,* 2002; Biffinger *et al.,* 2008; Choi & Chae, 2014). *Shewanella oneidensis* under strict anaerobic conditions can utilize lactate, but not acetate, for power production (Biffinger *et al.*, 2008; Kiely *et al.*, 2010). The inability of *Shewanella spp* to utilize acetate leads to the incomplete oxidation of organic acids to acetate and thus insufficient power is generated as most of the electrons available in the original substrate remain in acetate (Richter *et al.,* 2008).

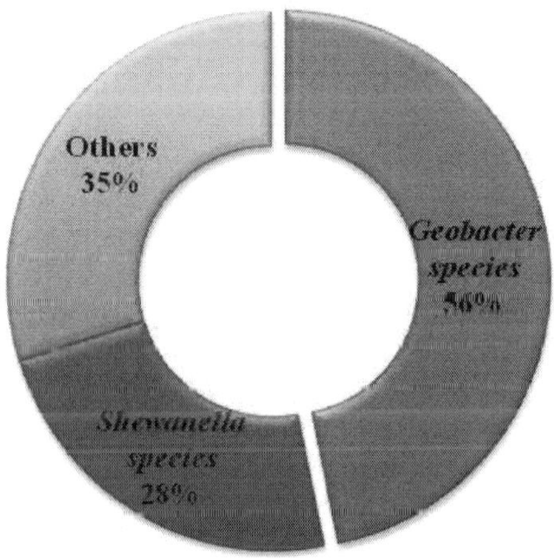

Fig. 3: - Microbial cultures used in MFC for the power generation.

5.3. Electron transfer in MFC biofilm

In the anode chamber generally it is observed that bacterial culture passes through a lag phase period after inoculation, followed by a rapid increase in current. This lag phase is explained to be associated with the time needed to establish initial bacteria-anode electron transfer (Choi *et al.*, 2013). A test done by Li *et. al.*, to correlate the substrate utilization (the substrate used was-sodium acetate) and current generation in MFC showed that during the growth period i.e. when the biofilm formation started in MFC the consumption of sodium acetate (substrate) in the anode chamber was fastest, but after the biofilm was mature or the current was constant, the consumption rate was slower. This indicated that the microbes consumed a large amount of organic substrate during the formation of biofilm (Li *et al.*, 2010).

It has been affirmatively accepted that both suspended and attached microbial cells can contribute to electron transfer, yet cells which are adhered on the anode in the form of biofilm are considered as the main contributor to current generation (Ringeisen *et al.*, 2006; Choi *et al.*, 2013). In an electroactive biofilm, microbes adapt different strategies of electron transfer depending upon the distance of that microbial cell from electrode and the type of species involved in the process. Three main pathways for electron transfer have been identified that include: (i) mediated electron transfer via electron shuttles, (ii) direct electron transfer via outer membrane c-type cytochromes (Bond, 2003) and (iii) long range electron transfer via electrical conductive pili or nanowires (Figure 4) (Reguera *et al.*, 2005; Lovley *et al.*, 2006; Lovley & Regan, 2006a; Lovley & Nevin, 2008; Lovley, 2008a; Lovley, 2008b; Logan, 2009; Franks & Nevin, 2010). The electron transfer pathways are identified through pure culture studies in MFC. These studies are primarily focused on *Geobacter spp.* and *Shewanella spp.*

5.3.1. Mediated electron transfer via electron shuttles

Mediators or electron shuttles are compounds which can undergo reversible redox reaction and transfer electron from one surface (microbial cell) to other (electron acceptor/ metal oxides/ electrode). Ideal mediator can function as an electron shuttle if it (i) displays reversible redox reaction; (ii) has appreciable solubility in an aqueous solution; (iii) stability; (iv) can facilitate the electron transfer (Sharma & Kundu, 2010; Raghavulu *et al.*, 2013). Addition of electrochemical mediators, which act as shuttles, can facilitate the electron transfer between bacteria and electrode (Park & Zeikus, 2000; Rabaey *et al.*, 2005). Electron mediator which has a potential close to the redox potential of $NADH/NAD^+$ can facilitate electron shuttling from microbial cell to terminal electron acceptor (metal or electrode) (Rahimnejad *et al.*, 2012). Artificial mediators are added to the medium if bacterial cultures like *Bacillus sp* or *Escherichia coli* are used. Common electron shuttles including thionine, benzylviologen, 2-hydroxy-1, 4-naphthoquinone and various phenazines, phenothiazines, iron chelates, methyl viologen, methylene blue, neutral red, etc., are used in MFC (Lovley, 2006). Whereas bacteria like *Shewanella oneidensis* can biosynthesis mediators which act as shuttle in electron transfer as depicted in Figure 4 (Biffinger *et al.*, 2008). Under this mechanism the electron is transferred by means of exogenous mediator or biosynthesized electron shuttles (Figure 4). For this type of electron transfer the microbial cell might not be in direct physical/electrical contact with the electrode (Rinaldi *et al.*, 2008). *Pseudomonas spp.*, are also reported to produce mediators (pyocyanin), that shuttle electrons from the bacteria through the biofilm matrix to the anode (Reguera *et al.*, 2005; Yong *et al.*,

2014). Outer membrane c-type cytochrome also plays a vital role in electron shuttle mechanism of electron transfer (Lovley, 2006).

5.3.2. Direct electron transfer via outer membrane c-type cytochromes

C-cytochromes are heme-containing proteins which are widespread in most bacteria. C-type cytochromes have been considered as one of the most important electron transfer strategies in current generation by exoelectrogens. The outer-membrane cytochromes and conductive pili were identified in *Geobacter* sp. and *Shewanella sp.* (Kim *et al.*, 2007). It was reported that in *Geobacter*, C-cytochromes are bound to the matrices of extracellular polymeric substrates (Richter *et al.*, 2009). As Cytochromes are outer membrane proteins, the bacterial cell here requires a physicl/electrical contact with the electrode (in Figure 4). It is being proved that the genome of *Geobacter sulfurreducens* has gene that encodes approximately 110 c-type cytochromes (Methe *et al.*, 2003, Kracke *et al.*, 2015).

5.3.3. Long range electron transfer via electrical conductive pili or nanowires

Bacterial appendages called nanowires were identified in both the exoelectrogens, *Shewanella* and *Geobacter*. Later in case of *Shewanella* it was discovered that the pili where actually a plasma membrane extension (Aracic *et al.*, 2014). The nanowires are known for the transport of electrons form distant cells to electrodes and also contain surface-located C-cytochromes. Gene expression studies have suggested that the production of microbial nanowires is important for long-range electron transfer through the *G. sulfurreducens* biofilms (Gorby *et al.*, 2006; Reguera, 2006; Debabov, 2008; Franks & Nevin, 2010; Bonanni *et al.*, 2012; Schechter *et al.*, 2014). Occurrence of pili in the biofilm is an indication that, a long range electron transfer process is followed by the microbial culture during current generation. It is well analysed and documented through genetic studies that pili help in long-range direct electron transfer from each microbe to the electrode (Reguera *et al.*, 2005; Reguera *et al.*, 2006; Zhao *et al.*, 2009; Schechter *et al.*, 2014).

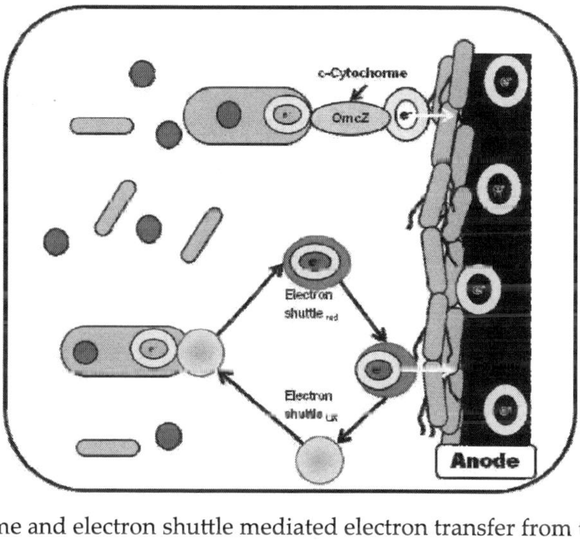

Fig. 4: Cytochrome and electron shuttle mediated electron transfer from the microbial cell to the electrode

6. Classic Examples of Electron Transport in Biofilm

The electron transport chain may vary from microbe to microbe depending upon the environmental conditions. Microbes have a general property to adapt for survival. Common catalyst that take part in this redox reactions are

- *Primary dehydrogenases:* - They catalyse the supply of high energy electrons from donor like NADH with simultaneous H^+ or Na^+ transport across the membrane.
- *Multi-protein complex:* - These are usually located on membrane like cytochromes and terminal reductase.
- *Co-factors:* - Electron carrying co-factors such as quinones, flavins, heme group, iron-sulfur cluster or copper ions are also important part of electron transport chain. Soluble lipophilic molecules (e.g., quinones) shuttle the electrons between enzymatic complexes within the membrane, while some co-factors are catalytic in nature (e.g., heme group of cytochromes) (Kracke *et al.*, 2015).

The model organism *Geobacter sulfurreducens* and *Shewanella oneidensis* are well studied for direct and indirect electron transfer mechanism. For both the bacteria outer membrane cytochromes are essential to smooth transfer of electrons. Other bacteria such as *Thermincola* and *Clostridium lijungdahlii* also exhibit electron transport (Kracke *et al.*, 2015), but in this review we will only discuss the model mechanisms of *Geobacter sulfurreducens* and *Shewanella oneidensis*.

6.1. Electron transfer in Shewanella spp.

Shewanella onedensis is a gram negative microbe well known for its property of reduction of metals by exoelectron transfer. Metal oxides like Fe (III) have very low solubility in water, due to which they cannot enter any microbial cell, where they can be completely degraded. To overcome this barrier bacterium like *Shewanella onedensis* transfer electron from inside the cell to the cell surface, where it can reduce Fe (III) oxide (Shi *et al.*, 2012).

The Mtr- pathway (Figure 5) is used by the microbe to overcome external barrier in electron transfer. In this mechanism decaheme cytochrome MtrA receives electrons from CymA via electron transport chain and further passes the electron to extracellular decaheme cytochromes MrtC. MtrC, transfers the electron to the extra cellular electron acceptors. It is prposed that there is a complex formation between MtrA MtrC and MtrB. MtrB is a porin molecule in the outer membrane. The complex MtrCAB, is formed so that the MtrA and MtrC are organized and stabilised for the electron transfer. One more decaheme OmcA has been found to be present in the outer membrane; it also facilitates the electron transfer to extracellular acceptor (Lovley, 2006; Rinaldi *et al.*, 2008; Shi *et al.*, 2012).

As the microbe prefers shuttles and mediators for electron transfer, these flavins/ shuttle can also take part in the extracellular electron transfer from microbe cell wall to electrode depending upon the experimental/environmental conditions (Kracke *et al.*, 2015).

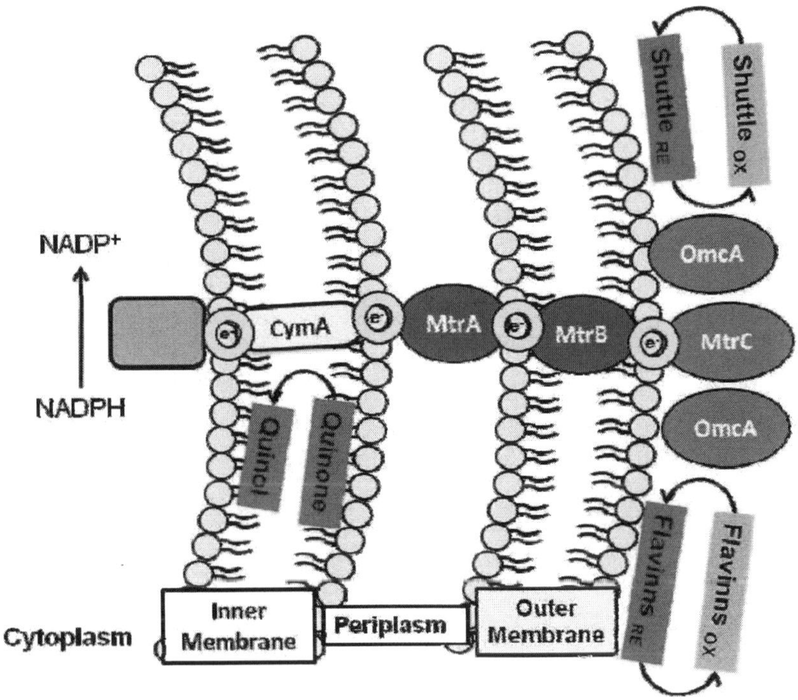

Fig. 5: Extracellular electron transfer from the *Shewanella* cell to the electrode.

6.2. Electron transfer in Geobatcer spp.

In Geobacter extracellular electron transport multiheme c-type cytochromes play an important role. The interaction between different cytochromes complex at different level is based on the redox potential difference between them. Cytochromes enable the transport of electrons from menaquinone pool (MQ) to extracellular metal oxides.

As illustrated in Figure 6, there are many cytochromes such as diheme cytochromes c peroxidase, generally known as 'metal reduction associated cytochromes (MacA) helps in the transfer of electron from inner membrane to triheme periplasmic c-type cytochromes (PpcA), which is in the periplasmic space. From the periplasmic space the PpcA transfer the electron to the outer membrane cytochromes, known as OMCs. These OMCs such as OmcB, OmcC, OmcS, OmcZ transfer the electron further to the extracellular acceptor. The OMCs system is very complex. Bacteria may express different OMCs as per the extracellular metals or electrodes available. Among all OMCs OmcZ is found to be expressed in large number by the microbial cell. The gene deletion studies revealed that the deletion of gene coding OmcZ (*omcZ* gene) decreases the current more than 90%, while there is no significant effect of deletion of other OMCs (Kim *et al.*, 2006a; Kim *et al.*, 2008; Nevin *et al.*, 2009; Richter *et al.*, 2009; Lovley & Nevin, 2011; Richter *et al.*, 2012). For example though the dodecaheme cytochrome OmcB is important for Fe (III) reduction, but when we delete of gene *omcB* the organism now termed as OmcB mutant can express its homologs like dodecaheme OmcC, which can facilitate the electron transfer to Fe(III) (Leang & Lovley, 2005; Lovley, 2006; Rinaldi, 2008; Shi, 2012).

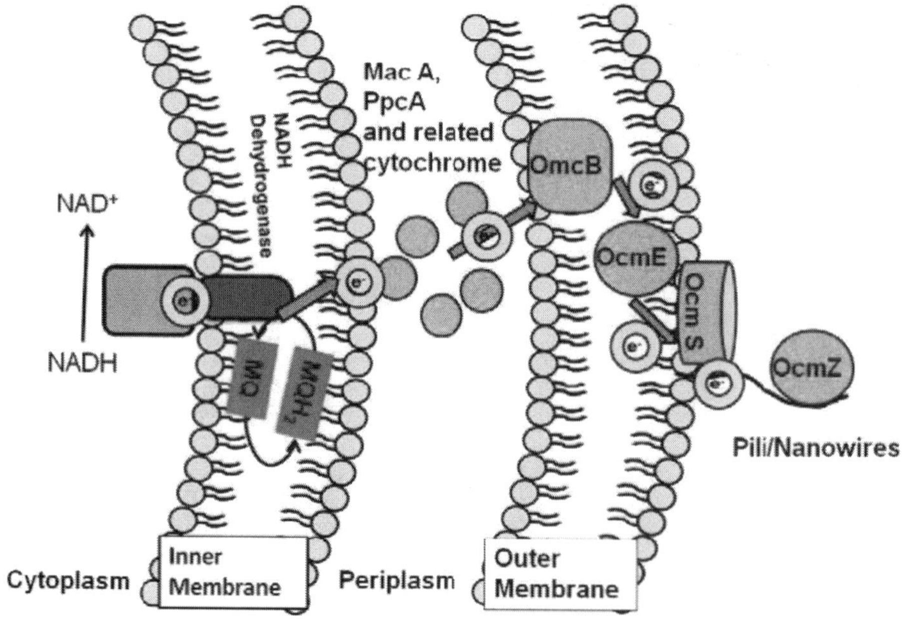

Fig. 6: Long distance extracellular direct electron transfer via Pili/Nanowire from the *Geobacter* cell to the electrode; MQH2- menaquinol, MQ- menaquinone.

Geobacter biofilms can conduct electrons via two mechanisms, identified as, mediator based in which the microbe secret mediators in the biofilm which can act as electron shuttle for transport of electrons; second one is through nanowires. The mechanism of electron transfer through nanowaires is not yet established, metal like conductivity and hopping electrons are the mechanism so far reported (Malvankar *et al.*, 2011; 2012; 2015).

7. Factors Affecting Biofilm Formation in MFC

The main location for biofilm formation in MFC is on the surface of electrodes. Different factors play crucial role in the biofilm formation on the electrode surface. As depicted in Figure 2 different structural composition of electrodes and experimental condition affect the biofilm formation on electrode surface. The composition and capability of biofilm formed under the influence of above said factors affect the performance of MFC (Fig 2).

7.1. Electrode

Electroactive biofilms formed on the electrode surface are the mediators for better electron transfer. The physiochemical composition of electrodes thus influences the biofilm formation and thereby performance of MFC. The ohmic losses in MFC are mainly due to the resistance of the electrode (Mustakeem, 2015).The positively charged and hydrophilic electrode surfaces are more favorable for electroactive biofilm formation (Guo *et al.*, 2013; Kumar *et al.*, 2016, Baranitharan *et al.*, 2015).

7.1.1. Material and structure of electrode

Most likely electrode materials are chosen on the basis of their electrical conductivity and cost affectivity. Electrode material has direct impact on the bacterial adhesion. Electrodes with more surface area favor more biofilm growth. Modification in the conventional carbon based electrode and use of material like graphite felt and graphite fiber brush increases the surface area of the electrode. An ideal electrode material should have (i) good electrical conductivity, (ii) low resistance, (iii) strong biocompatibility, (iv) chemical stability, (v) anti corrosion, (vi) large surface area, (vii) mechanical strength and toughness as per requirement (Rahimnejad *et al.*, 2015).

Structurally anodes can be classified under

a) Plane: - Carbon paper, carbon cloth, carbon mesh, graphite foil, graphite sheets and graphite plates are plane structured electrodes. These are generally used in laboratory level MFC studies. As compare to smooth graphite plate, rough graphite plate gave better results due to increase surface area (Wei *et al.*, 2011).

b) Packed: - To increase the surface area graphite and activated carbon are filled in the anode chamber in granular form. This increase in surface area is found to enhance the power output of MFC (Wei *et al.*, 2011).

c) Brush: - The brush type electrode is also a physical modification to increase the surface area and conductivity of the electrode, where graphite fibers are winded on two twisted, non-corrosive but conductive titanium wires (Logan, 2008). In one such effort Logan *et al.*, found that power density increased four times with the use of graphite fiber brush compare to carbon paper (Logan *et al.*, 2007).

Apart from the physical variation, different treatments on the conventional carbon, graphite and steel electrode material are also found to be effective in increasing bacterial adhesion. Treatments with ammonia (Cheng *et al.*, 2007), inorganic acid, heat (acid and heat treatment together also increases the roughness of the electrode surface) (Feng *et al.*, 2010) etc., promote the formation of functional groups on the electrode material which in turn increased positive charge on the surface and further bacterial adhesion (Mustakeem, 2015).

New material like Carbon nanotubes (CNTs) are recently investigated and found to be an effective electrode material due to its increased surface area, electrical conductivity, chemical stability, and biocompatibility (Mustakeem, 2015). Microbes when grown on CNTs developed the ð-ð stacking between the pili and carbon atoms of graphite, which resulted in excellent charge transfer between microbe and electrode (Erbay *et al.*, 2015).

Electrode used as cathode should have additional properties like high ionic conductivity and good catalytic activity. Low oxygen reduction rate is the major limitation in the performance of double chambered MFC. As carbon based materials have poor catalytic activity, a catalytic layer is generally coated on the electrode which has to be used as cathode in any MFC system. Platinum is the most preferred catalyst because of its high surface area and low over potential for oxygen reduction reaction (ORR) (Watanabe, 2008).

Due to the higher cost and non-environmental friendly nature of platinum; now biocathodes (where microbial biofilm on the cathode surface catalyses the ORR) are thoroughly studied for their possible use in the MFC system (Harnisch & Schroder, 2010).

7.2. pH

A change in pH has direct effect on bacterial growth. Bacterial cell possess membrane-bound proton pumps that help in the extradition of protons from the cytoplasm and generate a transmembrane electrochemical gradient, i.e. the proton motor force. A passive influx of protons in response to the proton motive force can create problem for cells when they try to regulate their cytoplasmic pH (Booth, 1985). Large variations in external pH can strongly affect such mechanisms and have a biocidal effect on the microorganisms (Garret *et al.*, 2008).

In any operational MFC system when oxidation of organic material is carried out by microorganism, both protons and electrons are produced. The electrons are transferred instantaneously through the conductive biofilm to the electrical circuit of the MFC and protons have to migrate from the biofilm to the cathode via proton permeable membrane. The later phenomenon occurs at a much slower rate and thus is one of the inhibiting factors in power production (Arends & Verstraete, 2011). For every electron produced which further contributes to current generation, a proton is also produced within the biofilm (Franks *et al.*, 2009).

During the power production analysis in MFC it was observed that, decrease in the pH of the bulk fluid contribute to decrease in power production (Torres *et al.*, 2008; 2008a). The specific production of current by the microbes in the MFC indeed increased the proton concentration, which can be equivalent to 1 pH unit (Franks & Nevin, 2010).

The effect of pH on biofilm is well documented by Yuan *et. al.*, (2011). They found that electron transfer rate constant and exchange current density were greater/ increased at alkaline pH (pH 9.0), whereas charge transfer resistance was smaller/ decreased at neutral (pH 7.0) and acidic pH (pH 5.0). At alkaline pH (pH 9.0), SEM analysis revealed better biofilm formation as compare to the biofilm formation at pH 7.0 and 5.0. These results showed that electrochemical interactions between bacteria and electrodes in MFCs are enhanced under alkaline conditions (Yuan *et al.*, 2011). In contradiction to the above mentioned studies, there are several studies which described that under neutral and acidic conditions the power production has increased. Whereas few studies also claim that the range of 6 to 9 i.e., both a little acidic up to alkaline pH are suitable for the biofilm growth, obtained from pH neutral waste water (He & Angenent, 2008; Patil *et al.*, 2011; Schechter *et al.*, 2014). Through their studies scientists have proved that, power production in MFC is dependent on the pH of anolyte and the correlation between pH and biofilm is depended on the bacterial species adherent to anode (Schechter *et al.*, 2014).

The studies discussed till now were the studies between the external pH and anodic biofilm, but one more level at which pH can affect the functionality of biofilm is the pH gradient within the biofilm. As it is very difficult to monitor activities within the biofilm without disturbing it; there are very few studies on the real time pH gradient within the biofilm. In studies it was found that the pH gradient within the biofilm is in the direction towards the anode surface from the exterior to the interior of the biofilm pillars in decreasing order. In one such study a pH-sensitive fluoroprobe was used to study pH gradient within the *G. sulfurreducens* anode biofilm and it revealed a strong pH gradient within the biofilm. Various controlled studies demonstrated that proton accumulation affects the pH and indirectly was associated with current production. Decreasing the pH of the culture medium from 7 to 6 limited the growth of *G. sulfurreducens*. (Franks *et al.*, 2009; Schechter *et al.*, 2014).

7.3. Temperature

At optimum temperature conditions, microorganisms increase their nutrient intake and achieve healthy growth with good nutrient metabolism. A healthy growing microbial community is a prerequisite for biofilm formation (Stepanovic *et al.*, 2003). Nutrient metabolism is directly associated and dependent on the presence of enzymes. So, a relation can be developed that the formation of a biofilm is dependent on the presence and reaction rates of enzymes. The enzyme reaction controls the development of many physiological and biochemical systems of bacteria. Temperature is an important variable in a bacterial life cycle and has direct correlation with the reaction rate of enzymes. Thus under adverse conditions; when the growth temperature is away from the optimum temperature, the enzyme reaction rate is adversely affected and this reduces the bacterial growth efficiency. The temperature variation may affect the adhesive properties required for the attachment of stationary phase cells which form a foundation for the growth of biofilm (Garret *et al.*, 2008). Temperature range from 5°C to 45°C was found to be suitable for the microbes from waste water. The trend of increasing temperature help in initial growth and also influence the bioelectrocatalytic activity of biofilm up to certain limit of upper temperature value (Patil *et al.*, 2010).

7.4. Stirring

Stirring in anode chamber can affect the biofilm and current production during MFC operation. In an attempt to understand the effect of stirring on the current production Li *et. al.*, (2010) stopped the stirring in a working MFC system when the current generation became stable in it. It was noted that as a result of stopping the stirring the current rapidly decreased from 0.89 mA to 0.82 mA and when stirring was restarted, the current returned to its previous value. The reason behind this observation was that stirring accelerates the ion transfer and decreases the internal resistance, which led to increase in current production (Li *et al.*, 2010). Stirring could cause dissociation in the biofilm due to shear force (*Fd*). A stable biofilm structure depend on how to balance the interaction between shear force (*Fd*) and growth force (*Fg*) (growth force rely on the penetration and permeability of the substrate). In earlier research the experiment of stirring rate showed that the two forces could influence the distribution of organic substrate in the anode chamber (Rittmann *et al.*, 1992; Liu & Tay, 2002).

7.5. Temporary intermittence

It is well known that the static force between bacteria and the anode or among other bacterial cells is not because of the potential difference between the electrodes, but is mainly due to the chemical bond among the bacterial cells. After the amount of bacterial deposition was enough, the biofilm would be formed through EPS secreted by bacteria (Costerton, 1999; Ghigo, 2003; Li *et al.*, 2010). To study the effect of intermittence on *Geobacter* biofilm the circuit between the anode and the cathode was turned off for 24 hours. When it was re-connected the current returned to the previous value. This suggested that the biofilm can withstand the unexpected interruption (Li *et al.*, 2010). This behavior was explained by Bonanni *et. al.*,(2012) during their study of *Geobacter*-biofilm. They found that since *Geobacter* can store electrons in the heme of the exocytoplasmic cytochromes, the biofilm respiration could continue after the interruption of electrode polarization. When the electrode was connected again, stored electrons were recovered as a current (Bonanni *et al.*, 2012).

While operating a MFC it can be noted that as long as the biofilm had been formed, the electron transfer could be recovered with in short interval of time after any kind of intermittence.

8. Genetic Studies of Electroactive Biofilm

The Genetic studies which were done to understand the role of certain protein in the conductive nature of biofilm or organisms were informative and helped the researcher to understand the factors governing the behavior of biofilms (Butler *et al.*, 2010, Bonanni *et al.*, 2012). Most of the gene deletion studies done were focused to understand the importance of cytochrome production, nanowire regulation and requirement of both under the given conditions (Myers *et al.*, 2002; 2002a; Qian *et al.*, 2007; Richter *et al.*, 2009; Butler *et al.*, 2010). The genetic engineering attempts in order to improve current production were not much successful (Izallalen, 2008). It is reported that neither the over production of cytochromes or the microbial nanowires nor the creation of an ATP drain increased the current/ power production (Mahadevan *et al.*, 2006). These observations underline the fact that current production by bacteria in a MFC is a complex process. The electron transfer mechanism within the biofilm is highly regulated. Few changes in genes might not be much effective but studies can be planned for more changes, in genes or changes in bacterial respiration rates to increase current production. In MFC adaptive selection has meet with more success at producing a strain capable of increased current density (Yi *et al.*, 2009; Franks & Nevin, 2010; Yong *et al.*, 2014).

9. Techniques for Structural and Biochemical Study of Biofilm in MFC

As a promising effort towards the improvement of power production in MFC technology, it is evident to understand the chemical, physical and biological characteristics of the biofilm. Study of these properties of a biofilm is foreseen as a challenge, due to the low concentration of bacterial cells. In addition to conventional methods such as scanning electron microscopy (SEM) and confocal laser scanning microscopy (CLSM), there exist modern methods such as Raman spectroscopy, Fourier transform infrared spectroscopy (FTIR) and atomic force microscopy (AFM) (Schechter *et al.*, 2014) which help us to study details about bioiflms.

Microscopic techniques are generally used to observe the morphology of any surface. These techniques are useful in imaging of biofilm. Confocal laser scanning microscopy (CLSM) is often used in optical imaging of biological samples as thin as 0.3 ìm. The most popular application of CLSM is for *ex situ* identification of live and dead bacteria after suitable staining.

CLSM helps to determine thickness, architecture, spatial distribution and viability profile of microbial biofilms. This technique is used to observe thicker biofilms and to correlate it with the increased current production (Reguera *et al.*, 2006; Pham *et al.*, 2008). Using CLSM, microcolonies of Gram-positive and Gram-negative bacteria have also been observed in an electroactive biofilm (Murphy, 2001; Kim *et al.*, 2006; Aracic *et al.*, 2014; Schechter *et al.*, 2014).

Scanning electron microscopy (SEM) analysis is a magnification technique. This analysis uses a condensed electron beam to scan a sampled object. SEM imaging provides morphological details of the surface, information on the three-dimensional topography of the sample through highly resolved images. Surface-conducting coating of sample is done before SEM to avoid local charging and heating effects (Niemantsverdriet, 2007; Schechter *et al.*, 2014). SEM requires dehydrated samples. The plasma membrane extensions were thought to be pili under SEM observation. Later these extensions were detected along with cytrochrome redox protein by using fluorescent staining via Fluorescence Microscopy. MtrC and OmcA cytochromes were also identifying in the outer and periplasmic membrane extensions via Fluorescence Microscopy (Aracic *et al.*, 2014; Pirbadian, 2014).

The Raman spectroscopy analysis is generally used to study solid, liquid and gaseous samples. This provides information on vibrational, rotational and other low frequency transitions at the molecular level. Fluorescence of the sample or impurities within the sample can mask the results produced in Raman spectrum. This technique is sparsely used in MFC biofilm (Niemantsverdriet, 2007; Ly *et al.*, 2013; Lebedev *et al.*, 2014; Schechter *et al.*, 2014).

Atomic force microscopy (AFM) generates information like topographic, conductive, magnetic, mechanical (friction forces) or potential images of the surface. AFM techniques can work in ambient air or in a liquid environment, including physiological conditions (Niemantsverdriet, 2007). It can be used to study the electrodes, biological samples, biomolecules and even living organism. AFM enables imagining of biofilms and the EPS distribution within the biofilm (Beech *et al.*, 2002). AFM imaging is non-destructive technique (Schechter *et al.*, 2014). The two techniques AFM and scanning tunneling microscopy (STM) were successfully used together for the identification of the pili on *Geobacter* species (Reguera *et al.*, 2005; Zhao *et al.*, 2009; Lebedev *et al.*, 2014; Schechter *et al.*, 2014).

Cyclic voltammograms investigate the electrochemical interactions of mixed or pure cultures with an anode in the form of electron transfer (Logan *et al.*, 2006; Fricke *et al.*, 2008; Richter *et al.*, 2009; Carmona-Martinez *et al.*, 2011; Friman *et al.*, 2013). Cyclic voltammetry (CV) techniques can differentiate direct and indirect electron transfer process that occur within the electrode-associated biofilms and also the electron transfer process that occur in the anodic biofilm depending upon the stage of biofilm development, the biofilm community and power generation by the electrode associated biofilm (Srikanth *et al.*,2008; Cheng *et al.*,2009). Cyclic voltammetery has been shown to only probe the biofilm closet to the electrode. Cyclic voltammetery cannot be used to probe the bulk biofilms as there may be a significant potential gradient within the biofilm. CV should be supported with other analytical methods to drive any conclusions regarding the functional aspects of biofilm and to understand the physiochemical nature of the mediator involved in the electron transfer process (Cheng *et al.*, 2009; Franks & Nevin, 2010; Carmona-Martinez *et al.*, 2011).

To measure the adhesion strength of bacterial biofilm it is necessary to remove them from a surface. Fowler and McKay, described two types of adhesion measurement: (a) adhesion number (the counting of cells before and after an event) and (b) critical force (measurements during an event). Adhesion number can be determined through imaging techniques such as environmental SEM, optical microscopy and CLSM. As these techniques are purely observational they do not measure directly the adhesion of bacterial populations. Critical force can be measured through techniques like AFM and micromanipulation. These techniques directly interact with bacteria so that a force required to remove bacteria can be determined. Of these techniques only one enables the direct measurement of biofilm adhesion, micromanipulation (Fowler & McKay, 1980; Garret *et al.*, 2008).

10. Conclusion

The microorganisms are the main driving force behind the substrate degradation and power generation in MFC's. The microbial composition of any MFC depends on the degradation reaction that will be taking place inside its chamber. The formation of a biofilm on the electrode surface is the most important step in MFC. Functionality and capability of biofilm has its impact on the work efficiency of MFC.

Thus biofilm formation and electronic nature of microbes dwelling in the biofilm can be used as a source of energy through MFC technology. There is a greater need to initiate studies for better understanding of electroactive biofilm and optimize implementation of the same to address the limitation of power generation in MFC.

Advanced analytical, biochemical and microscopic techniques can help us to understand the composition and morphology of biofilms. Periodic studies regarding the factors affecting the formation and function of biofilms can generate data to understand the behavior of different biofilms in different conditions. The observations and information generated through these research studies as well as investigative techniques can serve as an input for the future modeling of MFC.

11. Acknowledgement

The study was funded by Department of Science and Technology, New Delhi, India, under the project code DST-WOS-A (SR/WOS-A/ET-1054/2014(G)).

References

Anderson, R. T., Vrionis, H. A., Ortiz-Bernad, I., Resch, C. T., Long, P. E., Dayvault, R., Karp, K., Marutzky, S., Metzler, D. R., Peacock, A., White, D. C., Lowe, M. & Lovley, D. R. (2003). Stimulating the in situ activity of *Geobacter species* to remove uranium from the groundwater of a uranium-contaminated aquifer. *Applied Environronmental Microbiology. 69,* 5884–5891.

Aracic, S., Semenec, L. & Franks, A. E. (2014). Investigating microbial activities of electrode-associated microorganisms in real-time. *Frontiers of Microbioliology. 5,* 663- 670.

Arends, J. B. A. & Verstraete, W. (2012).100 years of microbial electricity production: Three concepts for the future. *Microbiology Biotechnology. 5,* 333–346.

Babauta, J., Renslow, R., Lewandowski, Z. & Beyenal, H. (2012). Electrochemically active biofilms: Facts and fiction a review. *Biofouling. 28,* 789–812.

Baranitharan, E., Khan, M. R., Prasad, D. M. R., Teo, W. F. A., Tan, G. Y. A. & Jose, R. (2015). Effect of biofilm formation on the performance of microbial fuel cell for the treatment of palm oil mill effluent. *Bioprocess Biosystem and Engineering. 38,* 15–24.

Barkay, T. & Schaefer, J. Metal and radionuclide bioremediation: Issues, considerations and potentials. *Current Opinions in Microbiology. 4,* 318–23 (2001).

Beech, I. B., Smith, J. R., Steele, A. A., Penegar, I. & Campbell, S. A. (2002). The use of atomic force microscopy for studying interactions of bacterial biofilms with surfaces. *Colloids and Surfaces B. Biointerfaces. 23,* 231– 247.

Beecroft, N. J., Zhao F., Varcoe, J. R., Slade, R. C. T., Thumser, A. E. & Avignone-Rossa, C. (2012). Dynamic changes in the microbial community composition in microbial fuel cells fed with sucrose. *Applied Microbiology Biotechnology. 93,* 423–437.

Biffinger, J. C., Byrd, J. N., Dudley, B. L. & Ringeisen, B. R. (2008). Oxygen exposure promotes fuel diversity for *Shewanella oneidensis* microbial fuel cells. *Biosensors and Bioelectronics. 23,* 820–826.

Bonanni, P. S., Schrott, G. D. & Busalmen, J. P. (2012). A long way to the electrode: How do *Geobacter* cells transport their electrons? *Biochemical Society Transactions. 40,* 1274–1279.

Bonanni, P. S., Schrott, G. D., Robuschi L. & Busalmen, J. P. (2012). Charge accumulation and electron transfer kinetics in *Geobacter sulfurreducens* biofilms. *Energy and Environmental Science. 5,* 6188–6195.

Bond D. R. & Lovley D. R. (2003). Electricity production by *Geobacter sulfurreducens* attached to electrodes. *Applied Environmental Microbiology. 69,* 1548–1555.

Booth, I. R. Regulation of cytoplasmic pH in bacteria. (1985). *Microbiology Reviews. 49*, 359–78.

Butler, J. E., Young, N. D., & Lovley, D. R. (2010). Evolution of electron transfer out of the cell: Comparative genomics of six *Geobacter* genomes. *BMC Genomics 11*. 40, 1–12.

Carmona-Martinez, A. A., Harnisch, F., Fitzgerald, L. A., Biffinger, J. C., Ringeisen, B. R., & Schroder, U. (2011). Cyclic voltammetric analysis of the electron transfer of *Shewanella oneidensis MR-1* and nanofilament and cytochrome knock-out mutants. *Bioelectrochemistry. 81*, 74–80.

Carmona-Martínez, A. A., Harnisch, F., Kuhlicke, U., Neu, T. R. & Schroder, U. (2013). Electron transfer and biofilm formation of *Shewanella putrefaciens* as function of anode potential. In Wlodzimierz Kutner (Ed.), *Bioelectrochemistry, 93*. Proceedings of the 6th International Workshop on Surface Modification for Chemical and Biochemical Sensing (SMCBS) (pp. 23–29). Lochow, Poland.

Catal, T., Li, K., Bermek, H., & Liu, H. (2008). Electricity production from twelve monosaccharides using microbial fuel cells. *Journal of Power Sources. 175*, 196–200.

Celmer-Repina, D., Hwangb, J. H., Cicekc, N. & Oleszkiewiczb, J. A. (2010). Autotrophic nitrogen-removing biofilms on porous and non-porous membranes. *Environmental Technology. 31*, 1391–1401.

Characklis, W. G., McFeters, G. A. & Marshall, K. C. (1990). Physiological ecology in biofilm systems. In W. G.

Characklis & K. C. Marshall (Eds.), *Biofilms* (pp. 341–94) New York, USA. John Wiley & Sons.

Cheng, K. Y., Cord-Ruwisch, R. & Ho, G. (2009). A new approach for in situ cyclic voltammetry of a microbial fuel cell biofilm without using a potentiostat. *Bioelectrochemistry. 74*, 227–231.

Cheng, S. & Logan, B. E. (2007). Ammonia treatment of carbon cloth anodes to enhance power generation of microbial fuel cells. *Electrochemical Communications. 9*, 492– 496.

Choi, S. & Chae, J. (2013). Optimal biofilm formation and power generation in a micro-sized microbial fuel cell (MFC). *Sensors and Actuators A. 195*, 206– 212.

Coppi, M. V., Leang, C., Sandler, S. J. & Lovley, D. R. (2001). Development of a genetic system for *Geobacter sulfurreducens. Applied Environmental Microbiology. 67*, 3180–3187.

Costerton, J. W. Introduction to biofilm. (1999). *International Journal of Antimicrobial Agents.11*, 217–221.

Costerton, J. W., Lewandowski, Z. & Caldwell, D. E., (1995). Microbial biofilms. *Annual Review of Microbiology. 49*, 711–745.

Dalton, H. M. & March, P. E. (1998). Molecular genetics of bacterial attachment and biofouling. *Current Opinion in Biotechnology*. 9, 252–5

De Weger, L. A., Vlugt, C. & Wijfjes, A. H. M., Bakker, P., Schippers, B. & Lugtenberg, A. B. (1987). Flagella of plant-growth-stimulating *Pseudomonas fluorescens* strain are required for colonization of potato roots. *Journal of Bacteriology. 169*, 2769–73.

Debabov, V. G. Electricity from microorganisms. (2008). *Microbiology*. 77, 123–131.

Dunne, W. M. (2002). Bacterial adhesion: Seen any good biofilms lately? *Clinical Microbiology Reviews. 15*,155– 66.

El Abed, S., Ibnsouda, S. K., Latrache, H. & Hamadi, F. (2012). *Scanning electron microscopy (SEM) and environmental SEM: Suitable tools for study of adhesion stage and biofilm formation.* Croatia, European Union. INTECH Open Access Publisher.

El-Naggar, M. Y., Wanger, G., Leung, K. M., Yuzvinsky, T. D., Southam, G., Yang, J., Lau W. M., Nealson, K. H.

Gorby, Y. A. (2010). Electrical transport along bacterial nanowires from *Shewanella oneidensis MR-1. PANS*.107, 18127–18131.

Erbay, C., Pu, X., Choi, W., Choi, M. J., Ryu, Y., Hou, H., Lin, F., de Figueiredo, P., Yu, C. & Han, A. (2015).

Control of geometrical properties of carbon nanotube electrodes towards high-performance microbial fuel cells. *Journal of Power Sources. 280*, 347–354.

Feng, Y., Yang, Q., Wang, X. & Logan, B. E. (2010). Treatment of carbon fiber brush anodes for improving power generation in air–cathode microbial fuel cells. *Journal of Power Sources. 195*, 1841– 1844.

Fowler, H. W. & McKay, A. J. (1980). *Microbial adhesion to surfaces*. Chichester Sussex, UK. Ellis Horwood Ltd.

Franks, A. E. & Nevin, K. P. (2010). Microbial Fuel Cells: A Current Review. *Energies. 3*, 899-919.

Franks, A. E., Nevin, K. P., Jia, H., Izallalen, M., Woodard, T. L. & Lovley, D.R. (2009). Novel strategy for three-dimensional real-time imaging of microbial fuel cell communities: Monitoring the inhibitory effects of proton accumulation within the anode biofilm. *Energy and Environmental Science.2*, 113–119.

Freguia, S., Teh, E. H., Boon, N., Leung, K. M., Keller, J. & Rabaey, K. (2009). Microbial fuel cells operating on mixed fatty acids. *Bioresource Technology. 101*, 1233 1238.

Fricke, K., Harnisch, F. & Schroder, U. (2008). On the use of cyclic voltammetry for the study of anodic electron transfer in microbial fuel cells. *Energy and Environmental Science.1*, 144–147.

Friman, H., Schechter, A., Ioffe, Y., Nitzan, Y. & Cahan, R. (2013). Current production in a microbial fuel cell using a pure culture of *Cupriavidus basilensis* growing in acetate or phenol as a carbon source. *Microbial Biotechnology. 6*, 425–434.

Galvez, A., Greenman, J. & Ieropoulos, I. (2009). Landfill leachate treatment with microbial fuel cells: Scale-up through plurality. *Bioresource Technology. 100*, 5085–5091.

Ganesh, R., Robinson, K. G., Reed, G. D. & Sayler, G. S. (1997). Reduction of hexavalent uranium from organic complexes by sulfate- and iron-reducing bacteria. *Applied Environmental Microbiology. 63*, 4385–4391.

Garrett, T. R., Bhakoo, M. & Zhang, Z. (2008). Bacterial adhesion and biofilms on surfaces. *Progress in Natural Science 18*, 1049–1056.

Ghigo, J. M. (2003). Are there biofilm-specific physiological pathways beyond a reasonable doubt? *Research in Microbiology. 154*, 1–8.

Gorby, Y. A., Yanina, S., McLean, J. S., Rosso, K. M., Moyles, D., Dohnalkova, A., ...Nealson, K. H., Fredrickson, J. K. (2006). Electrically conductive bacterial nanowires produced by *Shewanella oneidensis Strain MR-1* and Other Microorganisms. *PANS*. 103, 11358–11363.

Guo, K., Freguia, S., Dennis, P. G., Chen, X., Donose, B. C., Keller, J., Gooding, J. J. & Rabaey, K. (2013). Effects of surface charge and hydrophobicity on anodic biofilm formation, community composition, and current generation in bioelectrochemical systems. *Enviromental Science and Technology. 47*, 7563–70.

Hall-Stoodley, L. & Stoodley, P. (2002). Developmental regulation of microbial biofilms. *Current Opinions in Biotechnology. 13*, 228–33.

Harnisch, F. & Schroder, U. (2010). From MFC to MXC: Chemical and biological cathodes and their potential for microbial bioelectrochemical systems. *Chemical Society Reviews. 39*, 4433–4448.

He, Z., Huang, Y. L., Manohar, A. K. & Mansfeld, F. (2008). Effect of electrolyte pH on the rate of the anodic and cathodic reactions in an air-cathode microbial fuel cell. *Bioelectrochemistry. 24*, 78–82.

Heidelberg, J. F., Paulsen, I. T., Nelson, K. E., Gaidos, E. J., Nelson, W. C., Read, T. D., ...Fraser, C. M. (2002). Genome sequence of the dissimilatory metal ion-reducing bacterium *Shewanella oneidensis*. *Nature Biotechnology. 20*, 1118–1123.

Holmes, D. E., Bond D. R., O'Neil, R. A., Reimers, C. E., Tender, L. R. & Lovley, D.R. (2004). Microbial communities associated with electrodes harvesting electricity from a variety of aquatic sediments. *Microbial Ecology. 48*, 178–190.

Holmes, D. E., Chaudhuri, S. K., Nevin, K. P., Mehta, T., Methe, B. A., Liu, A., Ward, J. E., Woodard, T. L., Webster, J. & Lovley, D.R. (2006). Microarray and genetic analysis of electron transfer to electrodes in *Geobacter sulfurreducens*. *Environmental Microbiology. 8*, 1805–1815.

Houdt, R. V. & Michiels, C.W. (2010). Biofilm formation and the food industry: A focus on the bacterial outer surface. *Journal of Applied Microbiology. 109*, 1117–1131.

Izallalen, M., Mahadevan, R., Burgard, A., Postier, B., Didonato Jr, R., Sun, J., Schilling, C. H. & Lovley, D. R. (2008). *Geobacter sulfurreducens* strain engineered for increased rates of respiration. *Metabolic Engineering.10*, 267–275.

Jung, S. & Regan, J. M. (2007). Comparison of anode bacterial communities and performance in microbial fuel cells with different electron donors. *Applied Microbiology and Biotechnology. 77,* 393–402.

Kiely, P. D., Call, D. F., Yates, M. D., Regan, J. M. & Logan, B. E. (2010). Anodic biofilms in microbial fuel cells harbor low numbers of higher-power-producing bacteria than abundant genera. *Applied Microbiology and Biotechnology. 88,* 371–380.

Kim, B. C., Postier, B. L., Didonato, R. J., Chaudhuri, S. K., Nevin, K. P. & Lovley, D. R. (2008). Insights into genes involved in electricity generation in *Geobacter sulfurreducens* via whole genome microarray analysis of the OmcF-deficient mutant. *Bioelectrochemistry. 73,* 70–75.

Kim, B. C., Qian, X., Leang, C., Coppi, M. V. & Lovley, D. R. Two putative c-type multiheme cytochromes required for the expression of OmcB, an outer membrane protein essential for optimal Fe (III) reduction in *Geobacter sulfurreducens. Journal of Bacteriology. 188,* 3138–3142 (2006).

Kim, B., Park, H., Kim, H., Kim, G., Chang, I., Lee, J. & Phung, N. (2004). Enrichment of microbial community generating electricity using a fuel-cell-type electrochemical cell. *Applied Microbiology Biotechnology. 63,* 672– 681.

Kim, G. T., Webster, G., Wimpenny, J. W., Kim, B. H., Kim, H. J. & Weightman, A. J. (2006). Bacterial community structure, compartmentalization and activity in a microbial fuel cell. *Journal of Applied Microbiology 101,* 698-710.

Kim, J. R., Jung, S. H., Regan, J. M. & Logan, B. E. (2007). Electricity generation and microbial community analysis of alcohol powered microbial fuel cells. *Bioresource Technology. 98,* 2568–2577.

Klimes, A., Franks, A. E., Glaven, R. H., Tran, H., Barrett, C. L., Qiu, Y., Zengler, K. & Lovley, D. R. (2010). Production of pilus-like filaments in *Geobacter sulfurreducens* in the absence of the type IV pilin protein PilA. *FEMS Microbiology Letters. 310,* 62–68.

Kokare, C. R., Chakraborty, S., Khopade, A. N. & Mahadik, K.R. (2009). Biofilm: Importance and applications. *Journal of Biotechnology. 8,* 159-168.

Kracke, F., Vassilev, I. & Krömer, J. O. (2015). Microbial electron transport and energy conservation –the foundation for optimizing bioelectrochemical systems. *Frontiers in Microbiology. 6,* 1–18.

Kumar, R., Singh, L. & Zularisam, A. W. (2016). Exoelectrogens: Recent advances in molecular drivers involved in extracellular electron transfer and strategies used to improve it for microbial fuel cell applications. *Renewable and Sustainable Energy Reviews. 56,* 1322–1336.

Leang, C., & Lovley, D. R. (2005). Regulation of two highly similar genes, omcB and omcC, in a 10kb chromosomal duplication in *Geobacter sulfurreducens. Microbiology Microbiology. 151,* 1761–1767.

Lebedev, N., Strycharz-Glaven, S. M. & Tender, L. M. (2014). High resolution AFM and single-cell resonance raman spectroscopy of *Geobacter sulfurreducens* biofilms early in growth. *Frontiers in Energy Research. 2,* 1– 8.

Li, H. R., Feng, Y. L., Tang, X. H., Zhang, J. J., & Lianb, J. (2010). The factors affecting biofilm formation in the mediatorless microbial fuel cell. *Chemical and Biochemical Engineering Quarterly. 24,* 341–346.

Li, X., Wang, X., Wan, L., Zhang, Y., Li, N., Lic, D. & Zhou, Q. (2016). Enhanced biodegradation of aged petroleum hydrocarbons in soils by glucose addition in microbial fuel cells. *Journal of Chemical Technology and Biotechnology. 91,* 267–275.

Liu, H. & Logan, B. (2004). Electricity generation using an air-cathode single chamber microbial fuel cell in the presence and absence of a proton exchange membrane. *Environmental Science and Technology. 38,* 4040–4046.

Liu, Y. & Tay, J. H. (2002). The essential role of hydrodynamic shear force in the formation of biofilm and granular sludge. *Water Research. 36,* 1653–1665.

Liu, Y., Harnisch, F., Fricke, K., Schroder, U., Climent, V. & Feliu, J. M. (2010). The study of electrochemically active microbial biofilms on different carbon-based anode materials in microbial fuel cells. *Biosensors and Bioelectronics. 25,* 2167–2171.

Lobato, J., Canizares, P., Fernandez, F. J. & Rodrigo, M. A. (2012). An evaluation of aerobic and anaerobic sludges as start-up material for microbial fuel cell systems. *New Biotechnology. 29,* 415– 420.

Logan, B. E. & Regan, J. M. (2006a). Microbial fuel cells-challenges and applications. *Environmental Science and Technology. 40,* 5172–5180.

Logan, B. E. (2008). *Microbial Fuel Cells.* Hoboken, New Jersey, USA. John Wiley & Sons, Inc.

Logan, B. E. (2009). Exoelectrogenic bacteria that power microbial fuel cells. *Natures Review of Microbiology. 7,* 375–381.

Logan, B. E., Cheng, S., Watson, V. & Estadt, G. (2007). Graphite fiber brush anodes for increased power production in air-cathode microbial fuel cells. *Environmental Science and Technology. 41,* 3341–3346.

Logan, B. E., Hamelers, B., Rozendal, R., Schroder, U., Keller, J., Freguia, S., Aelterman, P., Verstraete, W. & Rabaey, K. (2006). Microbial fuel cells: Methodology and technology. *Environmental Science and Technology. 40,* 5181–5192.

Lovley, D. R. & Anderson, R. T. (2000). Influence of dissimilatory metal reduction on fate of organic and metal contaminants in the subsurface. *Hydrogeology Journal. 8,* 77–88.

Lovley, D. R. & Nevin, K. P. (2008). Electricity production with electricigens. In J. Wall, C. Harwood & A.

Demain (Eds.) *Bioenergy: Microbial contributions to alternative fuels* (pp. 295–306) Washington D.C., USA. ASM Press.

Lovley, D. R. & Nevin, K. P. (2011). A shift in the current: New applications and concepts for microbe-electrode electron exchange. *Current Opinion in Biotechnology. 22,* 441–448.

Lovley, D. R. (2006). Bug juice: Harvesting electricity with microorganisms. *Nature Review of Microbiology. 4*, 497–508.

Lovley, D. R. (2006a). Microbial fuel cells: Novel microbial physiologies and engineering approaches. *Current Opinions in Biotechnology 17*, 327–332.

Lovley, D. R. (2008a). The microbe electric: Conversion of organic matter to electricity. *Current Opinions in Biotechnology 19*, 564–571.

Lovley, D. R. (2008b). Extracellular electron transfer: Wires, capacitors, iron lungs, and more. *Geobiology. 6*, 225– 231.

Luo, H., Liu, G., Zhang, R. & Jin, S. (2009). Phenol degradation in microbial fuel cells. *Chemical Engineering Journal. 147*, 259–264.

Ly, H. K., Harnisch, F., Hong, S. F, Schroder U., Hildebrandt, P. & Millo, D. (2013). Unraveling the interfacial electron transfer dynamics of electroactive microbial biofilms using surface-enhanced raman spectroscopy. *ChemSusChem. 6*, 487 – 492.

Mahadevan, R., Bond, D. R., Butler, J. E., Esteve-Nunez, A., Coppi, M. V., Palsson, B. O., Schilling, C. H. & Lovley, D. R. (2006). Characterization of metabolism in the Fe (III)-reducing organism *Geobacter sulfurreducens* by constraint-based modeling. *Applied Environmental Microbiology. 72*, 1558–1568.

Malvankar, N. S., Tuominen, M. T. & Lovley, D. R. (2012). Comment on "On electrical conductivity of microbial nanowires and biofilms" by S.M. Strycharz- Glaven, R.M.Snider, A. Guiseppi-Elie, and L.M. Tender. Energy Environ. Sci. 2011, 4, 4366, *Energy and Environmental Science. 5*, 6247–6249.

Malvankar, N. S., Vargas, M., Nevin, K., Tremblay, P. L., Evans-Lutterodt, K., Nykypanchuk, D., Martz, E., Touminen, M. T., & Lovley, D.R. (2015). Structural basis for metallic-like conductivity in microbial nanowires. *mBio. 6*, e000841–10.

Malvankar, N.S., Vargas, M., Nevin, K.P., Franks, A.E., Leang, C., Kim, B. C., Inoue, K., Mester, T., Covalla, S. F., Johnson, J. P., Rotello, V. M., Tuominen, M. T. & Lovley, D.R. (2011). Tunable metallic-like conductivity in microbial nanowire networks. *Nature Nanotechnology 6*, 573–579.

Mathuriya, A. S. & Sharma, V.N. (2009). Bioelectricity production from various wastewaters through microbial fuel cell technology. *Journal of Biochemical Technology. 2*, 133–137.

Methe, B. A., Nelson, K. E., Eisen, J. A., Paulsen, I. T., Nelson, W., Heidelberg, J. F., ...Fraser, C. M. (2003). The genome of *Geobacter sulfurreducens*: Insights into metal reduction in subsurface environments. *Science. 302*, 1967–1969.

Morris, J. M. & Jin, S. (2008). Feasibility of using microbial fuel cell technology for bioremediation of hydrocarbons in groundwater. *Journal of Environmental Science and Health A: Toxic/Hazardous Substances and Environmental Engineering. 43*, 18–23.

Murphy, D. B. (2001). Confocal laser scanning microscopy. In *Fundamentals of Light Microscopy and Electronic Imaging*. New Jersey, USA (pp. 205–230). John Wiley & Sons.

Mustakeem. (2015). Electrode materials for microbial fuel cells: Nanomaterial approach. *Materials for Renewable and Sustainable Energy. 4,* 1–11.

Myers, C. R. & Myers, J. M. (2002a). MtrB is required for proper incorporation of the cytochromes OmcA and OmcB into the outer membrane of *Shewanella putrifaciens MR-1, Applied Environmental Microbiology. 68,* 5585–5594.

Myers, J. M. & Myers, C. R., (2002). Genetic complementation of an outer membrane cytochrome OmcB mutant of *Shewanella putrifaciens MR-1* Requires OmcB plus downstream DNA, *Applied Environmental Microbiology. 68,* 2781–2793.

Nevin, K. P., Kim, B. C., Glaven, R. H., Johnson, J. P., Woodard, T. L., Methe, B. A., DiDonato Jr, R. J., Covalla, S. F., Franks, A. E., Liu, A. & Lovley D. R. (2009). Anode biofilm transcriptomics reveals outer surface components essential for high density current production in *Geobacter sulfurreducens* fuel cells. *PLOS One. 4,* e5628 1 –11.

Nevin, K. P., Richter, H., Covalla, S. F., Johnson, J. P., Woodard, T. L., Orloff, A. L., Jia, H., Zhang, M. & Lovely, D. R. (2008). Power output and columbic efficiencies from biofilms of *Geobacter sulfurreducens* comparable to mixed community microbial fuel cells. *Environmental Microbiology. 10,* 2505–14.

Niemantsverdriet, J. W. (2007). *Spectroscopy in catalysis: An Introduction.* (3rd ed.), Weinheim, Germany. Wiley-VCH Verlag GmbH & Co KGaA.

Niessen, J., Schroder, U. & Scholz, F. (2004). Exploiting complex carbohydrates for microbial electricity generation – a bacterial fuel cell operating on starch. *Electrochemistry Communications. 6,* 955–958.

O'Toole, G., Kaplan, H. B. & Kolter, R. (2000). Biofilm formation as microbial development. *Annual Review of Microbiology. 54,* 49–79.

Pant, D., Bogaert, G. V., Diels, L. & Vanbroekhoven, K. (2010). A review of the substrates used in microbial fuel cells (MFCs) for sustainable energy production. *Bioresource Technology. 101,* 1533–1543.

Park, D. H. & Kim, B. H. (2001). Growth properties of the iron-reducing bacteria, *Shewanella putrefaciens IR-1* and MR-1 coupling to reduction of Fe(III) to Fe(II). *Journal of Microbiology. 39,* 273–278.

Park, D. H. & Zeikus, J. G. (2000). Electricity generation in microbial fuel cells using neutral red as an electronophore. *Applied Environmental Microbiology. 66,* 1292–1297.

Patil, S. A., Harnisch, F., Kapadnis, B., & Schroder, U. Electroactive mixed culture biofilms in microbial bioelectrochemical systems: The role of temperature for biofilm formation and performance. *Biosensors and Bioelectronics 26,* 803–808 (2010).

Patil, S. A., Harnisch, F., Koch, C., Hubschmann, T., Fetzer, I., Carmona-Martínez, A. A., Müller, S. & Schroder U. Electroactive mixed culture derived biofilms in microbial bioelectrochemical systems: The role of pH on biofilm formation, performance and composition, *Bioresource Technology 102,* 9683–9690 (2011).

Patil, S. A., Surakasi, V. P., Koul, S., Ijmulwar, S., Vivek, A., Shouche, Y. S. & Kapadnis, B. P. (2009). Electricity generation using chocolate industry wastewater and its treatment in activated sludge based microbial fuel cell and analysis of developed microbial community in the anode chamber. *Bioresource Technology 100*, 5132– 5139.

Percival, S. L., Walker, J. T. & Hunter, P. R. (2000). *Microbiological Aspects of Biofilms and Drinking Water*. Florida USA. CRC Press.

Pham, H. T., Boon, N., Aelterman, P., Clauwaert, P., DeSchamphelaire, L., Van Oostveldt, P., Verbeken, K., Rabaey, K. & Verstraete, W. (2008). High shear enrichment improves the performance of the anodophilic microbial consortium in a microbial fuel cell. *Microbiology Biotechnology. 1*, 487–496.

Pirbadian, S., Barchinger, S. E., Leung, K. M., Byun, H. S., Jangir, Y., Bouhenni, R. A., Reed, S. B., Romine, M. F., Saffarini, D. A., Shi, L., Gorby, Y. A., Golbeck, J. H., & El- Naggar, M. Y. (2014). *Shewanella oneidensis MR-1* nanowires are outer membrane and periplasmic extensions of the extracellular electron transport components. *PANS*. 111, 12883–2888.

Qian X., Reguera G., Mester T. and Lovley D. R. (2007). Evidence that OmcB and OmpB of *Geobacter sulfurreducens* are outer membrane surface proteins. *FEMS Microbiology Letters. 277*, 21–27.

Rabaey, K., Boon, N., Hofte, M., & Verstraete, W. (2005). Microbial phenazine production enhances electron transfer in biofuel cells. *Environmental Science and Technology 39*, 3401–3408.

Radwan, S. S., Al-Hasan, R. H., Salamah, S. & Al-Dabbous, S. (2002). Bioremediation of oily sea water by bacteria immobilized in biofilms coating macroalgae. *International Biodeterioration Biodegradation. 50*, 55–9.

Raghavulu, S. V., Modestra, A., Amulya, K., Reddy, C. N. & Venkata Mohan, S. (2013). Relative effect of bioaugmentation with electrochemically active and non- active bacteria on bioelectrogenesis in microbial fuel cell. *Bioresource Technology. 146*, 696–703.

Rahimnejad, M., Adhami, A., Darvari, S., Zirepour, A. & Oh, S-E. (2015). Microbial fuel cell as new technology for bioelectricity generation: A review. *Alexandria Engineering Journal. 54*, 745–756.

Rahimnejad, M., Najafpour, C. D., Ghoreyshi, A. A., Talebnia, F., Premier, G C., Bakeri, G., Kim, J. R., & Oh, S-E. (2012). Thionine increases electricity generation from microbial fuel cell using *saccharomyces cerevisiae* and exoelectrogenic mixed culture. *The Journal of Microbiology. 50*, 575–580.

Ramasamy, R. P., Ren Z., Mench M. M. & Regan, J. M. (2008). Impact of initial biofilm growth on the anode impedance of microbial fuel cells. *Biotechnology and Bioengineering. 101*, 101–108.

Read, S. T., Dutta, P., Bond, P. L., Keller J. & Rabaey, K. (2010). Initial development and structure of biofilms on microbial fuel cell anodes. *BMC Microbiology. 98*, 1 – 10.

Reguera, G., McCarthy, K. D., Mehta, T., Nicoll, J. S., Tuominen, M. T. & Lovley, D. R. (2005). Extracellular electron transfer via microbial nanowires. *Nature. 435*, 1098–1101.

Reguera, G., Nevin, K. P., Nicoll, J. S., Covalla, S. F., Woodard, T. L. & Lovley, D. R. (2006). Biofilm and nanowire production leads to increased current in *Geobacter sulfurreducens* fuel cells. *Applied Environmental Microbiology. 72*, 7345–7348.

Ren, Z., Steinberg, L. M. & Regan, J. M. (2008). Electricity production and microbial biofilm characterization in cellulose-fed microbial fuel cells. *Water Science Technology. 58*, 617–622.

Richter, H., McCarthy, K., Nevin, K. P., Johnson, J. P., Rotello, V. M. & Lovley, D. R. (2008). Electricity generation by *Geobacter sulfurreducens* attached to gold electrodes. *Langmuir. 24*, 4376–4379.

Richter, H., Nevin, K. P., Jia, H., Lowy, D. A., Lovley, D. R. & Tender, L. M. (2009). Cyclic voltammetry of biofilms of wild type and mutant *Geobacter sulfurreducens* on fuel cell anodes indicates possible roles of omcb, omcz, type iv pili, and protons in extracellular electron transfer. *Energy and Environmental Science. 2*, 506– 516.

Richter, K., Schicklberger, M. & Gescher, J. (2012). Dissimilatory reduction of extracellular electron acceptors in anaerobic respiration. *Applied Environmental Microbiology* 78, 913–921.

Rinaldi, A., Mecheri, B., Garavaglia, V., Licoccia, S., Di Nardoc, P. & Traversa, E. (2008). Engineering materials and biology to boost performance of microbial fuel cells: A critical review. *Energy and Environmental Science. 1*, 417–429.

Ringeisen, B. R., Hendeson, E., Wu, P.K., Pietron, J., Ray, R., Little, B., Biffinger, J. C. & Jones-Meehan, J. M. (2006). High power density from a miniature microbial fuel cell using *Shewanella oneidensis* DSP10, *Environmental Science and Technology. 40*, 2629–2634.

Rittmann, B. E., Trinet, F., Amar, D. & Chang, H. T. (1992). Measurement of the activity of a biofilm: Effects of surface loading and detachment on a three-phase, liquid-fluidized-bed reactor. *Water Science and Technology*. 585–594.

Rodrigo, M.A., Canizares, P., Lobato, J., Paz, R., C. Saez & Linares J. J. (2007). Production of electricity from the treatment of urban waste water using a microbial fuel cell. *Journal of Power Sources. 169*, 198–204.

Rooney-Varga, J. N., Anderson, R. T., Fraga, J. L., Ringelberg, D. & Lovley, D. R. (1999). Microbial communities associated with anaerobic benzene degradation in a petroleum-contaminated aquifer. *Applied Environmental Microbiology. 65*, 3056–3063.

Sandholm, T. M. & Wirtanen, G. (1992). Biofilm formation in the industry: A review. *Food Reviews International. 8*, 573–603.

Schechter, M., Schechter, A., Rozenfeld, S., Efrat, E. & Cahan R. (2014). Anode Biofilm, In Chin-Tsan Wang (Ed.), *Technology and application of microbial fuel cells* (pp. 57–75). Croatia, European Union. INTECH Open Access Publisher.

Sharma, V. & Kundu, P. P. (2010). Biocatalysts in microbial fuel cells. *Enzyme and Microbial Technology 47* 179–188.

Shi, L., Rosso, K. M., Clarke, T. A., Richardson, D. J., Zachara, J. M. & Fredrickson, J. K. (2012). Molecular underpinnings of Fe (III) oxidereduction by *Shewanella oneidensisMR-1. Frontiers of Microbiology. 3,* 1–10.

Shirtliff, M. E., Mader, J. T. & Camper, A. K. (2000). Molecular interactions in biofilms. *Chemistry and Biology. 9,* 859–71.

Singh, D., Pratap, D., Baranwal, Y., Kumar, B. & Chaudhary, R. K. (2010). Microbial fuel cells: A green technology for power generation. *Annals of Biological Research. 1,* 128–138.

Srikanth, S., Marsili, E., Flickinger, M. C. & Bond, D. R. (2008). Electrochemical characterization of *Geobacter sulfurreducens* cells immobilized on graphite paper electrodes. *Biotechnology and Bioengineering. 99,* 1065 – 1073.

Stepanovic, S., Cirkovic, I., Mijac, V. & Svabic-Vlahovic, M. (2003). Influence of the incubation temperature, atmosphere and dynamic conditions on biofilm formation by *Salmonella spp. Food Microbiology. 20,* 339–343.

Sun, J., Hu, Y.-Y., Bi, Z. & Cao, Y.-Q. (2009). Simultaneous decolorization of azo dye and bioelectricity generation using a microfiltration membrane air-cathode single chamber microbial fuel cell. *Bioresource Technology. 100,* 3185–3192.

Sung, Y., Fletcher, K. F., Ritalaliti, K. M., Apkarian, R. P., Ramos-Hernandez, N., Sanford, R. A., Mesbah, N. M.

Loffler, F. E. (2006). *Geobacter lovleyi sp nov strain SZ,* a novel metal-reducing and tetrachloroethene-dechlorinating bacterium. *Applied Environmental Microbiology. 72,* 2775–2782.

Teh, K. H., Flint S., Brooks, J. & Knight, G. (2015). *Biofilms in the Dairy Industry.* West Sussex, UK. John Wiley & Sons Ltd.

Teng, S. X., Tong, Z. H., Li, W. W., Wang, S. G., Sheng, G. P., Shi, X. Y., Liu, X. W. & Yu, H. Q. (2010). Electricity generation from mixed volatile fatty acids using microbial fuel cells. *Applied Microbiology Biotechnology. 87,* 2365–2372.

Torres, C. I., Kato Marcus, A. & Rittmann, B. E. (2008). Proton transport inside the biofilm limits electrical current generation by anode-respiring bacteria. *Biotechnology Bioengineering. 100,* 872–881.

Torres, C. I., Lee, H. S. & Rittmann B. E. (2008a). Carbonate species as OH- carriers for decreasing the pH gradient between cathode and anode in biological fuel cells. *Environmental Science and Technology. 42,* 8773– 8777.

Venkidusamy, K., Megharaj, M., Marzorati, M., Lockington, R. & Naidu, R. (2016). Enhanced removal of petroleum hydrocarbons using a bioelectrochemical remediation system with pre-cultured anodes. *Science of the Total Environment 539,* 61–69.

Wang, X., Feng, Y. J. & Lee, H. (2008). Electricity production from beer brewery wastewater using single chamber microbial fuel cell. *Water Science and Technology. 57,* 1117–21.

Watanabe, K. (2008). Recent developments in microbial fuel cell technologies for sustainable bioenergy. *Journal of Biosciences Bioengineering. 106,* 528– 536.

Wei, J., Liang, P. & Huang, X. (2011). Recent progress in electrodes for microbial fuel cells. *Bioresource Technology. 102,* 9335–9344.

Wen, Q., Wu, Y., Zhao, L. & Sun, Q. (2010). Production of electricity from the treatment of continuous brewery wastewater using a microbial fuel cell. *Fuel. 89,* 1381–1385.

Wilkins, M. J., Livens, F. R., Vaughan, D. J. & Lloyd, J. R. (2006). The impact of Fe (III) - reducing bacteria on uranium mobility. *Biogeochemistry. 78,* 125– 150.

Yi, H., Nevin, K. P., Kim, B. C., Franks, A. E., Klimes, A., Tender, L. M. & Lovley, D. R. (2009). Selection of a variant of *Geobacter sulfurreducens* with enhanced capacity for current production in microbial fuel cells. *Biosensors and Bioelectronics. 24,* 3498–3503.

Yong, X-Y., Shi, D-Y., Chen Y-L., Feng, J., Xu, L., Zhou, J., Wang, S-Y., Yong, Y-C., Sun, Y-M., OuYang, P-K.

Zheng, T. (2014). Enhancement of bioelectricity generation by manipulation of the electron shuttles synthesis pathway in microbial fuel cells. *Bioresource Technology. 152,* 220–224.

You, S. J., Zhao, Q. L., Jiang, J. Q., Zhang, J. N. & Zhao, S. Q. (2006). Sustainable approach for leachate treatment: Electricity generation in microbial fuel cell. *Journal of Environmental Science and Health Part A. 41,* 2721– 2734.

Yuan, Y., Zhao, B., Zhou, S., Zhong, S. & Zhuang, L. (2011). Electrocatalytic activity of anodic biofilm responses to pH changes in microbial fuel cells. *Bioresource Technology. 102,* 6887–6891.

Zhang, Y., Min, B., Huang, L. & Angelidaki, I. (2009). Generation of electricity and analysis of microbial communities in wheat straw biomass-powered microbial fuel cells. *Applied Environmental Microbiology. 75,* 3389–3395.

Zhao, F., Slade, R. C. & Varcoe, J. R. (2009). Techniques for the study and development of microbial fuel cells: An electrochemical perspective. *Chemical Society Review. 38,* 1926–1939.

Chapter 2

Nano in Fine Print

Suhani Patel, Sonal Bakshi*

Institute of Science, Nirma University, Ahmedabad-382 481, Gujarat, India.
E-mail: suhanipalkhiwala@gmail.com, sonal.bakshi@nirmauni.ac.in*

Abstract

The rapid increase in use and new applications of the engineered nanoparticles presents a challenge to the regulatory agencies in forming guidelines to ensure safety and avoid potential hazards to the users and environment at large. It's a paradox that the properties of nanoparticles that gives them an edge over other materials in terms of economic and scientific value are the same that raise concerns over safety, as these are potentially hazardous in nature. The regulatory framework concerning the manufacture and use of engineered nanoparticles is inadequate and the laws are not ubiquitously accepted. It is essential to address the newly emerging hazards that nanotechnology presents. Nanoparticle containing items are currently being regulated by a variety of federal agencies around the world. Organizations working on the safety aspects and the regulations of nanomaterials intended for daily use include International Standard Organisation, Organisation for Economic Co-operation and Development (OECD), U.S. Environmental Protection Agency (EPA), National Institute for Occupational Safety and Health (NIOSH), Europeon Commission are amongst a few of them. Also a few non government organisations have been making their presence felt regarding the risks and safety concerns of nanoparticles. Even though legal authority does exist, substantial regulatory changes in the existing laws are likely to be essential in order to effectively address the fundamental concerns related to the safety aspect of engineered nanoparticles. The current laws and regulatory systems must be adjusted and applied to the nanomaterials based on the knowledge regarding fate of nanoparticles entering the human body and eco system. There is an urgent need for sound laboratory data of safety assessment that takes into consideration the unique particokinetics properties of nanoparticles. Globally various research groups are contributing to this need. This will address the need for understanding cause and effect relation of exposure to various nanoparticles and potentially adverse biological effects.

Keywords: Nanoparticles, Biological effect, *in vitro* genotoxicity assessment, international regulatory guidelines, safety.

1. Introduction

In between all the controversies relating nanotechnology, the concept explained by Richard Feynman in his lecture is agreed by all. In his lecture entitled 'There's plenty of room at the bottom' he explains that '*A biological system can be exceedingly small. Many of the cells are very tiny, but they are very active; they manufacture various sub- stances; they walk around; they wiggle; and they do all kinds of marvelous things – all on a very small scale. Also, they store in- formation. Consider the possibility that we too can make a thing very small which does what we want – that we can manufacture an object that maneuvers at that level*' (Feynman, 1960). Nanotechnology can be generally explained as any technology, which on a Nano scale, can manipulate matter and has application in the real world. Over a period of time, researchers have developed a better understanding of matter at finer levels, and have come up with proposals for definitions (Lövestam *et al.*, 2010). International Organization for Standardization (ISO) Technical Committee on Nanotechnology (TC229) has developed a working definition for nanotechnology. A majority of jurisdictions currently define the 'nanoscale' as encompassing materials between 1 and 100 nanometers in size in at least one dimension. The term 'nanomaterial' refers to any material having one or more dimensions in the nanoscale or a material that is itself nano-structured. The term 'nanoparticle' refers to a minute piece of matter with defined physical boundaries, in which a particle can move as a unit. This general particle definition applies to nano-objects. The OECD has adopted the ISO definitions (ISO/TS 80004-4:2011). In October 2011 the EU Commission has presented a recommendation regarding the definition of nanomaterials. Commission Recommendation 2011/696/EU defined 'nanomaterial' as follows: *"Nanomaterial" means a natural, incidental or manufactured material containing particles, in an unbound state or as an aggregate or as an agglomerate and where, for 50 % or more of the particles in the number size distribution, one or more external dimensions is in the size range 1 nm - 100 nm* (EU Commission, 2011).

The manufactured nanomaterials referred to as the engineered nanomaterials are materials that typically possess nanostructure-dependent properties (e.g., chemical, mechanical, electrical, optical, magnetic, biological), which make them desirable for various commercial or medical applications. However, these same properties potentially may lead to nanostructure-dependent biological activities that affect the human body, since the behavior of nanoparticles is relatively different from bulk. While the applications and benefits are impressive, the information regarding the potential effects of their increasing and widespread use in consumer and industrial products are beginning to emerge (Hoet *et al.*, 2004). Nanoparticles are unique not simply due to their small size, but their large surface area relative to their small size. Research of nanoparticles is currently of prime importance due to the following reasons. (1) The increase in the ratio of surface area to volume dimensions below the critical wavelength renders them transparent, making them highly suitable for cosmetics, coatings and packing. (2) These are better than the conventional delivery systems because: (a) excellent performance via different routes such as oral, intravenous or dermal (b) enhanced bioavailability and high level of pharmacological action (c) applications in controlled and targeted delivery. (3) Used as drug carriers due to high stability, higher capacity, and feasibility of incorporation of both hydrophilic and hydrophobic substances. The attributes of nanoparticles due to which the physicochemical properties of a material can be altered, also create the opportunity for increased uptake and interaction with the biological tissue. And this can lead to adverse biological effects in the living cells, which would not otherwise happen with the same material in larger form (Shinde *et al.*, 2012). Thus the physical and chemical properties of nanoparticles have a very strong influence on the biological components or the environment, and also on the way they move, accumulate and clear in the body (The dose makes the poison, 2011). This concern has led to research investigations for safety of nanoparticles. A rapid identification of research priorities is needed long with a road map for nanosafety. This paper briefly describes current status of international government and nongovernment agencies which play a major role in addressing safety and regulations associated with the use of nanotechnology.

2. Government Institutions

2.1. US-EPA (Environmental Protection Agency)

The role of EPA is researching and developing the benefits of nanotechnology, along with the obligation and mandate to safeguard environment and protect human health. This is done by addressing potential risks and understanding the physicochemical parameters of the nanoscale materials (Morris and Willis, 2007). With passage of time, the EPA is shifting from a voluntary approach to a mandatory approach, along with regulating and collecting information on the potential risks from nanomaterials (Duvall and Wyatt, 2011). The Toxic Substances Control Act (TSCA) act is responsible for regarding many nanoscale materials as "chemical substances" (Control of Nanoscale Materials under the Toxic Substances Control Act, EPA). In the year 2014, EPA retains the prior plan "to require reporting and recordkeeping under TSCA section 8(a), which would require that persons who manufacture these nanoscale materials notify EPA of certain information including production volume, methods of manufacture and processing, exposure and release information, and available health and safety data" (Duvall and Wyatt, 2014). The information gathered is intended to enable EPA to evaluate the need for additional regulations under TSCA. The proposed rule is not yet public.

2.2. FIFRA (Federal Insecticide, Fungicide, and Rodenticide Act)

FIFRA and EPA implement regulations that provide an effective framework for regulating pesticide products containing nanomaterial. According to the report in June 2011, 3 components are included in the notice. Under the section 6(a)(2) existing information regarding which nanoscale material is present in a registered product and its potential effects on humans or the environment has to be made. Obtaining information on the nanoscale materials in pesticide products using data call in notices under FIFRA section 3(c)(2)(B). A new approach for how we will determine on a case-by-case basis whether a nanoscale active or inert ingredient is a "new" active or inert ingredient for purposes of FIFRA and the Pesticide Registration Improvement Act, even when an identical, non-nanoscale form of the nanoscale ingredient is already registered (Control of Nanoscale Materials under the Toxic Substances Control Act, EPA).

2.3. FDA (US Food and Drug Administration)

US FDA is a public health agency that uses scientific information to make regulatory decisions about products ranging from cosmetics to chemotherapy agents to food packaging. Recently, on June 24, 2014, FDA issued one draft and three final guidance documents related to the use of nanotechnology in regulated products (Nanotechnology Fact Sheet, 2014). Following are the guidelines.

2.3.1. Final Guidance for Industry: Considering Whether an FDA-Regulated Product Involves the Application of Nanotechnology

An affirmative finding to either of the points to consider might suggest the need for particular attention by the Agency and/or industry to the product to identify and address potential implications for safety, effectiveness, public health impact, or regulatory status of the product.

2.3.2. Final Guidance for Industry: Safety of Nanomaterials in Cosmetic Products

It describes FDA's current thinking on the safety assessment of nanomaterials when used in cosmetic products. The following are the conclusions:

1. Cosmetics and cosmetic ingredients (with the exception of color additives) are not subject to premarket approval; however, they must be safe for consumers under labeled or customary conditions of use, and they must be properly labeled.
2. Cosmetics manufactured using nanomaterials are subject to the same legal requirements as any other cosmetics. Companies and individuals who market cosmetics are legally responsible for the safety of their products.
3. In general, the framework currently in use for assessing safety of cosmetics is appropriate for cosmetics containing nanomaterials. However, data needed and the testing methods should be evaluated in light of the properties, behaviors, and/or effects that may be exhibited by nanomaterials used in cosmetic products.

2.4. NIOSH (National Institute for Occupational Safety and Health)

NIOSH leads the federal government nanotechnology initiative. Research and activities are coordinated through the NIOSH Nanotechnology Research Center (NTRC) established in 2004. On Oct 2, 2014 NIOSH signed a Memorandum of Understanding with the Colleges of Nanoscale Science and Engineering (CNSE) at SUNY Polytechnic Institute in Albany, New York. NIOSH and CNSE would be working together to advance research and guidance for occupational safety and health in the nanoelectronics industry and other settings where workers are potentially exposed to engineered nanomaterials (National Institute for Occupational Safety and Health (NIOSH), http://cdc.gov/niosh/).

2.5. NIST (National Institute of Science and Technology)

NIST nanotechnology research develops measurements, standards, and data crucial to a wide range of industries and Federal agencies. Labs at NIST develop advanced spectroscopic methods needed to increase efficiency in advanced photovoltaics, and the standard reference materials and data necessary to accurately quantify and measure the presence and impact of nanomaterials in the environment (National Nanotechnology Initiative. National Institute of Standards and Technology (NIST), US Department of Commerce, https://www.nano.gov//node/145).

2.6. OSHA (Occupational Safety and Health Administration)

As part of a government-wide coordination effort, OSHA is working with other federal agencies to address issues related to the impact of nanomaterials on human health and the environment. Nanomaterial use may fall under either OSHA General Industry or Construction standards. OSHA's Nanotechnology Safety and Health Topics Page highlights some of the OSHA standards that may apply to situations where workers handle or are exposed to nanomaterials. The General Duty Clause, Section 5(a)(1) of the *Occupational Safety and Health Act,* also may apply in situations where workers handle or are exposed to nanomaterials. States with OSHA-approved state plans may have additional standards that apply to nanotechnology (Occupational Safety and Health Administration (OSHA), 2013).

In April 2013, OSHA published Fact Sheet 3634, containing safety recommendations for the use of nanomaterials in the workplace. In summary, OSHA recommended that employers, identify nanomaterials and the processes in which they are used; conduct exposure assessments at the work site; use engineering and administrative controls and personal protective equipment (PPE) to reduce exposure to nano materials; develop emergency measures to take in the event of a nanomaterial spill or release; limit worker exposure to respirable carbon nanotubes and carbon nanofibers to less than 7.0 micrograms per cubic meter (μg/m3) on an 8-hour time weighted average; and limited worker exposure to nanoscale particles of titanium dioxide (TiO2) to less than .03 milligrams per cubic meter (mg/m3) on an 8-hour time weighted average (Occupational Safety and Health Administration (OSHA), 2013).

2.7. White House

Policy principles for U.S. Decision Making Concerning Regulation and Oversight of Applications of Nanotechnology and Nanomaterials.

The White House in U.S. published a memorandum for the heads of executive Departments and Agencies on the subject of Policy Principles for the U.S. Decision-Making Concerning Regulation and Oversight of Applications of Nanotechnology and Nanomaterials. President Obama addressed this issue on January 18, 2011 by saying *"Our regulatory system must protect public health, welfare, safety, and our environment while promoting economic growth, innovation, competitiveness, and job creation. It must be based on the best available science"* (Holdren *et al.*, 2011).

2.8. European Commission

The European Parliament together with several EU countries have called for more transparency, traceability and information for consumers regarding the use and possible exposure to nanomaterials, by the introduction of registers for products which contain nanomaterials or make use of nanotechnology, and/or by labelling of such products. Currently the EU legislation requires nanomaterials to be reported in the list of ingredients, with "nano" added in brackets after the substance name for food, cosmetics and biocides. Importantly, this labelling should be understood as risk-independent, as the nanomaterial presence does not automatically imply a risk. In addition, voluntary "nanoclaims" indicating the presence or absence of nanomaterials are sometimes added by manufacturers on different types of consumer products, mainly for marketing reasons (European Commission, 2014).

2.9. REACH (Registration, Evaluation, Authorization and Restriction of Chemicals)

The European chemicals legislation REACH (European Parliament and Council 2006) is based on the principle that manufacturers, importers and downstream users must ensure that the substances they manufacture, place on the market or use do not adversely affect human health or the environment (REACH, European Chemicals Agency (ECHA), 2006). Nanomaterials are covered by the substance definition of REACH, and the REACH provisions apply to them. Nanomaterials can be registered as nanoform(s) in the dossier of the corresponding non-nanoform of a substance or as distinct substance. Specific guidance for NM registration under REACH has been issued by ECHA. (European Chemicals Agency). A safety data sheet needs to be prepared for all substances, including nanomaterials classified as hazardous. The CLP (Classification, Labelling and Packaging) Regulation requires that hazardous properties of nanomaterials (as for any other substance or mixture) have to be communicated through the supply chain (any user or consumer). Those properties have to be indicated on the product label (above certain concentration limits). Cosmetic products containing nanomaterials need to be labelled (since July 2013 onwards) and notified to the European Commission before being placed on the market. The notification is done via the Cosmetic Products Notification Portal of the EC. The use of nanotechnology in food production is covered by the Novel Food Regulation. Nanomaterials used as novel food, food additives, food supplements or in food contact materials have to undergo an EU-wide authorization which is based on a risk assessment. Risk assessment and authorization for the macromaterial do not cover nanoforms. Engineered nanomaterials in food have to be indicated in the list of ingredients with the word "nano" in brackets (from the end of 2014). The Commission has adopted a proposal for a new Regulation on medical devices which explicitly addresses nanomaterials. It requires labelling of all medical devices which incorporate or consist of nanomaterials. Those devices that consist of nanomaterials are in class III, the highest risk class for medical devices. Only safe consumer products shall be placed on the EU market. Consumers have to be informed about risks associated with products and (dangerous) products have to be traceable. Currently there is no requirement in EU legislation to label consumer products in general (including textiles) for their content of nanomaterials (Aschberger et al., 2014).

2.10. OECD (Organization for Economic Co-operation and Development)

OECD is playing its part in coordinated approach to ensure that potential challenges are being addressed in parallel with the development and use of technology. Under the Committee on Scientific and Technological Policy (CSTP), a Working Party on Nanotechnology (WPN) was established in March 2007. The objective of the WPN is to advise on emerging policy-relevant issues in science, technology and innovation for the responsible development and use of nanotechnology. The work of the WPN complements the activities of other OECD committees and other organizations. The OECD Chemicals Committee Working Party on Manufactured Nanomaterials (established in 2006) is working on international co-operation in health-related and environmental safety-related aspects of manufactured nanomaterials (OECD Working Party on Nanotechnology (WPN): Vision Statement, 2007).

2.11. ISO (International Organization of Standardization)

With regard to nanotechnology ISO cooperates with the International Electrotechnical Commission (IEC) and with the European Committee for Standardization (CEN), in addition to having liaisons with several other organizations. In nanotechnology IEC's interest is primarily on electrical and electronic products and systems (IEC TC 113). CEN TC 352 is the European committee for nanotechnology standardization. In 2005 ISO established a technical committee (TC) for standardization in the field of nanotechnology. This TC currently consists of a Chairman's Advisory Group (CAG), four working groups (WGs) and three task groups. There are 34 participating (voting) member countries, 10 observing countries, and 8 liaison organizations (the EU, the OECD23, and other projects and organizations. TC 229 creates so-called 'anticipatory standards', creating the ground for development rather than simply harmonizing existing practices. In this situation ISO is in reality building a conceptual foundation for science and technology development. Therefore the first working groups (WGs) to be established – in addition to the working group on Health, Safety and Environmental Aspects (WG 3) - were on terminology and nomenclature (JWG 1) and measurement and characterization (JWG 2). These groups will allow the naming, describing and specifying of things, as well as measuring and testing things. Terminology and nomenclature standards are to provide a common language for scientific, technical, commercial and regulatory processes; and measurement and characterization standards are to provide an internationally accepted basis for quantitative scientific, commercial and regulatory activities (Forsberg, 2010).

3. Lawsuit against the FDA

In December 2011, ICTA filed the first lawsuit over the health and environmental risks of nanotechnology and nanomaterials on behalf of consumer and environmental groups with the U.S. Food and Drug Administration. The lawsuit demanded FDA to respond to a 2006 petition filed by ICTA requesting the FDA issue specific regulations for nanotechnology and properly regulate the use of nanoparticles in sunscreens. In its report, the panel criticized the National Nanotechnology Initiative, the coordinator of nano-funding and priorities across Federal agencies, with failing to connect research and research findings with the creation of strategies to prevent and manage risk at the Federal level. The report also notes that, "today's exposure scenarios may not resemble those of the future," making the need for immediate action by Federal agencies all the more necessary.

In 2008, ICTA and the Center for Food Safety (CFS) filed a legal petition with the EPA on behalf of a coalition of 14 public interest organizations calling on EPA to regulate nanosilver and other nano-pesticide products pursuant to its authority under the Federal Insecticide, Fungicide, and Rodenticide Act (FIFRA) (Hanson and O'Neil, 2012).

In November 2009, the EPA convened a Scientific Advisory Panel (SAP) to assess and evaluate the hazards and exposure risks associated with nanosilver and other nanometal pesticide programs. The SAP concluded that data gaps on potential exposure and hazards related to nanoparticles are broad; most existing models are not appropriate for use with nanomaterials and are unable to predict accurately nanomaterial exposure scenarios; additionally, existing data on current exposure and toxicity studies vary greatly with respect to metrics, particle size, etc. Ultimately, the SAP concluded that nanoparticles are fundamentally different substances from their larger scale cousins and that nanomaterials can create new and unique health and environmental risks that need new forms of safety testing.

In November 2010, ICTA and CFS filed a similar petition with the EPA to use its FIFRA authority to halt the sale of untested nano-copper products, providing yet another blueprint for how EPA should be treating and regulating nanomaterials.

In response to the suit, on April 20, 2012 the FDA responded to the petition and released the guidance. In its formal response to the groups' lawsuit, FDA acknowledged that there are differences between nanomaterials and their bulk counterparts, and that nanomaterials have potential new risks and may require new testing. However, the agency declined to enact mandatory regulations at this time. On May 2, 2012 several leading non-profits working on nanotechnology oversight— Center for Food Safety (CFS), Friends of the Earth (FoE), Institute for Agriculture and Trade Policy (IATP) and the International Center for Technology Assessment—issued a statement responding to recent steps taken by the Food and Drug Administration (FDA) that represent marginal progress toward regulation of products made with this new technology (Kimbrell *et al.*, 2012).

4. Nanotechnology in India

Regulation essentially relates to government action in the form of laws and notifications with the objective of directing private action for a specific purpose or with a certain aim (Brownsword, 2008). The Ministry of Science and Technology administers its functions through three departments – department of science and technology (DST), department of biotechnology (DBT) and department of scientific and industrial research (DSIR). Of these DST is the most important one with the objective of promoting new areas of science and technology and to play the role of a nodal department for organizing, coordinating and promoting S&T activities in India (The Energy and Resources Institute (TERI), 2009). Currently, DST is the most instrumental wing of government for providing a thrust to nanotechnology development. The Department, engaged with the agenda of promoting nanotech as a thrust area, has declared large investments for basic and applied research promotion, infrastructure support, education and international collaboration under the Nano Mission started in 2007. Nano Mission is an umbrella programme implemented by DST for capacity building towards overall development of the field of nanotechnology research in India. Given that nanotechnology is an enabling technology that finds its application at various levels and in different spheres, often in concomitance with other technologies, departments such as DBT and Department of Information Technology (DIT), which have an otherwise dedicated mandate, are also taking a plunge.

Even Defense Research and Development Organization (DRDO) and DSIR too have been fairly proactive in capturing the excitement around nanotechnology. DRDO, which has fullerenes & Nano tubes as one of the thrust areas in Materials research, has developed diagnostics tools for TB and typhoid, using nanotechnology. The Ministry of Commerce and Industry and especially the Department of Industrial Policy and Promotion (DIPP), aims at facilitating investment and technology flows in industrial development. Recently, the commerce secretary also has made a public statement emphasizing how 'India would not be able to do without it (nanotechnology), and Indian companies should be encouraged to get into it at the earliest'.

In reference to the research on the safety concern of engineered nanoparticles, our lab is involved in understanding the genotoxic potential of Zinc Oxide and Titanium dioxide nanoparticles on human peripheral blood lymphocyte culture. This requires assessment of the stability of nanoparticles in the nano form in culture and the DNA binding activity. The particokinetic analysis is done using Mansingh Survismeter, UV-visible spectroscopy and Fluorescence spectroscopy at a physiological temperature of 37°C.

Another interesting aspect is revisiting the ancient counterpart of nano which used traditional medicine i.e., *Bhasma.* There is a branch in ethnomedicine named '*Rasayana Shastra*' that deals with Bhasma. Bhasma are basically the metal compounds with size in nano dimensions. Since the attributes of engineered nanoparticles and Bhasma are similar, the evaluation of engineered nanoparticles in terms of Ayurvedic *Rasayana Shastra* norms for *Bhasma* in terms of various physico-chemical attributes can be useful. Our observations of few tests like '*Rekhapurtva*', '*Nirdhumtva*', '*Varitaratva*' for the engineered nanoparticles of ZnO, and TiO2 do indicate the similarity between the engineered nanoparticles and Bhasma (unpublished data). Apart from the tests regarding fineness, there are other chemical criteria for the engineered nanoparticles, which can be checked as compared to the conventional nanoparticles i.e. *Bhasma.* We propose that since Bhasma if prepared in authentic manner are known to have great medicinal value, the safety aspect of nanoparticles may be affected by the method in which they are manufactured. Our current study of in vitro assessment of genotoxicity of nanoparticles following particokinetics characterization is aimed to fill the gap of knowledge regarding biological effects.

Acknowledgement

Authors would like to thank Nirma University, Ahmedabad- 382 481, Gujarat, India for providing essential support.

References

Feynman, R. P. (1959). There's plenty of room at the bottom. *Miniaturization*, 282-296.

Lövestam, G., Rauscher, H., Roebben, G., Klüttgen, B. S., Gibson, N., Putaud, J. P., & Stamm, H. (2010). Considerations on a definition of nanomaterial for regulatory purposes. *Joint Research Centre (JRC) Reference Reports*, 80004-1.

Nanotechnologies: Vocabulary – Part 4: Nanostructured Materials. ISO; 2011. ISO/TS 80004-4: 2011.

EU Commission. (2011). Commission Recommendation of 18 October 2011 on the definition of nanomaterial (2011/696/EU). *Official Journal of the European Communities: Legis.*

Hoet, P. H., Brüske-Hohlfeld, I., & Salata, O. V. (2004). Nanoparticles–known and unknown health risks. *Journal of nanobiotechnology*, 2(1), 12.

Shinde, S. K., Grampurohit, N. D., Gaikwad, D. D., Jadhav, S. L., Gadhave, M. V., & Shelke, P. K. (2012). Toxicity induced by nanoparticles. *Asian Pacific Journal of Tropical Disease*, 2(4), 331-334.

The dose makes the poison. (2011). *Nature Nanotechnology*, *6*(6), 329-329.

Morris, J., & Willis, J. (2007). US Environmental Protection Agency nanotechnology white paper. *US Environmental Protection Agency, Washington, DC.*

Duvall, M., & Wyatt, A. (2011). Regulation of nanotechnology and nanomaterials at EPA and around the world: Recent developments and context. *Washington, DC: Beveridge & Diamond, PC.*

"Control of Nanoscale Materials under the Toxic Substances Control Act". *US Environmental Protection Agency (EPA).*

Duvall, M., & Wyatt, A. (2014). EPA Reworks Strategy for Regulation of Nanomaterials under TSCA; Proposed Rule Sent to OMB.

Nanotechnology Fact Sheet. (2014). *US Food and Drug Administration.*

National Institute for Occupational Safety and Health (NIOSH). http://cdc.gov/niosh/ .

National Nanotechnology Initiative. National Institute of Standards and

Technology (NIST), US Department of Commerce. https://www.nano.gov//node/145 .

Occupational Safety and Health Administration (OSHA). (2013). OSHA and Nanomaterials guidelines as of May 2013. http://www.nanotortlaw.com/2013/05/16/osha-and-nanomaterials-guidelines-as-of-may-2013/ .

Holdren, J. P., Sunstein, C. R., & Siddiqui, I. (2011). Nanotechnology regulation and oversight principles. *National Academic Press, Washington DC Huang Z, Chen HC, Yip A et al (2003) Longitudinal patent analysis for nanoscale science and engineering: country, institution and technology eld. J Nanopart Res, 5,* 333363.

European Commission. (2014). New JRC report discusses labelling and reporting schemes for nanomaterials in consumer products in the EU.

REACH, European Chemicals Agency (ECHA). (2006). http://echa.europa.eu/regulations/reach .

Aschberger, K., Rauscher, H., Crutzen, H., Rasmussen, K., Christensen, F. M., Sokull-Klüttgen, B., & Stamm, H. (2014). Considerations on information needs for nanomaterials in consumer products. *Discussion of a Labelling and Reporting Scheme for Nanomaterials in Consumer Products in the EU.*

OECD Working Party on Nanotechnology (WPN): Vision Statement. (2007). https://www.oecd.org/sti/nano/oecdworkingpartyonnanotechnologywpnvisionstatement.htm .

Forsberg, E. M. (2010). The role of ISO in the governance of nanotechnology. *Work Research Institute of Norway,* 1-76.

Hanson, J., O'Neil, C. (2012). Expert Panel Raises Red Flags on Risks of Nanomaterials. *International Center for Technology Assessment (ICTA).*

Kimbrell, G. A., Illuminato, I, Suppan, S, Hanson, J. (2012). Sustained Pressure by Non-Profits Forces Change in FDA Nanotech Policy. *International Center for Technology Assessment (ICTA).*

Brownsword, R. (2008). Rights, Regulation and Technological Revolution. New York, NY: Oxford University Press.

The Energy and Resources Institute (TERI). (2009). Regulatory Challenges posed by Nanotechnology Developments in India. TERI project: Capability, Governance, and Nanotechnology. Developments - a focus on India, New Delhi: The Energy and Resources Institute. [Project Report No. 2006ST21: D6].

Chapter 3

Resurgence of Organic Pigments and its application in Technical Textile Industry

Urvi Vachheta
Research Project Assistant
Gujarat National Law University, Gandhinagar
Email: urviv55@gmail.com

Abstract

Colour affects different aspects of our life whether it is clothes, home furnishings, food, etc. The colour also affects the mood of a person. The colouring agents obtained from sources like vegetables, fruits, seeds, roots and microorganisms are often called "Biocolors" due to their biological origin. The recent years has seen the resurgence of organic pigments in the market. The organic pigments are much more reliable due to their stability. There are numerous sources of organic pigments but very few are available in sufficient quantities. Biotechnology could allow the efficient mass production of such colourants.

Natural inorganic pigments have wide applications as colorants in pharma, food, textile, printing industries etc. According to a study on dyes and organic pigments, the worldwide demand for organic colourants was projected to increase from 4.9 % in 2003 to $10.6 billion in 2008. The demand of microbial pigments increased when people changed their perspective and started focusing on healthy, non-allergic and eco-friendly colours. This study will help the readers in understanding the development, market value and the current scenario of Technical Textiles globally as well as in India.

Introduction

Colour affects different aspects of our life whether it is clothes, home furnishings, food, etc. The colour also affects the mood of a person. The colouring agents obtained from sources like vegetables, fruits, seeds, roots and microorganisms are often called "Biocolors" due to their biological origin.[1],[2]. Natural organic pigments obtained from these sources are a part from historical pigments for bodily ornaments, cosmetic and textile dyeing. (Table-1) shows the Naturally derived pigments from plant sources. The commercial use of natural organic pigments reduced in 1900's when the chemically synthesized pigments were introduced. This was because the synthesized or inorganic pigments are known for their fastness, availability in a wide range of colours, low cost even at high concentration in low volumes and they are devoid of aroma and taste. It has been observed that inorganic pigments cause allergies and some are carcinogenic and teratogenic in nature.

The recent years has seen the resurgence of organic pigments in the market. The organic pigments are much more reliable due to their stability. They are also preferable because of their non-toxic and eco-friendly nature. There are numerous sources of organic pigments but very few are available in sufficient quantities. Biotechnology could allow the efficient mass production of such colourants. Plant cell and tissue culture, microbial fermentation and gene manipulation have all been investigated with respect to pigment production[2.] The pigments obtained from microorganism are in great demand worldwide. This growing interest in microbial pigments is due to several reasons like their natural character and safety to use, production being independent of seasons and geographical conditions and predictable yield[3]. The production of microbial pigments is controlled and the rapid growth of microorganisms helps in reducing the production time when compared to the production techniques of plant and animal sources. In the study of (Joshi *et al., 2003)* they have mentioned *that* a large number of different species of bacteria, molds, yeasts and algae are used to produce pigments. The ability to produce desired products cost efficiently through fermentation is a benefit of the microbial system. In addition, the collection of microbial organisms is sustainable and has no negative impact on the environment. (Table 2) shows the Naturally derived colours from microorganisms

Table 1: Naturally Derived Colours from Plants Sources[4]

Sr. No.	Plant Sources	Pigments	Colour/appearance
1	Turmeric	Curcumin	Bright lemon Yellow
2	Marigold and alfalfa	Lutein	Golden yellow
3	Palm oil	Natural mixed carotenes	Golden yellow to orange
4	Bixa orelana	Bixin/ nor-bixin	Orange
5	Paprika/capsicum annum	Capsanthin/ casorubin	Reddy Orange
6	Tomatoes	Lycopene	Orange red
7	Black grape skin, elderberries, black carrots, red cabbage	Anthocyanin	Pink/Red to mauve
8	Red table beet root	Betanin	Pink to red
9	Grass, nettle	Chlorophyll	Olive green

Table 2: Naturally Derived Colours from Micro-Organism [5,6]

Sr. No.	Micro-organisms	Pigments	Colour/appearance
1	*Staphylococcus aureus*	Zeaxanthin	Golden yellow
2	Serratia marcescens	Prodigiosin	Red
3	*Phaffia rohodozyma*	Astaxanthin	Red
4	*Blakesela trispora*	Lycopene β-carotene	Red Yellow Orange
5	*Flavobacterium* spp.	Zeaxanthin	Yellow
6	*Pseudomonas aeruginosa*	Pyocyanin Blue	Green
7	*Dunaliella Salina*	β-carotene	Cream
8	*Monascus* sp.	Monascorubramin, Rubropunctatin	Yellow, Orange, Red
9	*Rhodotorula* sp. *Rhodotorula glutinis*	Torularhodin	Orange-Red
10	*Monascus roseus*	Canthaxanthin	Orange-Pink

Application of Inorganic Pigments

Natural inorganic pigments have wide applications as colorants in pharma, food, textile, printing industries etc.

- **Pharmaceutical Industry**: Investigation of most of the microorganisms has shown the efficiency in potential clinical applications of secondary metabolites (pigmented) for treating various diseases. These have many properties like antibiotic, anticancer and immune-suppressive properties[7]. For e.g. the property of bacteria to produce bio pigments, is used to produce medically important products. *Adonirubin* and astaxanthin are the xanthophyll, which also act as nutraceuticals[8].
- **Food Industry**: The goal of food industry is to produce food which is appealing to the eyes. The natural food colours are preferable than artificial ones as the artificial ones leads to negative impacts when consumed. The natural food colours do not meet its demand in market. Many natural colours are available, in which microbial colorants play important role as food colouring agent.

  For e.g. *Penicillium oxalicum* is a fungus which produces red colour used in cosmetic and food industry [9].These colours are useful in different products like baby foods, breakfast cereals, pastas, sauces, processed cheese, fruit drinks, vitamin-enriched milk products, and some energy drinks and so on. Therefore, natural colours are environment friendly and moreover serve as the dual need for visually attractive colours and health benefits in food colorants of probiotic[10].Therefore, pigments from microbial sources are good alternative. The addition of natural or microbial colours in food products can also help to overcome the growing public concern over the adverse effects. In addition, natural colorants will not only be beneficial to human health but will also be helpful for the maintenance of biodiversity.

- **Textile industry:** The textile produces large amount of waste which mainly consist of synthetic dyes. These synthetic dyes are used in industries, due to their easy and cheap synthesis, stability towards light, temperature and advanced colours covering whole colour spectrum. However, these synthetic dyes have many drawbacks like toxicity, mutagenicity and carcinogenicity properties leading to various health problems like skin cancer and allergies[11,12].

The Indian textile industries now predominantly use synthetic organic dyes like direct dyes, processing dyes, reactive dyes, etc. The main reason of the use of artificial dyes and chemicals in Textiles is in attempt to make large spectrum of attractive popular shades of fabrics for a competitive market[13].The Textile materials and garments provide large surface area and absorb moisture required for microbial growth and so they are believed to be susceptible to microbial attack[14].

The reason for which the importance of natural pigments has increased in Textile garment industries is the improper treatment of effluents released after the cloth processing. The waste water from printing and dyeing units contain excessive colour, residues of reactive dyes and chemicals. Due to the harmful effect of chemical dye on environment pollution, a number of countries have issued stricter regulations so as to preserve our environment. Hence, by using natural pigments the concerns regarding environment pollution can be reduced[15].

Comparing the scenario of Organic pigments in the Indian and International Level

According to a study on dyes and organic pigments, the worldwide demand for organic colourants was projected to increase from 4.9 % in 2003 to $10.6 billion in 2008. Generally. the dyestuff industry comprises three sub-segments, *viz:* dyes, pigments, and intermediates.

The Asian region has seen the highest development in textile production, followed by North America, Latin America and Western Europe. This shows the change in the global textile industry towards Asia. Subsequently, Asia offers dyestuff production both in terms of volumes and value, with about a 42 per cent share of the global production; the US is next with 24 per cent and Europe has around 22 per cent. Due to a wide use of polyester and cotton-based fabrics, there has been a change towards reactive dyes, applied in cotton-based fabrics, and disperses dyes used in polyester. These two dyes have been leading in all the three-regional global market, particularly Asia.

The company called the De la Robbia, which began in 1992 in Milan, produces water extracts of natural dyes such as weld, chlorophyll, logwood, and cochineal under the Eco-Tex certifying system, and supplies the textile industry. In USA, Allegro Natural Dyes produces natural dyes under the Ecolour label for textile industry[16].

In Germany, Livos Pflanzenchemie Forschungs and Entwicklungs GmbH marked numerous natural products. In France, Bleu de Pastel sold an extract of woad leaves. Rubia Pigmenta Naturalia is The Netherlands company, which manufactures and sells vegetable dyes. There are several small textile companies using natural dyes. India is still a major producer of most natural dyed textiles[17]

Within India, the leading producers in the pigments industry are Colour Chem and Sudarshan Chemicals while in the dyestuff industry the major players in terms of market share are Atul, Clariant India, Dystar, Ciba Specialities and IDI. The Indian companies together account for nearly 6 per cent of the world production[18].

The global consumption of textiles is estimated at around 30 million tonnes, which is expected to grow at the rate of 3% per annum. The colouration of this huge quantity of textiles needs around 700,000 tonnes of dyes which causes release of a vast amount of unused and unfixed synthetic colourants into the environment[19].

The global demand for organic pigments and dyes is expected to reach almost 10 million tons by 2017 according to Global Industry Analysts. The global dye manufacturing industry originally dominated by suppliers from UK, Switzerland and Germany and later shifted to Asia over the past 20 years. The Textile industry is believed remain the largest consumer of organic pigments and dyes.

A new study from The Fredonia Inc., a Cleveland-based industry research firm presented in World Dyes & Pigments that the World demand for organic pigments is expected to grow 6.0 percent per year to $19.5 billion in 2019.Moreover, between 2001 and 2005, in Western Europe it was reported an annual production increase of antimicrobial textiles around 15%, being one of the fastest growing sectors of the textiles industry. In a recent issue of Performance Apparel Markets, the report "Antimicrobial fibres, fabrics and apparel: innovative weapons against infection" referred to the global market for antimicrobial agents being expected to increase by about 12% each year between 2013 and 2018.

Understanding the relation between Technical Textiles and Microbial Pigments

Technical Textiles is gaining recognition of the economic and strategic potential of textiles to the fibre and fabric manufacturing and processing industries of industrial and industrialising countries. In some of the most developed markets, technical products (broadly defined) already account for as much as 50% of all textile manufacturing activity and output. The economic scope and importance of technical textiles extends far beyond the textile industry itself and has an impact upon just about every sphere of human economic and social activity.

The definition of technical textiles adopted by the authoritative *Textile Terms and Definitions*, published by the Textile Institute, is 'textile materials and products manufactured primarily for their technical and performance properties rather than their aesthetic or decorative characteristics'.

The leading international trade exhibition for technical textiles, Techtextil (organised biennially since the late 1980s by Messe Frankfurt in Germany and also in Osaka, Japan), defines 12 main application areas (of which textiles for industrial applications represent only one group):

- agrotech: agriculture, aquaculture, horticulture and forestry
- buildtech: building and construction
- clothtech: technical components of footwear and clothing
- geotech: geotextiles and civil engineering
- hometech: technical components of furniture, household textiles and floorcoverings
- indutech: filtration, conveying, cleaning and other industrial uses
- medtech: hygiene and medical
- mobiltech: automobiles, shipping, railways and aerospace
- oekotech: environmental protection
- packtech: packaging
- protech: personal and property protection
- sporttech: sport and leisure[20]

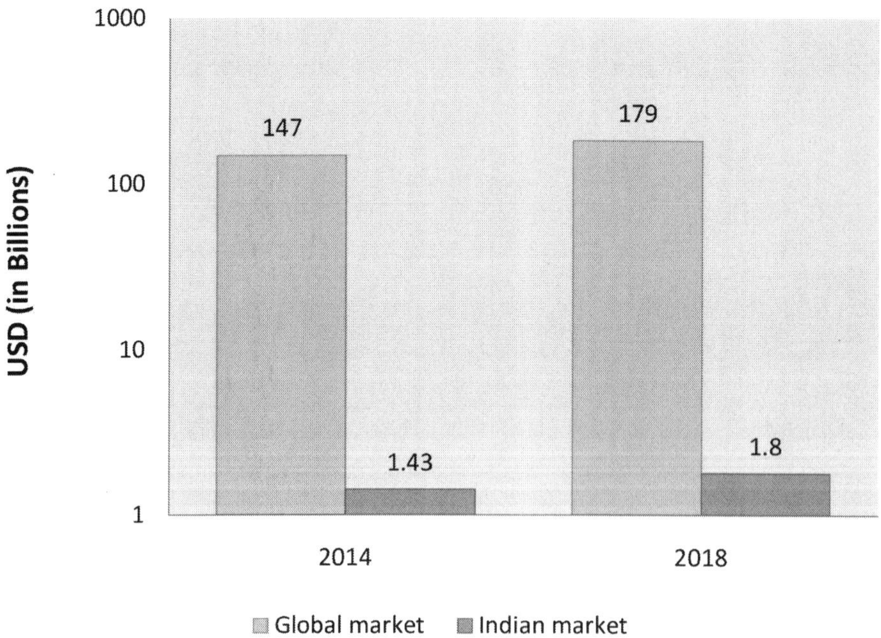

Fig. 1: Market value of Technical textile (data from Indian Textile Journal, April 2017)

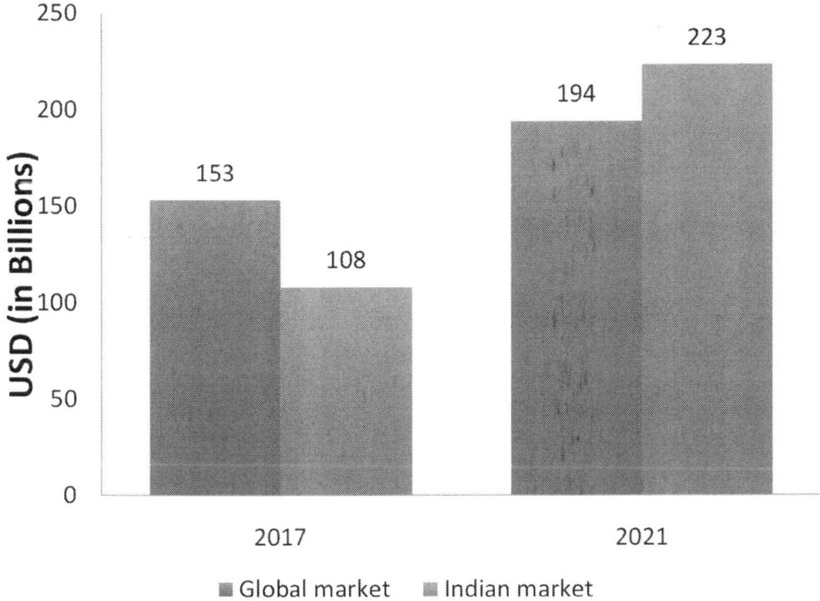

Fig. 2: Market value of Technical textile (data from Indian Textile Journal, April 2017)

The microorganism's growth on textiles causes a range of undesirable effects not only on the textile itself but also on the user. These effects include the generation of unpleasant odour, reduction in mechanical strength, stains and discoloration and an increased likelihood of user contamination. Therefore, due to the growing public health awareness of the pathogenic effects, over the last few years, intensive research and development have been promoted in order to minimize or even eliminate microbe's growth on textiles[21],[22].

The problems of hygiene are increasing day by day and it is now realised that a microbiocidal finish is very valuable in certain textiles for two reasons:

a) As a prophylactic measure to avoid infections

b) As a deodorant

Natural fibres have (keratin) and cellulose, etc., which provide basic requirements such as moisture, oxygen, nutrients and temperature for bacterial growth and multiplication. This often results odour and skin infection[23]. It is an utmost important now to control the growth of microorganisms on fabrics used in hospital, household furnishings, etc.

Few researchers have studied the antimicrobial activity on fabrics. Like (Han and Yang,2005)[24] studied the antimicrobial activity of wool fabric dyed with curcumin and found that the antimicrobial ability of curcumin finished wool is semi durable, more durable to home laundering than to light exposure. (Mariegold)[25] showed negative test against microbiological control for *E. coli* and *Salmonella*. (Singh et al,2005)[26] tested *acacia catechu, kerria lacca, quercus infectoria, rubia cordifora,* and *rumex maritimus* against pathogens like *E. coli, Bacillus subtilis,*

Klebsiella pneumoniae, Proteus vulgaris, and *Pseudomonas aeruginosa*. Minimum inhibitory concentration was found to vary from 5 μg to 40 μg. (Gupta et al,2004).[27] studied antimicrobial property of eleven natural dyes (acacia, indigo, lac, kamala, pomegranate, gall nuts, cutch, myrobolan, Himalayan rhubarb, Indian madder and golden dock) against three types of Gram-negative bacteria (*E. coli, Klebsiella pneumoniae* and *Proteus vulgaris*. Seven out of the eleven natural dyes (lac, kamala, pomegranate, gall nuts, cutch, myrobolan and Himalayan rhubarb) showed activity against one or more of the three bacteria studied.

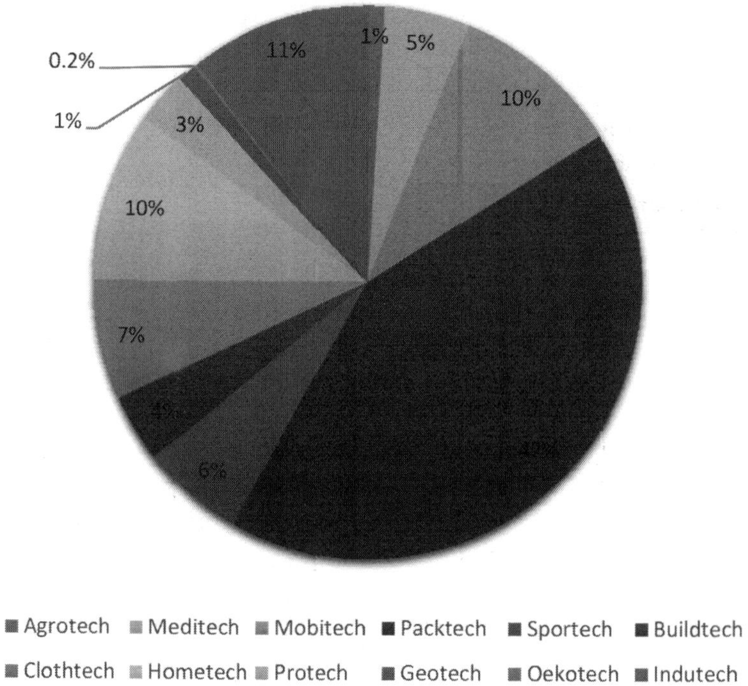

Fig. 4: Segment Wise Sharen Technical Textiles Market 2017-1018(P) [Indian Textile Journal, April 2017]

(Chen and Chang,2007)[28] studied the antimicrobial activity of cotton fabric pre-treated microwave plasma and dyed with onion skin and onion pulp extraction. (Dev et al.,2009)[29] studied the dyeing and antimicrobial characteristics of chitosan treated wool fabrics with henna dye.

There are only few reports on the dyeing of natural fibres for the improvement of deodorizing property with natural dyes. (Hwang *et al.*) reported deodorizing property of cotton, silk, and wool fabrics dyed with gardenia, coffee sludge, *Casia tora.* L., and pomegranate extracts[30]. (Nakamura *et al.*, 2003)[31] reported that violacein not only caused growth inhibition but also the death of bacteria. Furthermore, violacein is known to possess anti-fungal (Shirata *et al.*,1997)[32], antiviral (Andrighetti-Frohner et al.,2007)[33] and antiprotozoal activity (Costa et al.,2007[34]; Lopes et al.,2009[35]; Nakamura et al.[31]).

Endophytic fungal pigment was found to be superior to the commercial antibiotic Streptomycin against human pathogenic bacteria, Staphylococcus aureus, Klebsiella pneumoniae, Salmonella typhi and Vibrio cholera (Visalakchi and Muthumary,2010)[36]. Prodigiosin, a red colour pigment from Serratia marcescens was also shown as an antibacterial agent against gram+ve and gram -ve bacteria (Mekhael and Yousif,2009[37])

This enlightens on the fact that there is a need for antimicrobial finishes in fabric to be introduced in these areas to reduce the growth of microbes and protect skin from allergens.

The certain specification that are understood from the study done till now are that:

- Unlike synthetic dyes which are non-renewable, the natural dyes are renewable and biodegradable
- This is a labour-intensive industry, thereby providing job opportunities
- Some of the constituents are anti-allergens, hence it will prove safe for skin contact and mostly are non-hazardous to human health
- Natural pigments bleed but do not stain other fabric. The washing procedure will require less time and detergents
- Natural pigments can replace synthetic dyes in kids garments for safety[38]

Conclusion

The demand of microbial pigments increased when people changed their perspective and started focusing on healthy, non-allergic and eco-friendly colours. The use of microbial pigments in Textiles is just one example. There is diverse application of microbial pigments. There should be rigorous efforts to reduce the challenges due to high cost when compared with synthetic pigments. This study will help the readers in understanding the development, market value and the current scenario of Technical Textiles globally as well as in India.

References

1. Rymbai H, Sharma RR and Srivastav M: Biocolorants and its implications in health and food industry-A Review. International Journal of Pharm Tech Research. 2011; 3(4):2228-2244.

2. Pattnaik P, Roy U, Jain P: New Generation additives for ingredients. Beverage Food World. 1999; 26(3):36-40.

3. Francis, FJ. 1987. Lesser known food colorants. Food TechnoL, 41:62-68.

4. Joshi VK, Attri D, Bala A, and Bhushan S: Microbial pigments. Indian Journal of Biotechnology. 2003; 2:362-369.

5 Dufosse L: Pigments. Microbial Encylopedia Microbiol. 2009; 4:457-471.

6. Venil CK, Lakshmanaperumalsamy P: An Insightful Overview on Microbial Pigment, Prodigiosin. Electronic Journal of Biology. 2009; 5(3):49-61.

7. Venil CK, Zakaria ZA, Ahmad WA: Bacterial pigments and their applications. Article in Process Biochemistry. 2013; 48:1065-1079.

8. Kim HW, Kim JB, Cho SM, Chung MN, Lee YM, Chu SM: Anthocyanin changes in the Korean purple-fleshed sweet potato, Shinzami, as affected by steaming and baking. Food Chemistry. 2012; 130:966–72

9. Sardaryan H, Zihlova R, Strnad Z, Cermakoya C: Arpink Red– Meet a new natural red food colorant of microbial origin. In: Pigments in Food, More than Colours. Dufossé L. (ed) Université de Bretagne Occidentale, Quimper France. 2004; 207-08.

10. Nagpal N, Munjal N, Chatterjee S: Microbial Pigments with Health Benefits - A Mini Review. Trends in Bioscience. 2011; 4:157-60.

11. Srikanlayanukul M, Chartchai K, and Saisamorn L: Decolourization of Textile wastewater by immobilized *Coriolus versicolour* RC3 in Repeated-Batch System with the effect of Sugar Addition. CMU Journal. 2006; 5(3): 301-306.

12. Gurav A, Ghosh J, Girish K: Decolourization of anthroquinone based dye Vat Red 10 by *Pseudomonas desmolyticum* NCIM 2112 and *Galactomyces geotrichum* MTCC 1360. International Journal for Biotechnology and Molecular Biology Research. 2011; 2(6):93-97

13. Mathur, N. Bhatnagar, P. and Bakre, P. (2005): Assessing mutagenicity of textile dyes from Pali (Rajasthan) using Ames bioassay. *Applied ecology and environmental research,* 4(1): 111-118

14. Cardamone, J. M.: Proteolytic activity of aspergillus flavus on wool, *AATCC Rev*, vol. 2 (May 2002), pp. 30-35, ISSN 1532-8813.

15. http://express-press-release.com

16. Hwang, E. K., Lee, Y. H., & Kim, H. D. Dyeing, fastness, and deodorizing properties of cotton, silk, and wool fabrics dyed with gardenia, coffee sludge, *Cassia tora. L.*, and pomegranate extracts, *Fibers and Polymers,* Vol. 9 (2008) No. 3, pp. 334-340, ISSN 1875-0052.

17 Vankar, P. S.: *Handbook on natural dyes for industrial applications,* New Delhi: National Institute of Industrial Research, 2007, ISBN 8189579010

18. Doshi, G. (2006): Dyestuff Industry in India and China: http://EzineArticles.com/expert/Gaurav_Doshi/56873

19. Samanta, A. K. & Agarwal, P.: Application of natural dyes on textiles, *Indian Journal of Fibre & Textile Research,* Vol. 34 (December 2009) No. 4, pp. 384-399, ISSN 0975-1025.

20. A R Horrocks, and S C Anand (2000). Handbook of Technical Textiles. Cambridge, England

21. Shahidi, S.; Wiener, J. Antimicrobial Agents—Chapter 19: Antibacterial Agents in Textile Industry; Intech: Rijeka, Croatia, 2012. 7.

22. Gao, Y.; Cranston, R. Recent advances in antimicrobial treatments of textiles. *Text. Res. J.* 2008, 78, 60–72.
23. Thiry, M. C.: Small game hunting; antimicrobials take the field, *AATCC Rev*, Vol. 2 (November 2001), pp.11-17, ISSN 1532-8813
24. Hang, S. & Yang, Y.: Antimicrobial activity of wool fabric treated with curcumin. Dyes and Pigments, Vol. 64 (2005) No.2: pp. 157-161, ISSN 0143-7208
25. http://www.mdidea.com/products/herbextract/marigold/data.
26. Singh, R.; Jain, A; Panwar, S.; Gupta, D. & Khare, S. K.: Antimicrobial activity of some natural dyes, Dyes and Pigments, Vol. 66 (2005) No. 2, pp. 99-102, ISSN 0143-7208
27. Gupta, D.; Khare, S. K. & Laha, A.: Antimicrobial properties of natural dyes against Gram-negative bacteria, Coloration Technology, Vol. 120 (2004) No.4, pp. 167-171, ISSN 14784408
28. Chen, C. & Chang, W.: Antimicrobial activity of cotton fabric pre-treated microwave plasma and dyed with onion skin and onion pulp extractions. *Indian Journal of Fibre & Textile Research.* 32 (March 2007) No.1, pp 122-125, ISSN 0975-1025.
29. Dev, V. R. G.; Venugopal, J.; Deepika, G. & Ramakrishna, S.: Dyeing and antimicrobial characteristics of chitosan treated wool fabrics with henna dye, Carbohydrate Polymer, Vol. 75 (2009) No.4, pp. 646-650, ISSN ISSN 0144-8617.
30. Hwang, E. K.; Lee, Y. H. & Kim, H. D.: Dyeing, fastness, and deodorizing properties of cotton, silk, and wool fabrics dyed with gardenia, coffee sludge, Cassia tora. L., and pomegranate extracts, Fibers and Polymers, Vol. 9 (2008) No.3, pp. 334-340, ISSN 18750052
31. Nakamura Y, Asada C, Sawada T (2003) Production of antibacterial violet pigment by psychotropic bacterium RT102 strain. Biotechnol Bioprocess Eng. 8:37–40
32. Shirata A, Tsukamoto T, Yasui H, KatoH HS, Kojima A (1997) Production of bluish-purple pigments by Janthinobacterium lividum isolated from the raw silk and dyeing with them. Nippon Sanshigaku Zasshi 66:377–385
33. Andrighetti Frohner CR, Antonio RV, Creczynski-Pasa TB, Barandi CRM, Simo˜es CMO (2003) Cytotoxicity and potential antiviral evaluation of violacein produced by Chromobacterium violaceum. Mem Inst Oswaldo Cruz 98:834–848
34. Costa FTM, Justo GZ, Dura'n N, Nogueira PA, Lopes SCP: The use of violacein in its free and encapsulated form in polymeric systems against malaria. Brazilian Patent PIBr 2005, 056399 0
35. Lopes SCP, Blanco YC, Justo GZ, Nogueira PA, Rodrigues FLS, Goelnitz U, Wunderlich G, Facchini G, Brocchi M, Dura'n N, Costa FTM (2009) Violacein extracted from Chromobacterium violaceum inhibits Plasmodium growth in vitro and in vivo. Antimicrobial Agents Chemother 53:2149–2152

36. Visalakchi S, Muthumary J (2010) Antimicrobial activity of the new endophytic Monodictys castaneae SVJM139 pigment and its optimization. *Afr J Microbiol Res* 3(9):550–556

37. Mekhael R, Yousif SY (2009) The role of red pigment produced by Serratia marcescens as antibacterial and plasmid curing agent. *J Duhok Univ* 12(1):268–274

38. Ashis Kumar Samanta and Adwaita Konar (2011). Dyeing of Textiles with Natural Dyes, Natural Dyes, Dr. Emriye Akcakoca Kumbasar (Ed.), Intech, DOI: 10.5772/21341.

Available from: https://www.intechopen.com/books/natural-dyes/dyeing-of-textiles-with-natural-dyes

Chapter 4

Patenting Genes: From *Chakrabarty* to *Myriad* and Beyond

Aswini Anjana V.[1], Mariya Fatma[2]

[1]LL.M. II year, [2]Department of Intellectual Property Law,
The Tamil Nadu Dr. Ambedkar Law University M.G.R. Salai, Perungudi, Chennai, Tamil Nadu, India
Email: raveanju1993@gmail.com, huda.mariya@gmail.com

Abstract

Earth biosphere is an adobe to millions of living species which ranges in size from microscopic unicellular living organism to giant whales and huge elephants. The existence of variety of organisms with unique genotype and phenotype could be attributed to what have been acquired from the ancestral species and that which are carried down to their progeny's. The evolution and progress of gene research particularly involving DNA led a race to artificially change the DNA sequence using biotechnology tools to get new or desired characters. Scientists and the researchers have made successful attempts in isolating the genes from precise locations, which are found to produce useful results in the diagnosis of critical diseases. The genes are naturally occurring phenomena and any research oriented manipulation made to the genes using biotechnological tools could result in a useful product or process. The patenting of gene-based inventions have so far not raised any ethical concerns however they may develop in future due to the development of newer technologies. The balancing of scientific temper and maintaining ethics in the realm of public and private interest is thus the need of the hour.

Introduction

Earth biosphere is an adobe to millions of living species which ranges in size from microscopic unicellular living organism to giant whales and huge elephants. The existence of variety of organisms with unique genotype and phenotype could be attributed to what have been acquired from the ancestral species and that which are carried down to their progeny's. The carriers of these hereditary character lies within their cell called 'genes'. In 1865, the presence of genes was first discovered by the father of genetic biology, Gregor Mendel[1]. The existence of 'genes' as a

1 Torrance, A. W. (2010). Gene Concepts, Gene Talk, and Gene Patents.11 MINN. J. L. SCI. & TECH., 157-192.

chemical compound responsible for the hereditary character and variations among generations were confirmed over the years in 1944[2]. Finally in 1953, James Watson and Francis Crick, establishing the double helical structure of DNA (Deoxyribonucleic acid) substantiated that 'genes' are present in them[3] and Dr. Crick later decrypted and proposed the central dogma of the molecular biology that information encoded in the segment of DNA called 'genes' are transmitted to other parts of the cells through another molecule RNA (Ribonucleic acid) and then utilized to create the building block of protein[4].

The evolution and progress of gene research particularly involving DNA led a race to artificially change the DNA sequence using biotechnology tools to get new or desired characters. The process of traditional breeding and cultivationwhich was a lengthy and non-promising one was replaced by the Recombinant DNA technology (r-DNA). The process involves constructing and manipulating DNA sequences that do not occur naturally and combining the DNA fragments taken from different sources. The r-DNA technology allows genes and gene fragments to be excised from a precise location in the gene sequence. The identified gene or the gene fragment is spliced and placed in a different genomic location of the same, or even in a different type of organism. The technique involves three steps: (a) isolation of the gene coding for a protein of interest; (b) cloning (i.e. transfer) of this gene into an appropriate production host; (c) improving gene and protein expression by using stronger promoters, improving fermentation conditions[5]. The r-DNA technology thus serves the purpose of gene manipulation and new kind of characters have been invented which are useful in developing drugs, food, health and other industries.

The quest to develop newer kinds of characteristics involving gene manipulation and designing the genetic makeup was not merely restricted to animals and plants. Researchers in the field had gone to the extent of knowing and manipulating the genetic makeup of humans. This led to the inception of specialized projects concerning the research on human genes. In 1990, the Human Genome Project was launched by the US Government which was collaborated with many research programmes.After the completion of the project in 2003, it was confirmed that there are 25000 genes in the human body which are responsible for different characters in the human-beings[6]. Several other organizations across the world had then started to conduct researches based on human genes leading to newer innovations useful to the health industries.

2 *ibid*

3 *ibid*

4 *Association of Molecular Pathology* v.*United States Patent and Trademark Office, ET Al.*, (2009) http://www.patents4life.com/wp-content/uploads/2010/03/MyriadDecision.pdfaccessed on 12 Oct. 2017.

5 Introduction to molecular biology and genetic engineering, module http://www.fao.org/docrep/014/i1905e/i1905e00.pdf,accessed on 15 Oct. 2017.

6 National human genome research institute, https://www.genome.gov/12011238/an-overview-of-the-human-genome-project/, accessed on 15 Oct. 2017

Scientists and the researchers have made successful attempts in isolating the genes from precise locations, which are found to produce useful results in the diagnosis of critical diseases. Various genes have been codified and patents have been granted for the same. The development of new technologies has been of incredible support.The technologies and methods used for gene research includes old methods like Zinc-Finger Nucleases (ZFNs), Transcription Activator-like Effector Nucleases(TALENs) and the latest being Clustered Regularly Interspaced Short Palindromic Repeats (CRISPR/Cas9) technology[7].

Inventions based on gene research involve huge efforts of scientists and research fund organizations. The use of biotechnologies and recombinant technologies to invent gene based products or process, be it a new kind of microorganism, or a new cell at a prokaryotic or eukaryotic level are a breakthrough to a variety of problems faced by the society. The technologies may involve gene-editing or manipulation, causing new inventions to be created in the field resolving a long-pending problem in the society. New kinds of medications and therapeutic breakthrough have evolved this way. While such inventions are useful to the society and the inventors are striving to cater to the long-felt needs of the society, there also arises a need to provide legal protection to such inventions. Patents fit the purpose.

Patenting 'gene-based' inventions Possible?

Patent[8] is a kind of intellectual property right granted to the inventor for his useful invention, to commercially exploit such inventions without unauthorized third-party interventions for a limited and fixed period of time. Though the right is not absolute, it seeks to incentivize the inventor to further innovate and benefit the society. Any infringements against such inventions can be sued and the inventor can enjoy the monopoly till the patent term expires. The legislations dealing with patents have been long-existing in different countries, however the minimum standards for granting patent protection and the kind of legal protection has been standardized during the emergence of World Trade Organisation [WTO]. The trade was not merely restricted to goods and services, but also extended to patented products or processes.

The Agreement on Trade Related Aspects of Intellectual Property Rights [TRIPS, shortly] which came into effect from January 1, 1995, mandates the member nations to grant patents only if the inventions are patent eligible. Article 27 of the TRIPS Agreement 1995 is significant to be satisfied for the inventions to be patent eligible[9]. The invention could be a product or a process from any field

---

7 New Science Could Sharpen Crispr's Gene-Editing Scalpel, https://www.wired.com/story/new-science-could-sharpen-crisprs-gene-editing-scalpel/ accessed on 26 Oct, 2017, see also Deborah Ku, (2016)The Patentability of the CRISPR-CAS9 GenomeEditing Tool, Chi.-Kent J. Intell. Prop 16: 408, 439

8 Article 27 and 28 of TRIPS Agreement, 1995. https://www.wto.org/english/docs_e/legal_e/27-trips.pdf accessed on 17 Oct. 2017.

9 Art 27.1 – *" Subject to the provisions of paragraphs 2 and 3, patents shall be available for any inventions, whether products or processes, in all fields of technology, provided that they are new, involve an inventive step and are capable of industrial application….."*

of technology and it should not be contrary to the public order or morality or cause harmful effects on the environment or living beings[10]. In India, the existing legislation on patent is the Patent Act, 1970 while to be in compliance with the TRIPS Agreement, it was thereafter amended in 1999, 2002, and 2005 which brought in the major changes to patent laws in India.

The patent-eligibility of inventions involving genes in different countries is a question to be pondered to. The position in the United States regarding patent eligibility is contained in 35 U.S.C. § 101.[11] The inventions involving genes or genetically engineered mechanisms could fall under any of the categories mentioned in the section, *i.e., could be a product, process, method or composition of matter*. However, the standards "new" and "useful" need to be satisfied. In European Union, Article 52of the European Patent Convention 1973 [EPC] deals with patent-eligible subject matter and that stresses upon the invention to be new, involve industrial step and capable of industrial application.Biological inventions are also falling under the patentable subject matter[12]. However, an invention may not be granted patent if opposed to public order or morality[13]. It also raises a bar on patenting plants or animal varieties or essentially biological processes while the provision shall not apply to microbiological processes or the products thereof. There is no bar to obtain patents for biological inventions and Directive 98/44 deals with "Biotech Inventions[14]".

The position in India regarding patentability of biotech and gene based inventions, after incorporating all the major amendments in 1999, 2002 and 2005 in accordance with the TRIPS Agreement 1995 stands clear. The major provisions dealing with the patent eligibility in India are Sections 2(j), 2(ja) and 3 of the Patent Act, 1970. For an invention to be patentable it must be new and useful. It must also show some inventive step with technical advancement or economic significance and not be obvious to the person skilled in the art. The inventions which are not patentable had been dealt under Section 3 and it bars patentability of inventions involving natural phenomenon, or against public morality or causing ill effects on

10 Art 27.2- *"Members may exclude from patentability inventions, the prevention within their territory of the commercial exploitation of which is necessary to protect ordre public or morality, including to protect human, animal or plant life or health or to avoid serious prejudice to the environment, provided that such exclusion is not made merely because the exploitation is prohibited by their law."*

11 *"Whoever invents or discovers any new and useful process, machine, manufacture, or composition of matter, or any new and useful improvement thereof, may obtain a patent therefor, subject to the conditions and requirements of this title."*

12 *"Biotechnological inventions" are inventions which concern a product consisting of or containing biological material or a process by means of which biological material is produced, processed or used."*

13 http://www.epo.org/law-practice/legal-texts/html/epc/2016/e/ar53.html accessed on 18 Oct. 2017.

14 European Union (EU) Directive 98/44/EC of the European Parliament and of the Council of 6 July 1998 on the Legal Protection of biotechnological inventions http://www.wipo.int/wipolex/en/text.jsp?file_id=126956accessed on 20 Oct, 2017.

the environment or living beings. In particular, Section 3(j) disallows patentability of *plants and animals in whole or any part thereof other than microorganisms but including seeds, varieties and species and essentially biological processes for production or propagation of plants and animals.* A bare reading of the sectionmakes it clear that the patenting of genetically modified microorganism and anything derived essentially from non-biological processes are patentable. However inventions relating to human gene for therapeutic or diagnostic purpose[15] and discovery of any living or non-living substance[16]are not patentable.

Gene-based inventions whether 'Product of Nature'?

The genes are naturally occurring phenomena and any research oriented manipulation made to the genes using biotechnological tools could result in a useful product or process. However, the genes so manipulated are still considered to be naturally occurring phenomena as they have the inherent ability to multiply, reproduce and exist biologically. If biological inventions are patentable, they are to show significant improvement and advancement than the naturally occurring phenomenon. The standards of novelty, inventive step and industrial application apply and the resultant product should also remain significantly different from the natural occurring phenomenon. This is challenging to researchers as their efforts in invention may go in vain if the resultant invention does not surpass the "Product of nature" test.

The Court in the light of the "Product of nature" test has been critical in granting or rejecting patents to inventions involving genes or genetic engineering. The judicial interpretations seem to overcome the "product of nature" test with strictness to involve human intervention that significantly differentiates from the naturally occurring phenomenon. The "product of nature" was held to be freely available to all men on the earth and no person is entitled to enjoy ownership over the naturally occurring phenomenon. In *Funk Bros. Seeds Co.* v. Kalo*Inoculant Co.*, 1948[17], the Court held that the said invention did not create inhibition or non-inhibition in the bacteria. They were products of nature, not manmade. In the words of the Judge, "*The qualities of these bacteria, like the heat of the sun, electricity, or the qualities of metals, are part of the storehouse of knowledge of allmen. They are manifestations of laws of nature, free to all men and reservedexclusively to none. He who discovers a hitherto unknown phenomenon of nature hasno claim to a monopoly of it which the law recognizes. If there is to be invention from such a discovery, it must come from the application of the law of nature to anew and useful end.*"

15 Section 3(i) of Patent Act, 1970.

16 Section 3(c) of Patent Act, 1970.

17 *Funk Brothers Seed Co.* v. *Kalo Inoculant Co.*, 333 U.S. 127 (1948). Facts in brief, through some mysterious process, the leguminous plants were able to take nitrogen from the air and fix it in the plant for conversion to organic nitrogenous compounds. The ability to fix the nitrogen was due to the bacteria from a genus called Rhizobium which fixes nodules on the roots of the plants. There were six species of these bacteria and they were synthetically cultured at the laboratory for use by agriculturalist. The patents (Bond Patents) were related to use of these bacteria to fix the nitrogen.

In the United States, the first case which dealt with the gene-based patent was *Diamond* v. *Chakrabarty, 1980*[18]. The invention was relating to a Pseudomonas Bacterium which is a human made genetically engineered bacterium capable of breaking down the multiple components of crude oil. The question involved was whether the process of producing the bacteria and the bacteria itself is a patentable subject matter under 35 U.S.C. § 101of the US Patent. The Supreme Court has held that the pseudomonas bacterium is a "composition of matter" where that bacterium has got the special character of breaking down the multiple oil spills, which it otherwise cannot perform naturally. The court concluded that the Congress intention while enacting the Section to promote the useful art and progress the scientific temper. In this connection, the Chakrabartys' genetically modified Pseudomonas bacterium, was considered as a non-naturally occurring, which attained the character of breaking the oil spills by human intervention. The invention was held to be patentable overcoming the "Product of nature" test. The decision opened the gate for patenting biotechnological and life form patents.

The European Patent Office [EPO] had to deal with the patentability of a transgenic organism in the *Harvard OncoMouse, 2004*[19] case where the rodent was genetically engineered to be resistant to breast cancer and could facilitate earlier diagnosis. As per Article 53 (b) of the European Directive patents shall not be granted to plants or animal varieties or those of essentially biological processes for the production of plants and animals. On this basis, the patent was rejected by the EPO. On appeal, the human-engineered Oncomouse was granted patent as it was not naturally found and cannot be considered a 'variety of animal'. In another instance, the patentability of human genes was dealt. The *Relaxin*[20] *case* involved the patentability of relaxin which is a hormone produced in body to relax the uterus during childbirth. Howard Florey Institute in Australia isolated the nucleotide sequence that coded for relaxin and by cloning process using r-DNA techniques could ascertain a second type of relaxin hormone. The court held the patent to be valid because the new kind of relaxin hormone was itself novel and not to be found anywhere in the nature. In both the cases, the court has not suggested any moral or ethical issues that could arise from patenting transgenic varieties or the human genes itself.

The "Product of nature" test has been used to determine whether such bio-tech or gene based inventions could fall under the patentable subject-matter. However, when they surpass the test, they are to prove that they possess novelty and utility benefitting the mankind. In *re Fisher*[21], the Court had to decide upon the patentability of purified gene sequence extracted from maize plants. The five claimed Express Sequence Tags [ESTs] were used for different purposes

---

18 *Diamond* v. *Chakrabarty*, 447 U.S. 303 (1980)

19 Case T 0315/03, *President and Fellows of Harvard Coll.* v. *British Union for the Abolition of Vivisection* (EPO Boards of Appeal, 2004).

20 *Howard Florey Institute Of Experimental Physiology And Medicinev.Aglietta, Amendola et al.* ECLI:EP:BA:2002:T027295.20021023

21 *In re Fisher,* 421 F.3d 1365

such as (1) serving as a molecular marker for mapping the entire maize genome, which consists of ten chromosomes that together include about 50,000 genes; (2) measuring the level of mRNA in a tissue sample by way of microarray technology to provide information about gene expression; (3) providing a source for primers for use in the polymerase chain reaction (PCR) process to enable rapid and inexpensive duplication of specific genes; (4) identifying the presence or absence of a polymorphism; (5) isolating promoters by way of chromosome walking, controlling protein expression; and locating genetic molecules of other plants and organisms. The Court of Appeals for the Federal Court ruled that the invention lacked utility and failed to show enablement. Reason being, the claimed purposes are only general and does not claim anything specifically.

In India, the patent Act did not facilitate the patenting of genetically modified organism or genes but prior to the 2002 amendment, the Calcutta High Court[22] had to rule on the patentability of the invention relating to the process of preparing infectious Bursitis Vaccine which contained a live virus.As per the erstwhile Patent law, Section 2(i) (i) defined an 'invention' to be a new and useful art, process, method or manner of manufacture. The Patent examiner rejected the grant of patent as the process involved a living entity and the process cannot be regarded as a "manufacture". However on appeal before the Court, it was held to be patentable applying the "Vendibility Test", where the claimed process as undergone a process to be vendible in the market. In this light, the said invention would tantamount to a "manufactured" process.

Turning point decisions

The patent-eligibility of inventions based on gene research and use of biotechnology researches to medicines was influenced by two major decisions. In 2012, the US Supreme Court dealt with the case of Mayo Collaborative Services V. Prometheus Laboratories, Inc[23]. In this case the patent was pertaining to administration process of "Thiopurine drug" dosage to treat anti-immuno diseases. The issue involved was whether the said process is patent eligible under Section 101. The Supreme Court rejected the patent and compelled that for the invention to be patentable, particularly when it is applying an abstract idea or a 'principle of natural law', it is not sufficient if it is merely on the lines of conventional or pre-solution activity. Purely conventional or obvious pre-solution activity is normally not sufficient to transform an un-patentable law of nature into a patent-eligible application of such a law. Thus, the court stressed on significant post-solution activity for it to be patentable. The *Mayo*ruling had a considerable effect on the case dealing with human isolated gene patents.

The patent-eligibility of isolated human genes and their sequencing was in question before the US Supreme Court in*Association of molecular pathology* **v.** *Myriad Genetics, Inc. Et Al* in, 2013. Myriad Genetics Inc., obtained patent in 1994 for the process of isolation and sequencing of genes BRCA-1 and BRCA-2 whose

22 https://spicyip.com/wp-content/uploads/2013/11/Dimminaco-A.G.-v.-Controller-of-Patents-Designs.pdf accessed on 12 Oct. 2017.

23 *Mayo Collaborative Services* v. *Prometheus Laboratories, Inc*566 US _ (2012)

mutations caused the increased risk of breast and ovarian cancer. The Court had to interpret Section 101 to deal with the question. After rounds of legal battle in front of lower courts and in the Supreme Court[24], the Court relied on the *Mayo* decision which stressed for significant post-solution activity. The court tried to differentiate between the c-DNA and g-DNA and held that the isolated genes were not markedly different from the chromosomal genes. Hence the Myriad's patent was revoked. The court also gave directions to the USPTO to stop granting patents over genes if they are not markedly different from the naturally occurring genes. However c-DNA with advanced characteristics and post-solution effect may be eligible for patent protection.

Myriad and the road forward

The Supreme Courts' ruling in the Myriad has posed an important question before the legal and scientific fraternity regarding gene patentability. Before *Myriad's* ruling, a number of patents had been granted over the isolated genes, but the judgment reversed the process. The emergence of CRISPR/Cas 9 technology has made the gene editing technology easier and convenient.[25] Not only the non-human genes but even the human genes can be precisely spliced and new gene could be replaced in the sequence to get a changed character. The replacement of genes with new characteristics, though having the ability to develop biologically had posted a greater challenge to their patentability. The newly-edited genes could be granted patent in the light of *Chakrabarty* ruling or could be denied for not showing marked difference in the light of *Myriad.*

Over a period of time, it has been argued that materials, characters and organisms that are substantially similar to the organism already existing in nature should not be patentable. But the issue here is that in a biological world it would be difficult to demarcate a purely biotechnological product and naturally occurring product[26]. *For instance, under the Minimal Genome Project*[27]*, researchers created a partially synthetic species bysynthesising thegenome of the Mycoplasma mycoidesbacterium and transplanting the synthesized genome into the existing cell of a Mycoplasma capricolumbacterium that had its DNA removed*[28]. The bacteria, that was synthetic in origin, is capable of naturally propagating, thus leaving a thin line to decide if it can be categorized similar to a naturally occurring bacteria or a synthetic compound substantially different from its natural counterpart[29].

The *Myriad's* ruling though not clearly demarcated a naturally occurring DNA (g-DNA) from the synthetic DNA (c-DNA), havekept the patent- eligibility

24 *Association of molecular pathology* **v.** *Myriad Genetics, Inc. Et Al*569 U. S. ____ (2013)

25 Benjamin C. Tuttle, 2016. The Failure to Preserve CRISPR-Cas9's Patentability Post Myriad and Alice, 98 J. Pat. & Trademark Off. Soc'y 391, 405

26 Stephanie Constand, 2013, Patently a Problem – Recent Developments in Human Gene Patenting and Their Wider Ethical and Practical Implications, 13 QUT L. Rev. 100, 125

27 Henry T. Greely, 1998, Legal, Ethical, and Social Issues in Human Genome Research, Annual Review of Anthropology, Vol. 27 (1998), pp. 473-502

28 *Id at* Fn. 8

29 *ibid*

of c-DNA open if they show marked difference from the naturally occurring one. The use of new technologiessuch as CRISPRenables editing of human genes hence the edited genes could result in a new kind of gene, obviously different from the naturally occurring human genes. However, the patentability of human genes falls contrary to many of the national legislations, which strictly prohibit patenting of genetically edited human genes.

The patent-eligibility of human genes is not only a legal issue. There are ethical and social issues attached to the patent-eligibility of genes. Patent protection does not merely secure the invention alone but also secures the investment efforts of the inventor. Inventions in gene researches involve huge amount of money and time of the researches. If the inventor is not granted patent it would result in non-incentivizing further research. Patent assure the return of the economic benefit, which further induces interest and money in such researches. However, the notion of incentivizing the researches is not the only criteria but it should satisfy the statutory conditions. Gene based inventions particularly involving purification and isolation of a gene, are free to all men in the public domain. So it is generally criticized that the isolation of gene is more of a discovery rather than invention, where the gene was already present in nature in public domain[30].

The case against Myriad has reflected that researches were not able to conduct study or further research on the genes that were granted patents. There have been complaints that the researchers are not allowed to work on the patented genes and conduct clinical trial[31]. This can pose serious threat to the health care industry asthese isolated genes bring information that are useful in diagnosis of different genetic diseases caused by gene mutations. The patents are exclusive rights and when granted to such isolated genes or inventions pertaining to the genes, the patent holder will have rights to stop anybody from conducting such diagnostic test even using alternative techniques[32]. The abusive use of monopoly is a matter of concern and ultimate sufferings would be caused to the humankind.Infact, the techniques likes CRISPR might also help in editing the genes of a foetus before implantation in the womb to get a child of desired characters. No doubt the technology will help in removal of genetic and hereditary disease, but there are high chances that such technology won't be limited to the curative purpose, but shall start a race of getting off springs having enhanced characters. The patent granted on such genetically edited genes would then effectively lead to patent on humans per se, which is not allowed as per TRIPS Agreement.

Another major ethical issue arising out of gene patent is the question of *informed consent*[33]. The doctrine of prior informed consent derives from medical ethics, where it concerns the patient's right to agree, or refuse, certain medical

30 JauharA .And Narnaulia S. Jan 2010, "Patenting Life The America, European And Indian Way, JIPR 15(1) 55-56 See Also KumarAbhijeetAnd MishraAdrija Nov 2015, Gene patenting vis a vis notion of patentability. JIPR 20(6) 349-362.,

31 id

32 *Association of molecular pathology* v. *Myriad Genetics, Inc. Et Al*569 U. S. ____ (2013)

33 JauharA .And Narnaulia S. Jan 2010, "Patenting Life The America, European And Indian Way, JIPR 15(1) 55-56

treatment after being informed by the practitioner about the risks and benefits.[34] Scientist and Researchers conducts research on the discarded body parts or cells of person and in course of time come up with new inventions and get patents. The person, whose body parts were used for the research is not adequately informed about such research or invention. This is against the rightsof that person who has all the right to know about his body and parts thereof. The court in the*Jhonmoore* case[35] has severely admonished such an act, where an act of uninformed research was being conducted.No research in the fields of biology and medicine should prevail over respect for human rights and human dignity.[36]*Thus the 'informed consent' approach appears to require a patient's express consent in the event that samples taken in the course of the medical intervention are used for research purposes.* The 2005 UNESCO Declaration on Bioethics and Human Rights provides that *both scientific research and medical interventions "should only be carried out with the prior, free, express and informed consent of the person concerned."*[37]

When it comes to patenting of genetically modified human organ, gene or other parts, the US Congress passed Section 33 of the America Invents Act ("AIA")[38] in 2011, resulting in, among other things, a prohibition on patents for inventions "directed to or encompassing human organisms."[39] Unfortunately, the AIAnever expressly defines any of the terms in the provision, so it is not entirely clear what specific subject matter would fall under the prohibition[40].In Europe, the text of European human rights found in a Council of Europe treaty for human rights and biomedicine, prohibits introduction of any modification in the genome of the descendants[41].

There are prohibitions on genetically modifying human genes however they did not stand as a hindrancewhen it comes to genetic modification of plants and animals or micro-organism. It is notable that while dealing the *Onco mouse* case, the court did not consider the genetically edited mouse as an animal but was considered as an article. The mouse which is a living organism was induced

34 Bioethics and Patent Law: The Cases of Moore and the Hagahai People, Sept 2006. http://www.wipo.int/wipo_magazine/en/2006/05/article_0008.html accessed on 13 Oct. 2017.

35 Moore v. Regents of the University of California51 Cal. 3d 120

36 The United Nations Universal Convention on Human Genome and Human Rights, 1997 (63), says that research on the human genome shall respect the ethical standards of society; see also http://ijme.in/articles/patenting-of-human-genetic-material-v-bioethics-revisiting-the-case-of-john-moore-v-regents-of-the-university-of-california/?galley=html

37 http://www.wipo.int/wipo_magazine/en/2006/05/article_0008.html accessed on 22 Oct. 2017.

38 Leahy-Smith America Invents Act, Pub. L. No. 112-29, 125 Stat. 284 (2011) (codified as amended in scattered sections of Title 35 of the U.S. Code).

39 Id. § 33(a), 125 Stat. at 340.

40 Amanda H. Russo, 2014, "Association for Molecular Pathology v. Myriad Genetics, Inc. and Its Impact on the Patentability of Designer Genes," 4 NYU J. Intell. Prop. &Ent. L. 37, 66

41 Art. 13 of the Council of Europe treaty for human rights and biomedicine,Also see , Hillary Chua, "Designer Babies and the Law: A Legal Analysis of Human Germline Editing in Light of the UK's
Human Rights Obligations" , 8 King's Student L. Rev. 68, 87 (2017)

to change so that it can be patented.The animal rights activists have condemned such experiments and patent thereof, which involves pain and suffering to a living creature. The genetic modification also causes environmental threats as it leads to dilution of genetic diversity. Similarly, the genetic modification of seeds also causes huge threat to the environment in the form of genetic pollution, genetic uniformity and affects the traditional breeder's rights. The patent-eligibility criterions are scientific and procedural but the ethical and social concerns are factors to be considered before the grant of monopoly rights.

Conclusion

The recombinant DNA technologies and latest biotechnological tools have led to new kinds of gene based inventions. The patent laws across the world provide protection to new and useful inventions irrespective of the field of technology. Genomics as a field of science has led the man to discover and invent scientific and therapeutic breakthroughs to fulfil societal needs. The legal protection to inventions based on genes, their manipulation and the final outcome could be grantedonly if they surpass the 'product of nature' test. While the courts have stressed upon human intervention in creating useful products and services beyond the creation of nature, the recent trends have shifted in increasing the magnitude of human intervention to such inventions. Apart from satisfying the 'product of nature' test, the inventions must show significant post-solution activity with advanced characteristics non-existent in the nature.

The history of gene patenting although formally began from 1980 in the *Chakrabarty*decision, the standards have been constantly raised and set high by the legal system in the subsequent rulings. The *Myriad* decision in 2013 has now put-forth the latest standards to enable patenting of synthetically created DNA not naturally occurring and markedly different from the chromosomal DNA. In this light, new kinds of inventions in the field of genomics are expected to arise whose patent-eligibility would largely depend on *Myriad's* ruling. At present the ethical and moral concerns over patenting of genes have not been strictly considered by the courts. The patentability as per Article 27.2 of the TRIPS Agreement, 1995 has excluded inventions that are contrary to the public order or morality and harmful to environment or living beings. The patenting of gene-based inventions have so far not raised any ethical concerns however they may develop in future due to the development of newer technologies. The balancing of scientific temper and maintaining ethics in the realm of public and private interest is thus the need of the hour.

Chapter 5

Going the Unconventional Way- Gene Patents in India

Jai Shanker Bajpai and Smriti Gandhi

College of Legal Studies, University of Petroleum and Energy studies, Dehradun, Uttrakhand, India

Email: jaibajpai7@gmail.com

Abstract

The proper use of patents and other IPRs in relation to genetic research has created an absorbing and difficult debate. Ethical arguments are invoked but from perspectives which may embrace normative standards of many societies. They may derive from religious teaching, philosophical idealism, environmental imperatives, social and cultural specificities, economic and other utilitarian desiderata or the experience embodied in rules and procedures of legal systems.

One of the characteristics of gene-based industry is that it is highly unpredictable and immature, as most of the inventions are based upon trial and error, this makes it harder to mould patent laws according to the needs of the field as patentability requisites such as novelty, non-obviousness, and enablement and utility are based on predictability of the field.

Patent laws are always being customized and fine-tuned by governments to meet the ever changing needs of progressing technologies. Basic principles pertaining to patents have developed to cater to the needs of traditional fields of science. However, these principles fail when it comes to modern biotechnology and specifically gene-based inventions. This has given rise to ambiguities and confusion among biotechnology companies. Moreover, this would bring investment into the biotechnology sector in India, thus giving a boost to the Indian economy.

The scientific evidence of cryonics is indeed promising. In certain cases of mammals such as cats, which were neuro-preserved, frozen brains did show electrical activity upon being thawed. Also, LTP persists in tissue slices, and that nematode worms retain long-term memories after revival is evidence that significant information remains upon reanimation.

Genetic Patents and Bioethics

The proper use of patents and other IPRs in relation to genetic research has created an absorbing and difficult debate. Ethical arguments are invoked but from perspectives which may embrace normative standards of many societies.

They may derive from religious teaching, philosophical idealism, environmental imperatives, social and cultural specificities, economic and other utilitarian desiderata or the experience embodied in rules and procedures of legal systems.

Section 3(b) of the Indian Paten Act stipulates that an invention, the primary or intended use or commercial exploitation of which would be contrary to public order or morality or which causes serious prejudice to human, animal, or plant life or health or to the environment is not patentable.[1] The Manual of Patent Practice and Procedure stipulates that any biological process or material or method of making the same which can cause prejudice to human, animal or plant life or health or to the environment including the use that would be against public morality and order are not patentable. The *Manual* further stipulates that processes pertaining to cloning of animals or human beings or altering the genetic makeup of a human being or an animal are not patentable on the ground of being against public order and morality.[2]

The Indian patent law has strict prohibitions against patenting of gene based inventions based on morality and public order. The *Manual* even prohibits patenting of genetically modified animals which experimented on for finding the cure for fatal disease such as cancer, inducement of such a disease would be prejudicial to its health. Furthermore, gene modifications in human beings are considered to be immoral as India has an age old cultural heritage, it also has strong belief in religions and customs. In this sense, gene related inventions have always received strong resistance from the Indian public.

Europe and India have the same position with regard to provisions governing morality in patent regime. While USA on other hand does not have such provisions which govern an invention on moralistic grounds. So, the chances of a gene-based invention being rejected based on moralistic grounds is very high in Europe or India, when compared to USA.

Patentable Subject Matters in India and Genetic Inventions

The Indian Patent Act, stipulates that any product or process is patentable subject matter.[3] It prohibits patents on discovery of anything living or occurring in nature.[4]In one such instance, the Controller of Patent rejected a patent application relating to vaccine for bursitis virus, stating that it is a living organism and thus cannot be patented.[5] However, it provides for patenting micro-organisms and microbiological processes.[6] The Calcutta High Court was then approached and it reversed the decision stating that a living micro-organism is a patentable subject matter as a manufacture. This judicial ruling has cleared that genetically modified micro-organisms are allowed to be patented as per the interpretation of Section 3(c) of the patent act.

---

1 Indian Patent Act, 1970, Section 3(b).

2 Manual of Patent Practice and Procedure, Examination Guidelines for Patent Applications relating to Inventions in the field of Chemicals, Pharmaceuticals and Biotechnology-Annexure I (2005).

3 Indian Patent Act and 35 USC, Section 101.

4 Indian Patent Act, 1970, Section 3(c).

5 Dimminaco A.G. v Controller General of Patent, Designs and Trademarks (2002) accessed at http://www.tifac.org.in/do/pfc/case/microbio.htm visited on 21 October, 2017.

6 Indian Patent Act, 1970, Section 3(j).

The Manual of Patent Practice and Procedure talks of DNA, plasmids, and processes of manufacturing are patentable if they have been produced with human intervention. Thus, it provides that mere discovery of a living organism would not be successful in getting a patent but a living organism which is produced as result of substantive human intervention can be patented. Gene sequences having clear and disclosed functions are allowed to be patented in India. However, inventions pertaining to medicinal, surgical, diagnostic, therapeutic or like treatments of human beings or animals are not allowed to be patented.[7]

Comparative Analysis: USA, Europe and India

Table 1: Patentability of gene-based inventions in USA, Europe and India

Subject Matter	USA	Europe	India
Genes	Patentable	Patentable	Patentable
Genetically modified Unicellular Organisms	Patentable	Patentable	Patentable
Genetically Modified Humans	Not Patentable	Not Patentable	Not Patentable
Genetically modified Multicellular organisms	Patentable	Patentable	Not Patentable
Genetically Modified Animals (not including humans)	Patentable	Not patentable (Except Mammals)	Not Patentable
Gene Therapy	Patentable	Not Patentable	Not Patentable
Genetically Modified Plants	Patentable	Patentable	Not Patentable

Table 2: Number of Patents filed and granted to gene-based inventions in USA, Europe and India[8]

Company	USA	Europe	India
Council of scientific and Industrial Research	22	2	0
Dabur Research Foundation	2	2	1
National Institute of Immunology	2	0	1
Ranbaxy Laboratories Limited	3	1	0
Reliance Life Sciences Pvt. Ltd.	1	0	0
Wockhardt Limited	1	1	1

Novelty and Gene-based Inventions

In India, if an invention has to patented it has to satisfy the requirement of newness stipulated under Section 2(j) of the Patent Act, 1970, which states that a 'new invention is any invention or technology which has not been anticipated or predicted by publication in any document or used in country elsewhere in the world.

7 Indian Patent Act, 1970, Section 3(b).

8 *Genetic Patent Law and Strategy* (I ed., First), Manupatra.

In determining novelty of any invention in India, the following three parameters/steps may be considered:[9]

1. What is the invention about?
2. What is the information disclosed by the prior art?
3. Is the invention new?

The term 'prior art' means a body of information restricted by a point of time. It pertains to the material known before the date of filing of the patent application with the complete specification. Once the material is ascertained, the nature of information disclosed can be found out. Novelty depends upon various constituents concepts, such as 'the state of the art', 'publicly known', 'publicly used', 'published' etc, which have been statutorily defined or judicially interpreted and understood by patent laws of other countries. The problem that gene-based inventions face passing the novelty test is that these critical concepts have not been defined under the Patents Act. The practice of introducing phrases which can have multiple connotations without rendering appropriate definition will have an undesirable effect of relying on patent practices of other jurisdiction in search of meanings for the same.

Section 2(ja) of the Patent Act stipulates that an 'inventive step' means a distinct feature of an invention that includes technically advancing as opposed to existing knowledge, or having economic value, or both, making an invention not obvious to a person skilled in that particular field.[10] Indian law gives importance to economic value in determining the inventive step, any gene-based inventions would easily satisfy this test as most gene sequences and like inventions have great significance in the biopharma market because of the multiple uses that they provide.

The US law on this subject provides the list of non-extensive conditions and parameters that negate the novelty of an invention.[11] These requirements override the subject matter requirements in USA. The patent system recognizes the fact that most biotech inventions are related to naturally existing products, determination of their novelty overrides the provision for exclusion within the products of nature category under the subject matter requirement.[12] While the subject matter clause checks for human intervention in any given product, the novelty clause goes a step ahead and checks if the product which is so invented is new and different from the existing products.

In Europe, article 54 of the European Patent Convention deals with novelty.[13] It stipulates that an invention will be considered as new if it does not form the state of anything which includes everything made available to the public by means of

9 Bently, Lionel, *Intellectual Property Law*, (2000).

10 Indian Patent Act, 1970, Section 2(ja).

11 35 U.S. Code - Conditions for patentability; novelty, Section 102.

12 Courtney, J. M, 'Patent Law and Human Genomics', 26 CAP. U.L. REV. 893 911 (1997)

13 Convention on European Patents, Article 54 (1973), text as amended by the act revising Article 63 EPC of 17 December, 1991 and by decisions of the Administrative Council of the European Patent Organization of 21 December, 1978, 13 December, 1994, 20 October 1995 and 10 December, 1998.

written or oral description, by use, or in any other form or way, before the filing of the patent application.[14] The current regulations as provided by the convention stipulate that biological material, which is isolated from its environment or produced by the means of technical process even if it occurred in nature in the past, is patentable. It provides that even an element excluded from the human body or produced by means of an industrial process, including partial or whole sequence of gene, may be patented and the ground that the structure of that element is identical to that a natural element will not hold good, this is done in order to prevent such grounds cast a shadow on the patentability of genetic inventions. In brief, a general principle with regard to genetic patents emanates, that is, a gene sequence removed from nature would be considered as novel with respect to what exists in nature even if its structure or make resembles the one already existing in nature. Novelty of genetic inventions is still uncertain in Europe. Europe is struggling to define tests for determining novelty clearly. There have been number of precedents with regard to this subject, which provide different interpretation of the test, and thus there is ambiguity surrounding patentability of genetic inventions in Europe.

Non-Obviousness and Gene-based Inventions

Non-obviousness means that an invention must be non-obvious to a person who is ordinarily skilled in the field pertaining to that invention. It is the ultimate test that an invention has to clear in order to get patented.

In USA, non-obviousness is given under Section 103 of the United States Code.[15] It stipulates that an invention will be considered as 'non-obvious' if it is non-obvious to a person with ordinary skill in the given field of the invention.[16] To make an invention obvious, there must be a reasonable inference that the elements in any prior inventions are present in the invention which is brought forward for patenting. [17]An invention will not be considered obvious if its invention was an attempt to bring about the effect of a previous invention.[18]

In Europe, Article 52 of the European Patent Convention states that European Patent Convention stipulates that inventions containing an 'inventive step' meaning human intervention for bringing about a product is necessary. Both US and Europe consider the reasonable non-obviousness from the point of view of an ordinary skilled person in the given field. Furthermore, gene inventions pertaining to other species and existence of general methods of isolating genes will not make other isolated genes 'obvious' in USA but in Europe this would be considered as 'obvious' if it could have been found or invented by a person having ordinary skill in the given field.

In India, Section 2(ja) of Patent Act provides that 'inventive step' means that an invention involves technical advance when compared to already existing knowledge on the subject or economic importance of the invention or both that

14 European Patent Convention, Article 54(1)-54(2) (1973).

15 35 U.S. Code - Conditions for patentability; Non- Obviousness, Section 103.

16 Graham v. John Deere Co., No. 383 U.S. 1 slip op. at 17-18, 86 (U.S 1986).

17 Locite Corp. v Ultraseal Ltd., No. 781 F.2d 861 (Fed. Cir. 1985)

18 Merck & Co. v Biocrafts Labs., 874 F.2d 804, 807, (Fed. Cir. 1989)

makes the invention not obvious to a person having reasonable skill in the given field.[19] Here, due to lack of definitive history, the terms 'technical advance' and 'economic significance' have not been defined. However, the Manual of Patent Practice and Procedure, it can be interpreted that isolated gene sequences are considered as to contain an inventive step when compared to other naturally existing counterparts. It is pertinent to note that the Indian Patent Act is adamant upon the 'economic significance' of an invention, it is easy for genetic inventions to pass this test as they have great economic significance in biopharma sector. In this light, it is clear that gene-based inventions would pass through the test of having an inventive step much easily in India when compared to USA or Europe, which desist from giving importance to commercial standing of an invention. Written description makes it easy to evidence the filing date as the date of invention by pointing out that the applicant was in full possession of the subject matter on the given date when application was submitted.[20]

Written-Description and gene-based inventions.

Patent law in US, Europe and India makes it compulsory for any invention to have a 'written description' meaning that the invention must be disclosed to the public in the form of a disclosure (written), which stipulates for making use of the invention through enablement and defines the boundaries of its use while considering the claims that the invention makes.

In USA, Section 112 of the Patent Act stipulates that a written description or specification shall contain a lucid written description of the invention and the process of making and using it, so as to enable any person who is reasonably skilled in the field to make and use the invention.[21]It also stipulates that the written description shall also point out the distinct features of the invention, indicating that it is not similar to other inventions in the same field.

On the same lines, Article 83 of European Patent Convention stipulates that the patent application must in itself clearly disclose the invention in such a manner that it could be made and be used by a person having reasonable skill in the field pertaining to the invention.

In India, principles on the same have been stipulated under Section 10 of the Patent Act.[22] It stipulates that specification of every invention must clearly describe the invention and operation or use and the method which is used to bring about the effect of the given invention.[23] The law provides that if a patent application is granted for a biological material, it should be deposited in a recognized depository so as to make it available to public from the date of filing. The applicant is also required to specify the origin and source of biological material. The manual in this regard states that complete legal document should be submitted disclosing the invention fully so that a person skilled in the same field can produce the given

19 Indian Patent Act, 1970, Section 2(ja).

20 Lockwood v American Airlines, Inc., No. 107 F3d 1565 (Fed. Cir. 1997)

21 35 U.S. Code - Section 112.

22 Indian Patent Act, 1970, Section 10.

23 Indian Patent Act, 1970, Section 10(4).

invention.[24]

There are huge similarities in written description clauses of India, Europe and USA. These three countries require a disclosure that would enable a person with reasonable skill in the subject to carry out the invention easily without giving rise to ambiguities in the path. As far as gene based inventions are concerned, this clause does not portray or introduce any problem, as an accurate description of any gene based invention can be given in written form. However, the process involved in such inventions are very technical in nature and the person so producing them following the written description has to take care of the technical requirements given in the description, otherwise the reproduction of such an invention might fail.

A claim in a specification will not be ambiguous merely because some part of it is capable of more than one construction[25], which is a pertinent feature of description of many gene-based inventions. In such cases, the court should prefer the sensible construction and would read the claim in such a manner so as to avoid an absurd result. Ambiguous claims are drafted so that the patentee may claim the widest possible for the invention. The courts have cautioned not to interpret the claims so as to give a patentee the widest possible scope.[26]

Lack of clarity is a ground for revocation of a patent under the Patents Act.[27] Similarly, if the scope of any claim of the any claim of the complete specification is sufficiently or clearly defined, it could also be a ground for revocation. But the mere fact that a word, phrase or other provision in a patent claim is not wholly clear will not automatically lead to the conclusion that the claim is objectionable, as this would set an unrealistic standard for drafting in any field. A claim needs to be as clear as the subject matter reasonably permits.[28]

The purposive method for construction will not permit the introduction of any additional requirement over and above the ones stipulated by law. However, it is permissible for the court to introduce the requirements stated in section 10 of the Patents Act, the ingredients of which court may introduce by way of construction, the requirements that the claim must be fairly based on the matter disclosed in the specifications.[29]

TRIPS Agreement and Gene-based inventions.

'The Agreement on Trade-Related Aspects of Intellectual Property Rights' TRIPs agreement covers most forms of intellectual property including patents, copyright, trademarks, geographical indications, industrial designs, trade secrets, and exclusionary rights over new plant varieties. It has been observed that the TRIPs agreement has been a little ambiguous when it comes to patent laws.

24 Manual of Patent Practice and Procedure, 2005, Sufficiency of Disclosure, 2.6.

25 Henriksen v Tallon Ltd (1965) RPC 434, p 443, [1965] FSR 215 (HL).

26 Kirin-Amgen Inc v Hoechst Marion Roussel Ltd (2005) RPC 9.

27 Indian Patent Act, 1970, Section 64(1)(h).

28 LG Philips LCD Co Ltd v Tatung (UK) Ltd [2006] EWCA Civ 1774, para 20.

29 Indian Patent Act, 1970, Section 10(5).

The broad language of the TRIPs agreement signifies that it grants allowance to individual member states to enact their own intellectual property laws to remove ambiguities.[30]

By becoming a member of the World Trade Organization (WTO), India had agreed to conform its intellectual property laws to the requirements of the TRIPS Agreement. Accordingly, the Patent Act was amended in 1999, 2002 and 2005 to meet India's international obligations. The TRIPS Agreement offers patent protection for any invention, whether products or processes, in all fields of technology, provided that they are new, involve an inventive step, and are capable of industrial application. India had undertaken to align its patent laws with TRIPS by 1 January 2005. A 10 year period was granted to developing countries like India to align their patent laws so as to provide patent protection for inventions previously not covered by the Indian law.

The TRIPs agreement exclude naturally occurring genetic material but includes researched and modified genetic material for patentability which in turn prevents research and has a detrimental effect on consumer prices for products produced using gene based technology.[31]Supporters of gene patenting maintain that there is no evidence which suggests that gene patents prevents innovation or unnecessarily restrain trade by inflating costs or enabling predatory pricing.[32] Yet while the purpose of patents was to incentivize innovation, evidence indicates that patents do not increase innovation 6 and there are significant numbers of outspoken opponents to patenting genes.[33]Gene patents supporters argue that exclusive rights create so called "legal monopolies" or monopolies in name only, which do not dominate the market.[34] Moreover, while supporting these view they accept the fact that patentees holding exclusive rights to their invention does not meant that they do not compete with similar products that may produce the same functions and meet the same demand. However, the very process of information gathering and innovation would cease to exist if researchers were entirely unable to share knowledge and build upon it in the hopes of creating new inventions.

TRIPS provides four filters from which an invention must pass through in order to be granted a patent. These four filters are related to subject matter which includes process, novelty, inventive step and industrial application.[35] However, the agreement does not allow for inventions going against public order, morality, or animal/plant life.[36] It is pertinent to note that it allows member countries to exclude medical methods, plants or animals, except micro-organisms and essential

30 Christopher M. , H. (2007). Impact of Human Gene Patents on Innovation and Access: A Survey of Human Gene Patent Litigation (rev. 295 ed., Vol. 76, p. 34).

31 Johanna , G. (2009). Intellectual Property, Medicine and Health: Current Debates (p. 18).

32 Gregory , C.E. (2008). Emerging Biotechnologies Demand Defeat of Proposed Legislation that Attempts to Ban Gene Patents (5 ed., Vol. 1, p. 1). RICH. J. L. & TECH.

33 Michele, B. LEVINE, D.K. (2008). Against Intellectual Monopoly. (p. 186-18).

34 NunoPires De, C. (2008). The Trips Regime of Antitrust and Undisclosed Information. (p. 13).

35 TRIPS Agreement, 1994, Article 27, Para 1.

36 TRIPS Agreement, 1994, Article 27, Para 2.

biological processes except microbiological processes.[37] The member countries are allowed to amend their patent laws but those amendments are subjected to the aforementioned requirements provided in TRIPS. However, these filters have not been defined in detail, and thus are too broad in nature. In this sense, the standards defined under TRIPS are an inadequate and vague means of establishing standard criteria for patentability.

Business strategy and genetic patents

Among the three countries discussed, USA has the widest patent protection system for gene-based inventions. The law pertaining to patents in US is attentive to the needs of ever growing fields of science such as biotechnology, genetic engineering and likes of it. It also provides very narrow scope for getting a 'research exemption' meaning that a person can be exempted from patent laws if he or she uses it for research purposes, while doing so it provides better protection to the patented inventions. In this sense, it could be said that US law favours gene-based inventions. The presence of such patent regime has given US has given encouragement to progress in the field of genetic sciences. The patent laws provide adequate protection to the investors, who invest large amounts into the research and development of such inventions. As a result, US attracts many investors and researchers, even from other countries.

Europe when compared to USA has narrow patent protection regime. As discussed previously, not many gene based inventions are allowed to be patented and the patentability filters are too narrow to let pass any invention easily. However, the European patent regime is adamant upon granting research exemptions. This results in a framework which is not supportive of inventors as any researcher could use the invention without permission from the patent holder.

The patent regime in Europe is not encouraging genetic-based inventions, the biotechnology sector did not develop as much as in USA, partly because of its patent laws not favouring gene-based inventions. One major problem that inventors face is that of morality, many inventions are tested upon the touchstone of morality and are not granted patent. It has led to investors and researchers being overly speculative of their inventions in order to get it patented.

India when compared to USA has a very narrow genetic patent protection system. Moreover, the research exemptions are very broad when compared to USA or Europe. The patent laws in itself exclude plethora of genetic inventions and materials. Furthermore, the filter tests like utility, novelty and non-obviousness are broad, but the subject matter being very narrow makes the patentability requirements very strict. The clauses which define 'written description' are still not developed and the dearth of legislative history on the same, makes the clause ambiguous. Due to narrow patent regime and large and flexible public domain, the patent system in India does not encourage or support development of gene-based companies in India. This is a drawback as many industries want to set up industries in India because of its flourishing economy. However, with the presence of such a weak patent regime, many biopharma companies avoid to conduct any

37 TRIPS Agreement 1994, Article 27, Para 3.

business in India. This in turn hampers the economic growth and the benefits that come along with it such as employment, development, increase in standard of living etc.

The problem of morality is still persistent in the Indian patent regime. There is only a clause (Section 3, sub-clause b) defining morality and there is no legislative history or judicial pronouncements on the same defining the limits or extent of morality. This has given rise to ambiguity and the patent offices in India have retained the whip to define such ambiguous clauses according to their own whims and satisfaction.

In USA, the patent regime favours the genetic companies whereas in India the genetic patent regime is more inclined towards the public. Though an Indian company cannot get a patent in India on most gene-based inventions, it can get a patent for the same in USA very easily. It is because of such a patent regime in USA that Indian companies who are involved in genetic-based inventions and research turn to USA for patent protection. Due to broad research exemptions, a company in India can use technology patented in both USA and India without incurring any liability in order to help and encourage research.

Despite the benefits given to Indian companies by the differences in patent regime of USA and India, there are problems which relate to the incentive mechanism. As the incentives are the outcome of patents in USA and their commercialization in the US market, the Indian companies are directed to serve the needs of US market. So, that research benefits USA more than India. If the US patent regime could encourage research progress in India, a patent system suited to genetic inventions in India would help to promote the progress of biotechnology sector.

Conclusion

Patent laws are always being customized and fine-tuned by governments to meet the ever changing needs of progressing technologies. Basic principles pertaining to patents have developed to cater to the needs of traditional fields of science. However, these principles fail when it comes to modern biotechnology and specifically gene-based inventions. This has given rise to ambiguities and confusion among biotechnology companies. This greatly hampers the incentive and business advantage that the biotechnology sector could have had. In the absence of an effective regime, investors are not interested in investing large amount of sums into research and development as the research output could be exploited by anybody. In this sense, gene-based inventions is one such field which assumes high importance when it comes to patent laws.

One of the characteristics of gene-based industry is that it is highly unpredictable and immature, as most of the inventions are based upon trial and error, this makes it harder to mould patent laws according to the needs of the field as patentability requisites such as novelty, non-obviousness, enablement and utility are based on predictability of the field.

Gene-based inventions many a times challenge morality and ethics of a country, which are embedded in it through customs. As a result, morality and ethics has long been intertwined with progress in the field of biotechnology and the legislature faces a tough call when it is faced with making laws which go against the ethics and values which a country cherishes. However, the time calls for updating patent laws while balancing the other side consisting of moral and ethics. India has always been an admirer of US when it comes to law, it can make its patent laws on the US model of patent laws, this would result in a patent regime which caters to the less attended field of sciences such as biotechnology. Moreover, this would bring investment into the biotechnology sector in India, thus giving a boost to the Indian economy.

Chapter 6

Cryonics in India-Fulfilling the Ardent Desire to Live

Hatim Hussain[1], Prateek Srivastava[2]

[1]III Year, B.Com.L.L.B. (Hons.) Gujarat National Law University

[2]III Year, B.A.L.L.B. (Hons.) Gujarat National Law University

Email: hatimhussain110@gmail.com

Abstract

The desire for immortality, to defeat death- humanity's one and only greatest fear, has enticed human mind and thought since centuries. So much so that Rig Veda has imbued in it the famous 'Mrityunjaya Mantra' (RV, 7/59/12), a verse usually chanted to conquer death.

Modern world religions and even primeval cultures have often offered solace by promising life beyond death, proving the ardent desire of man to escape its physical form and consequently, become immortal. The idea of cryonics was first conceived by Robert Ettinger, also called as the father of cryonics movement and coined by Karl Werner. Though the idea of freezing dead bodies to reanimate them in future has been devoured since decades before him. Ettinger in his book *The Prospect of Immortality* in 1964 gave a renewed vigour to it, establishing the process and methodology in detail. The lack of legislative action will only be detrimental to interests of both science and general public welfare. Hence, a pre-emptive step in this regard may as well do wonders for humanity.

1. Introduction

Overview

The desire for immortality, to defeat death- humanity's one and only greatest fear, has enticed human mind and thought since centuries. So much so that Rig Veda has imbued in it the famous 'Mrityunjaya Mantra' (RV, 7/59/12), a verse usually chanted to conquer death.[1] Modern world religions and even primeval cultures have often offered solace by promising life beyond death, proving the ardent desire of man to escape its physical form and consequently, become immortal.[2]

1 Kumar, S. (n.d.). *Morality, Trans-Mortality and Immorality In Vedic Thought*. Retrived from http://www.sanskrit.nic.in/svimarsha/V6/c4.pdf

2 Platt, C. (1994). *A Short of Cryonics and a long, hard look at the lessons we can learn from it.*

The *Rig Veda*[3] mentions this desire for immortality aptly-

येच्चिद्धिमृत्युबंधवआर्दित्यामनंव: स्मसि।
प्रसून आयुंर्जीसेंतिरेतन।।

Not long ago, defeating death would have formed the premise of a good science fiction story, today technological triumphs have enabled humans to fight incurable diseases, discover undiscovered places in universe and generally do impossible things. Our superior biological knowledge has indeed enabled us to come as close to conquering mortality than ever before. In this attempt to supersede biological process with technological process, law becomes the primary tool to ensure that humanity does not interrupt the delicate balance of health and justice. Cryonics, the technological process of prolonging the life of humans by advanced methods is science poses one such formidable challenge to the entire institution of law.

The idea of cryonics was first conceived by Robert Ettinger, also called as the father of cryonics movement[4] and coined by Karl Werner. Though the idea of freezing dead bodies to reanimate them in future has been devoured since decades before him[5], Ettinger in his book *The Prospect of Immortality* in 1964 gave a renewed vigour to it, establishing the process and methodology in detail.[6] A book similar to this titled *Immortality: Physically, Scientifically, Now* was written by E Y Cooper in which he described how cryogenically freezing the human body creates "a possibility for eventually defeating death."[7] He eventually went on to found the first cryonics organization in the world Life Extension Society in 1963.[8] Subsequently, the Cryonics Society of New York, the Cryonics Society of Michigan and the Cryonics Society of California were founded.[9] Dr. James Bedford was the first person to be cryogenically preserved in 1967 by the Cryonics Society of

---

Retrieved from http://www.cs.cmu.edu/afs/cs/user/tsf/Public-Mail/cryonics/213

3 *"Courteously lengthen our lives so that we may live"* Verse 8.018.22 (n.d.), In *Rig Veda* (8th ed., Vol. Mandala). Retrieved September 28, 2017, from https://www.aurobindo.ru/workings/matherials/rigveda/08/08-018.htm

4 Ballard, M. (2009, November 7). *Life After Death.* Retrieved from https://www.theguardian.com/science/gallery/2009/nov/07/cryonics

5 The earliest known case of the idea of cryonics being brought forth was in 1773, when Benjamin Franklin discussed if it was possible to be 'immersed' in madeira and wake up in future. *See Letter from Benjamin Franklin to Barbeu Dubourg* (Albert Henry Smyth ed., Vol. 6) THE WRITINGS OF BENJAMIN FRANKLIN. (Apr. 1773). The scientific evidence of cryonics was first provided in 1940 by biologist Basil Luyet who published his work relating to freezing of living cells. *See* Luyet, B., & Gehenio, M. P. (1940). *Life and death at low temperatures.* Normandy, Missouri: Biodynamica. https://archive.org/details/lifedeathatlowte00luye.

6 Ettinger, R. C. (1964). *The Prospect of Immortality.* Ria University Press. Retrieved October 28, 2017, from https://www.cryonics.org/images/uploads/misc/Prospect_Book.pdf.

7 Duhring, N. (1962). *Immortality: Physically, Scientifically, Now.* Retrieved from http://depressedmetabolism.com/pdfs/cooper_immortality.pdf

8 Perry, M. (1992). *For the Record: Unity and Disunity in Cryonics.* Retrieved from http://www.alcor.org/cryonics/cryonics9208.txt;

9 Kent, S. (1983). *The First Cryonicist.* Retrieved from http://www.alcor.org/cryonics/cryonics8303.txt

California, now known as Alcor Life Extension Foundation, and remains frozen today.[10]

Process of Cryonics

The process of cryonics is generally executed at low temperature (achieved at a rate of 1° C per hour till it attains the temperature of -196° C) as metabolism gets slowed and chemical changes taking place in the body gets stopped. The method of *vitrification* is used to avoid disruption of cells due to ice formation. Remarkably, health condition which are currently incurable can be anticipated to be curable in future and this is the basis on which cryonics stands. In fact, human embryos can already be frozen and thawed safely, and adult non-mammals have also undergone the process successfully.[11] The feat of first human babies (twins) successfully being born from a previously frozen embryo was already achieved in 1983.[12] In 1987, Berkley scientists have also successfully performed a cryogenic preservation experiment using a domestic dog.[13] All these evidences present an optimistic picture of future of cryonics. Already achievements in reverse aging through use of nanotechnology are being experimented with remarkable success by scientists across the world.[14] This concept of arrested ageing involves stopping ageing entirely, or even reversing it, as would be achieved by taking a dip in the mythical fountain of youth. Yet, it must also be noted that based on the current state of play in biogerontology, arrested ageing like cryonics remains a very remote possibility.[15] The procedure of cryonics is currently performed by five major organisations across the world, although none of them is in India. These include- Alcor[16], Trans Times[17], Oregon Cryonics[18], KrioRus[19] and the Cryonics institute[20].

Currently, cryonic preservation procedures begin after legal death has been pronounced.[21] Once this has occurred, medications to maintain sedation, reduce

---

10 Perry, M. (1992). *For the Record: Unity and Disunity in Cryonics*. Retrieved from http://www.alcor.org/cryonics/cryonics9208.txt;

11 Gerard, H. (1984). Two Pregnancies Following Transfer of Intact Frozen: Thawed Embryos. *Fertility & Sterility*, 293, 295.

12 Bagch, A. (2008). Cryopreservation and Vitrification: Recent Advances in Fertility Preservation Technologies. *Expert Rev. Med. Devices*, 359.

13 *Dog 'Spunky' After It's Frozen in Test.* (1987). Retrieved from http://articles.latimes.com/1987 03-31/news/mn-1527_1.

14 Kurazweil, R. (2007, November 22). *Bring on the nanobots, and we will live long and prosper*. Retrieved from https://www.theguardian.com/commentisfree/2007/nov/22/comment.comment

15 Blumenthal, H. T. (2003). The aging-disease dichotomy: true or false? *J. Gerontol. A Biol. Sci. Med. Sci.* 58, 138-145.

16 Alcor (n.d.). Retrieved from https://www.alcor.org/

17 Trans Time (n.d.) Retrieved from http://www.transtime.com/index.html

18 Oregon Cryonics (n.d.). Retrieved from http://www.oregoncryo.com/index.html

19 KrioRus (n.d.). Retrieved from http://www.kriorus.com/en/

20 Cryonics Institute (n.d.). Retrieved from http://www.cryonics.org/

21 George P. Smith, II. (1996). Pathways to Immortality in the New Millennium: Human Responsibility, Theological Direction, or Legal Mandate. *St. Louis University. Public Law Review*, 15, 447.

metabolism, prevent blood clotting, reduce ischemia/ reperfusion injury, etc. are administered through circulation, while blood circulation and respiration are restored as far as possible to keep tissues alive. Injected medication is circulated through chest compressions through a process called Cardiopulmonary support.[22] The anticoagulant heparin is injected to keep the circulatory system free of blood clots.[23] The patient is cooled using ice water to bring down body temperature below 108°C, at which point perfusion with *vitrification* solution begins. Temperatures are then gradually lowered until the body reaches a storage temperature of -196°C. Such temperature is required to prevent preservation injury. At this point, nearly indefinite storage in liquid nitrogen with no change is possible.[24]

Firstly, the practitioners make an attempt to preserve the brain because it is the brain where neurological information that makes up the identity is stored. The brain is cooled and medicated through circulatory system of the body.[25] Metabolic support is provided to the brain cells by supplying oxygen through intubation and glucose through intravenous injections. Since time slot to execute the preservation is very less in most of the cases, a suspension team is often placed on location at the hospital in order to expedite the process and ensure immediate cooling if imminent death is known in advance.[26] Severely damaged brain is not fit for future reanimation which is the reason why the practitioner advocates that chances of successful reanimation are more when process is initiated before disease progression causes the body to deteriorate too far.

Vitrification

After performing the preliminary steps, the cryonics specialists executes the process of "*vitrification*."[27] The temperature is cautiously maintained so as to avoid freezing of water inside the cells which can crush the fragile cell membranes and cause irreparable damage to the organs. Another method to prevent this is by replacing the water in the cells with a "cryoprotectant" after removal of the blood.[28] It is a glycerol based substance which functions as an antifreeze for the human body. When the temperature of the body reaches approximately - 120° Celsius, the process of *vitrification* gets completed.[29] At last, the body is inserted into a large metal tank filled with liquid nitrogen where the body is cooled to its

22 Best, B. P. (2008). Scientific Justification of Cryonics Practice. *Rejuvenation Res,* 493-94.

23 Platt, C. (n.d.). *General Introduction to Procedures for Alcor Transport Technicians.* Retrieved from http://www.alcor.org/Library/pdfs/intro.pdf

24 Shaw, D. (2009). Cryoethics: Seeking life after death. *Bioethics*, 23(9), 515–521.

25 Platt, C. (n.d.). *General Introduction to Procedures for Alcor Transport Technicians.* Retrieved from http://www.alcor.org/Library/pdfs/intro.pdf

26 Cryonics Institute. (n.d.) *Outline of CI Cryopreservation Procedures for Human Patients.* Retrieved from http://www.cryonics.org/phases.html.

27 Ettinger, R. C. (1964). *The Prospect of Immortality*. Ria University Press. Retrieved October 28, 2017, from https://www.cryonics.org/images/uploads/misc/Prospect_Book.pdf.

28 Best, B. P. (2008, March) *Cryoprotectant Toxicity.* Retrieved from http://www.cryonics.org/immortalist/march08/cryoprotectant.pdf

29 Cryonics Institute. (n.d.) *Outline of CI Cryopreservation Procedures for Human Patients.* Retrieved from http://www.cryonics.org/phases.html.

long-term storage temperature of approximately -196° Celsius.[30] Liquid nitrogen has a tendency of getting boiled off with passage of time which makes it essential to replenish it regularly. When this is done, the body is inserted vertically with head-first so that it is ensured that the brain remains preserved even if others portions of the body gets accidentally thawed.

2. Religious, Ethical and Judicial Decisionmaking

Cryonics and Religion

The contrast between science and religion, two of the greatest forces which influence men, cannot be more aptly defined than the classic distinction between black and white. Some theorists view this disparity by a limited view which symbolizes science as a progressive force and religion as rather regressive school of ideologies.[31] Nevertheless, religion and science are as intertwined as DNA.[32] As a famous writer once said, *science is a child of magic*- the same element which propels faith and forms the bedrock of religion. Much akin to a child who upon reaching an age becomes resentful of his parents, science has grown vary of religion, but it doesn't distort the fact that they share a lot in common. It is in this context the theological and ethical aspects of cryonics have to be considered, particularly in Indian milieu which stands at the crossroads of this *liberative-oppressive* divide.

Indeed, the practice of cryonics raises more sceptics than optimists, possibly because of the impracticality and weak promise of the science governing it.[33] Nevertheless, much like Artificial Intelligence, cloning and other scientific developments which were once impracticable too, it is necessary to discuss the socio-legal issues that cryonics raises. We note here that a deep dive into the viability of cryonics as per religious and ethical jurisprudence is not within the objectives of this paper. But a broad overview of the same would certainly prove to be helpful in considering the viability of cryonics in India- a land of holy beliefs.

The idea of cryonics questions the concept of death which is a certain eventuality in almost all religions. The established beliefs that prevails in various religious teachings such as the life after death, salvation of soul, heaven and hell etc. have all been central to this debate. The Islamic medical jurisprudence does not recognize this concept, which rejects any denial of death (nafyu al-mawt) as being outside the purview of Islam. Qur'an says-

> *"Every soul will taste death, and you will only be given your [full] compensation on the Day of Resurrection."*[34]

30 *Ibid*

31 Fleming, F. (2016). *The Truth about Science and Religion from the Big Bang to Neuroscience.* Retrieved August 30, 2017, from http://www.pages.drexel.edu/~fff27/FlemingExcerpt.pdf

32 *Ibid*

33 Shemer, M. (2002). Nano Nonsense and Cryonics. *Scientific American,3*(285). Retrieved September 17, 2017, from https://www.ncbi.nlm.nih.gov/pubmed/11524966.

34 *Verse 3:185,* Qu'ran. Retrieved from https://quran.com/3/185.

As per Islam, *Allah* is the sole giver of life and death (*hifz al nafs)*[35] and revival of dead bodies is hostile to this basic idea. Further, since cryonics is a speculative science, any certainty or *yakin* (of death) is not capable of being replaced by uncertainty of cryo-suspension.[36]Notably, Christianity adopts a dualist approach to immortality with an immortal soul and a physical body, where the soul is considered as a form of body.[37] Unlike the ancient Hebrew scriptures which hailed physicalism (i.e. no life after death or immortal soul), this dualism is found in post-biblical teaching and is mostly based on Platonic philosophy.[38]However, the recent developments in cryonics and neuroscience question the function of soul by stating that man is an *informational being,* with identity established by the brain and not the soul.[39] Christianity therefore adopts a liberal approach to immortality and is concerned mostly with bodily and spiritual state. Matthew 10:8 states- *"Heal the sick, raise the dead, cleanse those who have leprosy, drive out demons. Freely you have received; freely give.*[40]

Even in Hinduism and Buddhism, the soul, being imperishable and separate from the mortal body, reincarnates upon death to another body which is related to the consciousness endowed into it until it attains salvation or *moksha.* This belief of body as a mere vessel for an immortal soul is in line with principles of cryonics.[41]

Ethical Issues and Medical Integrity

It might happen that there emerges a conflict between patient's right to self-determination and integrity of medical professionals.[42] It is a compelling state interest to protect their integrity.[43] Two of the cardinal principles of medical ethics are Patient Autonomy and Beneficence.[44] Autonomy means the right to self-determination, where the informed patient has a right to choose the manner of his treatment. Beneficence is acting in what is (or judged to be) in patient's best interest. Acting in the patient's best interest means following a course of action that is best for the patient, and is not influenced by personal convictions, motives or other considerations. It has to be noted that in case of cryonics preservation after a person his exercise right to refuse medical treatment, there is no such conflict there

35 Oseni U. A. (2009). Islamic Perspective of Cryonics: A Critical Appraisal. *Journal of Islamic Law Review* 5, 45-63.

36 *Ibid. See also,* A., Abdul Rahman, A., & Jumuah, A. (2001). *Al-Qawa'id al-Fiqhiyyah.* Saudi Arabia: Dar Ibn al-Qayyim, 272–273.

37 Murphy, Nancey (2011). Immortality versus resurrection in the Christian tradition. *New York Academy of Sciences*, 1234(1), 76-82. doi:10.1111/j.1749-6632.2011.06132.x

38 *Ibid*

39 Derek. (1990, December). Cryonics and Religion [Blog Post] Retrieved from http://alcor.org/Library/html/religionandcryonics.html

40 Matthew. (n.d.). In *New International Version*, Verse 10:8.

41 The authors' would like to state here that the above is a mere opinion based on limited knowledge and may not be the correct position.

42 Cruzan v. Mo. Dep't of Health 497 U.S. 261, 280 (1990).

43 Suresh Kumar v. Naz Foundation (2014) 1 SCC 1.

44 Aruna Ramchandra Shanbaug v. Union of India and Ors. (2011) 4 SCC 454.

is no deliberate and intentional act taken by the professional there.[45] Legislation reserves the power to make a law on active euthanasia[46] and such law for cryonics would not be in conflict with medical integrity or compelling state interest as the underline goal of cryonics is to preserve life. This is essentially similar to the goal of medical field.

Judicial Decision-making in the era of technology

In establishing legal principles governing medical science, the legislator may often be unable to anticipate and react to the uncertain developments. Owing to this incompetency, the role of courts in judicial decision-making and setting a path for the legislature to follows becomes more important than ever. This decision-making lays down a path for stability and predictability upon which societies can function seamlessly.[47]Previous trend of Indian courts in areas of *in vitro* fertilisation, euthanasia, privacy, sterilisation, artificial insemination, intellectual property etc. presents a promising picture of the future of technology in India. In rendering the landmark privacy law judgment in *Justice K.S.Puttaswamy (Retd.)*[48], the court while noting the importance of judicial decision making in the age of technology observed-

> *"The meaning of the Constitution cannot be frozen on the perspectives present when it was adopted.* ***Technological change has given rise to concerns which were not present seven decades ago and the rapid growth of technology may render obsolescent many notions of the present.*** *Hence the interpretation of the Constitution* ***must be resilient and flexible to allow future generations to adapt its content*** *bearing in mind its basic or essential features."*

Cryonic suspension raises legal issues that challenges the most basic assumptions of legal systems of today.[49] Even though that may be the case, cryonics is not an entirely novel idea, and certainly not the first to pose a judicial challenge.[50] For a common law country where courts are supposed to react and not proact[51], judiciary acts as scientific gatekeeper of technological development to ensure innovation and development is protected and preserved. In context of cryonics, more important than legal innovation is judicial innovation, with requirement of analysis and interpretation of laws that are already present to

45 Aruna Shanbaug, *Ibid.*

46 Aruna Shanbaug, *Ibid.*

47 Smith, J. P. II. (1999). Judicial Decision making in the Age of Biotechnology, *Notre Dame Journal of Law, Ethics & Public Policy* 13, 120.

48 Justice K S Puttaswamy (Retd.) and Anr. v. Union of India and Ors. Writ Petition (Civil) No. 494 of 2012.

49 Friedman, D. D. (2002). Does Technology Require New Law? *Harvard Journal of Law, & Public Policy* 25, 71

50 There have been cases where individuals have reappeared after being legally declared dead. One such case in US was Martin v. Phillips, 514 So. 2d 338, 339 (Miss. 1987), where a person declared dead in 1976 reappeared in 1983 and subsequently claimed property rights.

51 Smith, J. P. II. (1999). Judicial Decision making in the Age of Biotechnology, *Notre Dame Journal of Law, Ethics & Public Policy* 13, 120.

account for new developments. It is hoped that courts will proactively discharge their duty in shaping existing policies and laws by giving them meaning in light of medical, legal, scientific, technological and philosophical considerations.

3. Legal Issues

Essentially, every legislation must be pre-emptive of the innovation succeeding it, or at the very least, provide some scope for it. However, technology is by nature unpredictable, and hence legal issues are bound to arise. In India, there is currently no legislation which directly or indirectly addresses legal issues pertaining to cryopreservation of either human bodies or brains. That said, the jurisprudence concerning the subject is also limited and very conservative. Such conservatism is primarily a result of various ethical and religious issues concerning cryopreservation, dealt earlier in this article.[52] Nevertheless, the practice of preserving bodies have gained considerable interest in recent years, across the globe[53] and lately, in India.[54]This part discusses in detail, the current legislations dealing with cryonics and the wide gamut of legal issues concerning its practice in India.

A. Constitutional Issues in practice of suspended animation

A.1. Expanded scope of Article 21- Can it encompass Cryonics?

The Constitution of India provides a fundamental right of life to every person[55] which is in line with the mandate of International Conventions such as Universal Declaration of Human Rights[56] and UN Covenant on Civil and Political Rights.[57] In the opinion of the Supreme Court, it embodies a constitutional value of supreme importance in a democratic society as it concerns the sanctity of human life and has always strived to expand the scope of this right ever since *Maneka Gandhi* judgment.[58] Afterwards, the right has evolved as the Indian version of the American concept of "due process of law" and has become the source of many substantive rights and procedural safeguards which were not discussed in the Constitution.

Unwritten rights not mentioned in the Constitution but identified by the court are covered under substantive due process of law.[59] Justice Bhagwati, in *Maneka Gandhi v UOI* held that widest amplitude should be given to Article 21 along with giving additional protection under Article 19. Now, right to life is not merely equivalent to protection from death, or physical injury, but also includes

52 *See* Part II.C- Religious, Ethical and Judicial Decision-making.

53 O'Connell, M. (2017, February 9). 600 Miles in a Coffin-Shaped Bus, Campaning agsinst Death Itself. *The New York Times Magazine.* Retrieved from https://www.nytimes.com/2017/02/09/magazine/600-miles-in-a-coffin-shaped-bus-campaigning-against-death-itself.html?_r=0

54 Ramnath, N.S. (2010, June 9). Cryogenic Technology: The India Story. *Forbes India.* Retrieved from http://www.forbesindia.com/article/hindsight/cryogenic-technology-the-india-story/14012/1

55 § 21, Constitution of India.

56 § 6, Universal Declaration of Human Rights.

57 § 9, United Nations Covenant on Civil and Political Rights.

58 Maneka Gandhi v. Union of India 1978 AIR 597.

59 Massey. (2005). *American Constitutional Law: Powers and Liberties* (2nd ed.). Aspen Publishers.

right to lead a life with human dignity which would include all those aspects of life which would go to make a man's life meaningful and worth living.[60] As per former Chief Justice of India Hon'ble J.S.Verma, the right to live with dignity is a recognized fundamental right under Art. 21 of the Constitution of India and it is a basic human right inherent in human existence which is not a gift of any law.[61] The law merely recognized an inherent right and is not its source.

A.2. Cryonics, Euthanasia and Right to Die with Dignity

Notably, the Preamble in International Covenant as Civil and Political Rights, 1966 and International Covenant of Economic, Social and Cultural Rights, 1966 proclaims recognition of the inherent dignity.[62] The 'right to life' including the right to 'live with human dignity' would mean the existence of such a right up to the end of a natural life. This also includes the right to dignified life up to the point of death including a dignified procedure of death.[63] Right to dignity and fair treatment is not only available to a living man, but also to his dead body.[64] Though it can be contested that 'right to die' an unnatural death curtailing the natural span of life is not comparable to dying with dignity,[65] such an *arguendo* can be discussed more clearly analysed through the lens of legality of euthanasia. It is pertinent to note that passive euthanasia is permissible in India after the judgment of Aruna Ramachandra Shanbaug v. UOI.[66] Position previous to it was that right to life does not include the right to die.

The Supreme Court in *Gian Kaur v. State of Punjab*[67] held that the position of law in *P. Rathinam v. UOI*[68] which said 'right to life includes right to die' was not correct. Previous decisions had ruled that the right to life embodied in Art. 21 also embodied in it a "right not to live" a forced life, to his detriment, disadvantage or disliking, when a case exploring the relation between § 309 of IPC and Article 21 came up. Also, guidelines were prepared by the court by exercising power under Art. 142 of the Constitution till Parliament makes a law on the subject.

In *Gian Kaur* case, the Court reasoned that though right to life' is a natural right embodied in Art. 21, suicide is an unnatural termination or extinction of life and, therefore, incompatible and inconsistent with the concept of "right to life". The court ruled that S. 309, I.P.C., is not unconstitutional. By implication, § 306, I.P.C., was also been held to be constitutional. The Constitution Bench of the Supreme Court has upheld the constitutional validity of S. 309, I.P.C., in *Lokendra Singh v. State of Mahdya Pradesh.*[69]

60 P. Rathinam v. UOI (1994) 3 SCC 394.

61 Verma, J.S. (2004). *The New Universe of Human Rights*. Universal Publishing Co.

62 International Covenant as Civil and Political Rights, 1966 International Covenant of Economic, Social and Cultural Rights, 1966

63 Betts v. Brady (1942) 316 US 455.

64 De Jonge v. Oregon (1937) 299 US 353.

65 Gian Kaur v. State of Punjab 1996 AIR 946.

66 Aruna Ramchandra Shanbaug v. Union of India and Ors. (2011) 4 SCC 454.

67 Gian Kaur v. State of Punjab 1996 AIR 946.

68 P. Rathinam v. UOI (1994) 3 SCC 394.

69 Lokendra Singh v. State of Mahdya Pradesh (1996) 2 SCC 648.

The case of *Gian Kaur* is an important judgment in analysing the constitutional validity of cryonics since Supreme Court in this case explained Euthanasia and differentiated it from attempt to commit suicide, an issue which is continuously raised in practice of cryonics. In that case, the court concluded that Euthanasia is termination of life of a person who is terminally ill, or in a persistent vegetative state. In such a case, death due to termination of natural life is certain and imminent. When the process of natural death has commenced; Euthanasia only reduces the period of suffering. Euthanasia will only serve as an action to accelerate the conclusion of the process of natural death which has already begun and not as the one extinguishing life. However, the Court did not conclude on the point that whether this was covered under the concept of right to live with human dignity.

Subsequently, in the landmark *Aruna Shahbaug* judgment, the Court differentiated between Active Euthanasia & Passive Euthanasia and permitted only the latter. Passive euthanasia entails withholding of medical treatment for continuance of life *e.g.*, withholding of antibiotics where without giving it, a patient is likely to die or removing the heart-lung machine from a patient in coma. Passive euthanasia is legal without legislation provided certain conditions and safeguards are maintained. The core difference between them remained that an action was required to execute Active Euthanasia while one refrain from taking a medical action to execute Passive Euthanasia.

The decision of reanimation through cryonics would be one such decision where a person would be exercising his Right of Self-determination. This facet of Right to Privacy is inhibited in the combination of Article 19(1)(d), 19(1)(e) and 21 of the Constitution.[70] Right to privacy is a part of the right to "life" and "personal liberty" enshrined under Article 21 of the Constitution.[71] After the judgment in *Justice Puttuswamy (Retd.)*, it is now a fundamental right,[72] this facet has to stand the test of Golden Triangle of the Constitution.[73] Compelling interest of state when in conflict with right to privacy can let the invasion into privacy justified.[74]

It is also worth mentioning that the practice of cryonics is prevalent both pre-death and post-death of the individual. When it is executed before death, it is not heading towards unnatural death curtailing the natural span of life, since it is a temporary suspension or a pause owing to the fact that a person might be suffering from a disease, cure of which is not available.[75] In the judgment of Dalip Kumar Jha v. State of Punjab,[76] the Division Bench of Punjab & Haryana High Court refused to invade into the sacred territory of personal beliefs and faiths when a question of disposal of a person in samadhi came up. It went on to hold that this can be only

70 Kharak Singh v. State of MP 1963 AIR 1295.

71 People's Union of Civil Liberties v. Union of India AIR 1997 SC 568.

72 Justice K S Puttaswamy (Retd.) and Anr. V. Union of India and Ors. Writ Petition (Civil) No 494 of 2012.

73 Maneka Gandhi v. Union of India 1978 AIR 597.

74 Suresh Kumar v. Naz Foundation (2014) 1 SCC 1.

75 Minerva F., Sandberg A. (2017). Euthanasia and Cryothanasia. *Bioethics* 31, 526–533.

76 Dalip Kumar Jha v. State of Punjab AIR 2015 (NOC 562) 209.

done when there is a threat to public health, morality and order and ordered the government to examine the body to make sure that it remains preserved in a good state. Through cryonics, when the cure would be available in future, the person can resume and lead a healthy life. Body preserved through cryonics is not against compelling state interest. It is argued that this is essentially in the true spirit of Right to Life under Article 21 of the Constitution.

B. Clinical Death v. Biological Death- The legal conundrum underlying death process

Death of a person occurs when body of that person reaches such stage where it is not possible to reverse it.[77] It happens due to irreversible cessation of either functioning of the entire brain, including the brainstem; brainstem function; the capacity for consciousness; functioning of the circulatory and respiratory systems. There are basically two types of death; clinical and biological.[78] When the heart stops functioning and there is no evidence of circulation, breathing, and brain function but rescue is still possible, a person is clinically dead.[79] It is determined by the medical practitioner as per the *ordinary standards of medical practice* in each community, and the laws and customs of each state.[80] The World Medical Association is also in favour of determination of clinical death on the basis of clinical judgement supplemented by diagnostic aids instead of a precise medical definition.[81] Brain death, on the other hand, is the complete deprivation of oxygen to the brain, and is not reversible.[82] Clinical death precedes biological death. After Clinical death, pupils of the eye gets fixed and become dilated. Then tendon reflexes cease and in the absence of oxygen, Brain death immediately follows.[83] Even after a recognition of clinical death, certain biological activities occur and preservation has to be executed between this duration.[84]

Through cryonics, the practitioner would be attempting to reanimate the person from information-theoretic account of death.[85] This is a relatively new concept according to which, one is not dead as long as information encoded within one's brain is not corrupted to the point that it can never be recovered.[86] Only a pre-suspension or suspension injury which obliterates the structures encoding human memory and personality beyond recognition can cause information

77 Aruna Ramchandra Shanbaug v. Union of India and Ors. (2011) 4 SCC 454.

78 George P. Smith, II. (1996). Pathways to Immortality in the New Millennium: Human Responsibility, Theological Direction, or Legal Mandate. *St. Louis University. Public Law Review*, 15, 447.

79 Donaldson v. Lungran, 4 Cal Rptr. 2d. 59 (Cal. Ct. App. 1992)

80 Perlin, A. A. (2007). "To Die In Order To Live": The Need for Legislation Governing Post-Mortem Cryonic Suspension. *SW. U. L. REV.* 33, 37.

81 *Ibid*

82 Korein, J. (1979). Brain Death: Interrelated Medical and Social Issues.

83 K. Schuyter. (1968). The New Biology and the Rule Against Perpetuities. *U.C.L.A. L. Rev.* 15, 420.

84 Ettinger. (1968). Cryonic Suspension and the Law. *U.C.L.A. L. Rev. 15*, 414.

85 Eberl, J. T. (2008). Potentiality, possibility, and the irreversibility of death. *The Review of Metaphysics* 61–77.

86 Moen, O. M. (2015). The case for cryonics. *Journal of medical ethics* 41(8), 677–681.

theoretic death. Our consciousness is made up of physical structures like the rest of the body due to which the mind and memories can be restored just like other body parts after the body is thawed.

The scientific evidence of cryonics is indeed promising. In certain cases of mammals such as cats, which were neuro-preserved, frozen brains did show electrical activity upon being thawed.[87] Also, LTP persists in tissue slices,[88] and that nematode worms retain long-term memories after revival[89] is evidence that significant information remains upon reanimation. In fact, a non-mammal has already been reanimated through cryogenics and all this heads toward a positive sign that cryonics can yield good results for humans as well.[90]

C. Current Legislations affecting cryonics in India

1. Transplantation of Human Organs Act, 1994

In 1994, with the object of streamlining the organ transplantation procedure and prohibit unlawful trade, the Parliament enacted the Transplantation of Human Organs Act, 1994 ("THOA")[91]. The Act was further amended in 2011 with significant changes, based on the report submitted by THOA Review Committee constituted as a result of the renowned 2004 judgment in *Balbir Singh*[92]case. It is the foremost law affecting cryonics, albeit to a very limited extent. While the purpose of the Act as derived from its preamble is the 'regulation of removal, storage and transplantation of human organs and tissues for therapeutic purposes'[93], it does not include within its ambit anatomical donations (whole body donations) essential for the practice of cryopreservation. However, since cryonics also permits neuro-preservation[94], analysing THOA for the purpose of cryo-suspension of brain becomes essential.

THOA provides crucial insight into laws pertaining to death of an individual[95], a fundamental issue in the cryonics process. It defines a 'deceased person' in a rather interesting and vague manner, meaning an individual in whom all evidence

87 Suda, I., Kito, K., & Adachi, C. (1966). Viability of long term frozen cat brain. *Vitro. Nature* 212, 268–270.

88 Fahy, G. M., Guan, N. & de Graaf, I. A., Tan, Y., Griffin, L., & Groothuis, G. M. (2013). Cryopreservation of precision-cut tissue slices. *Xenobiotica* 43(1), 113–132.

89 Vita-More, N., & Barranco, D. (2015). Persistence of long-term memory in vitrified and revived caenorhabditis elegans. *Rejuvenation Research* 18(5), 458–463.

90 Darwin, M. (2011). *Does personal identity survive cryopreservation?* Retrieved from http://chronopause.com/chronopause.com/index.php/2011/02/23/does-personal-identity-survive-cryopreservation/

91 Transplantation of Human Organs Act, 1994, Act of Parliament, No.42 of 1994.

92 Balbir Singh Vs. The Authorisation Committee and Ors. AIR 2004 Delhi 413.

93 Statement of Objects and Reasons, Transplantation of Human Organs Act, 1994, Act of Parliament, No.42 of 1994.

94 Neuropreservation is preservation of the brain of a cryonics patient by the best means possible. *See* Neuropreservation FAQs, Alcor Life Extension Foundation, http://alcor.org/Library/html/neuropreservationfaq.html. For more discussion on this topic, refer Part I- Process of Cryopreservation.

95 This issue has been dealt in detail in II.B. *See* Part II.B- Clinical Death v. Biological Death.

of life has disappeared at any time after live birth occurs.[96] It also recognizes brain stem death and cardio-pulmonary failures[97], without specifically defining what would constitute a conclusive proof of death. The Act makes certification of death necessary for removal of organs or tissues in cases of brain stem death, and prescribes a board of medical experts for certification procedures.[98]Since healthcare is a subject matter of State list, THOA has been passed by a majority of Indian states, with exception of only two states, those being Andhra Pradesh and Jammu and Kashmir.[99]

Both the THOA and the subsequent Amending Act of 2011 make it very difficult for a foreign national to receive organ/ tissue donations, subject to prior approval of Authorisation Committee.[100] This is important considering the fact that currently there does not exist any cryopreservation centres within India that can sufficiently perform suspension process.[101] To make matters worse, for removal of organs/tissues from the body of the donor before his death, such donor must be a near relative[102] of the recipient.[103] If, however, the donor has expressed his desire for removal of organs for transplantation into the recipient not being a 'near relative', it is subject to the approval of Authorisation Committee, as established by Central/ State Governments from time to time.[104] Given the time sensitive nature of cryonic processes[105], it is argued that seeking approval of Authorisation Committee is both totally undesirable and unfeasible. Further, considering the narrow definition of the term 'recipient' in THOA[106], it is sufficiently clear that institutions preserving bodies for cryonic procedures cannot be considered as donees for the purpose of the Act.

96 §2 (e), Transplantation of Human Organs Act, 1994, Act of Parliament, No.42 of 1994. (Hereinafter, "THOA")

97 *Ibid.*

98 The format for brain-death certification is given in Form 8 of the THO Act, 1994. Furthermore, as per § 3(6), the board of medical experts consists of registered medical practitioner in charge of hospital, an independent specialist appointed by such registered practitioner, a neurologist/neurosurgeon or even a surgeon/physician/ anesthetic and the registered practitioner treating the patient.

99 Awadhoot, S. (2017, April 3). Practical, legal Issues with brain death situation in India vis-à-vis Transplantation of Organs Act [Blog Post]. Retrieved from https://counterview.org/2017/04/03/practical-legal-Issues-with-brain-death-situation-in-india-vis-a-vis-transplantation-of-organs-act/#_ftn7

100 §9(1-A), THOA Act, 1994.

101 Weaver, C. (2015, December 15). Inside the weird world of cryonics. *The Financial Times.* Retrieved from https://www.ft.com/content/d634e198-a435-11e5-873f-68411a84f346

102 The Act defines a near relative under § 2(i) to include spouse, son, daughter, father, mother, brother, sister, grandfather, grandmother, grandson or granddaughter.

103 § 9, THOA Act.

104 § 9(3), THOA Act.

105 Alcor Procedures. (n.d.) Retrieved from http://alcor.org/procedures.html

106 § 2 (m) defines a 'recipient' as a person into any human organ or tissue is proposed to be transplanted.

2. Anatomy Act, 1949

As discussed above, THOA restricts the scope of donation to human organs and tissues.[107] For purpose of full-body cryopreservation, since donation of entire human body is not covered under the THOA[108], one has to look into Anatomy Act of 1949 to determine whether whole body donation can be done for cryonic processes. Anatomy Act specifies that any person can direct his body to be donated for anatomical purposes, unless any relative of the deceased requires the body to be disposed off otherwise.[109] Generally, anatomical purposes include 'teaching, studying, or researching into, the gross structure of the human body.[110] An anatomical examination can only be carried out at an authorized school of anatomy as specified as per § 3 of the Act.[111] The Act remains silent on whether a Cryonics Institute falls within the definition of authorized school of anatomy. Arguably, there is little scope for such institutes to fall within the definition, as anatomical purposes are generally associated with medical examination or research and not preservation/procurement of bodies.[112] Furthermore, by virtue of § 9 of the Act, the preference of the deceased is not considered binding on relatives, even though it may have been given through testamentary disposition. As unfortunate as it may be, it leaves the donors without *any* protection under law, especially in India where the family there is high chance the family might be influenced by religious considerations.

3. Indian Penal Code, 1860 ("IPC") and Code of Criminal Procedure, 1973 ("CrPC")

While criminal legislations in India hardly deal with cryonics, in considering a potential struggle between individual rights to cryonic preservation and vested state rights in public interest, it is necessary to discuss the current position of law[113]. One such issue pertains to right of the State to order an examination of victims' body (post-mortem or autopsy) under §174 and §176 of Code of Criminal Procedure to determine the cause of death during the purpose of investigation.[114] An

107 The Report of Transplant of Human Organs Act Review Committee Directorate General of Health Services Ministry of Health & Family Welfare. Retrieved from http://www.prsindia.org/uploads/media/Organ%20transplantation/The%20Report%20of%20the%20transplantation%20of%20human%20organs%20act%20review%20committee.pdf

108 It is essential to note that in contrast to entire bodies, cryopreservation of human brain is also possible, which will be governed by THOA itself and not Anatomy Act, 1949. This is because a negative interpretation of organ' or 'tissue' to include donation of the entire human body is not possible due to restricted scope of the act.

109 § 9, Anatomy Act, 1949.

110 Acceptance of donor consent for anatomical examination (n.d.). Retrieved from https://www.hta.gov.uk/policies/acceptance-donor-consent-anatomical-examination

111 § 3 of Anatomy Act, 1949 states that- The Minister may from time to time authorize the establishment of schools of anatomy where the study and practice of anatomy may be carried out.

112 Legal Protection of Cryonic Patients: Part I. (2012, February 23). Retrieved October 01, 2017, from http://www.evidencebasedcryonics.org/2012/02/23/legal-protection-of-cryonics-patients-part-1/

113 Issues pertaining to Criminal Law are discussed in detail in Part II.E- Issues under Criminal Law.

114 § 174 & § 176 Code of Criminal Procedure, 1973. Such a demand for post-mortem can be made only through a police officer/magistrate/court.

autopsy is generally defined as a detailed external examination of one's body and frequently involves dissection of internal organs.[115]In circumstances where 'post-mortem' is ordered for a patient who wishes his body to be cryo-preserved, the body of patient is required to be intact meaning post-mortem essentially destroys *any* possibility of cryonic preservation. Could the patient then plead violation of fundamental right to reanimation of his body after death under Article 21? Unlike United States which allows objections to post mortem on certain grounds[116], India does not recognize any such right to object autopsies under any law. Hence, even though individuals have a right to preserve their bodies, such right is limited by considerations of state interest and public welfare.

D. Issues under Property Laws

In India, property laws are mainly governed by personal laws of the citizens. The significance of a discussion on cryonics and property rights is crucial since the practice of suspended animation raises interesting questions on estate of the cryo-suspended being, the right to his bodily property for purpose of maintenance during *deep freeze*, ownership of property after revival etc. Essentially, the article discusses property rights in two key aspects- (i) right to property in dead corpse and (ii) ownership of estate of suspended being.

D.1. Right to property in dead corpses- Do the dead have rights?

The question whether a property right in a dead corpse exists with a person wanting his property to be cryogenically preserved is central in the long-held debate on the legality of cryonics. Historically, the view of the courts as stipulated in *Williams v Williams*[117]was that an individual does not have a right to dispose of his body after the death. This view has now been overruled by courts. Today, the right to donate individual organs/tissues is legal and covered under THOA.[118] In fact, the unrestricted right to one's own body is so embedded that it is now an inherent right[119], except in certain cases where there exists conflict with state interest in its exercise. Thus, though an individual can dispose of the body post-death in a manner he/she desires[120], it is not clear whether the disposed body can be owned as 'property' for cryonic purposes. One reason for this is that in the

115 Ayoub, T. & Chow, J. (2008). The conventional autopsy in modern medicine. *Journal of the Royal Society of Medicine, 101*(4). Retrieved from https://www.ncbi.nlm.nih.gov/pmc/articles/PMC2312379/

116 The Uniform Anatomical Gift Act of 1987 in five states of USA (California, New York, New Jersey, Ohio and Rhode Island) recognize the right to religious exception to post mortem. *See* N.J. STAT. ANN. § 52:17B-88.2 (West 2001); N.Y. PUB. HEALTH § 4210-c (McKinney 2002); OHIO REV. CODE ANN. § 313.131(B), N.J. STAT. ANN. § 52:17B-88.1(b).

117 Williams v Williams (1882) 20 CH. D. 659.c.

118 Mujeeb Bhai v. State of U.P. and Ors. Civil Misc. Writ Petition No.38985 of 2004.

119 The fundamental right to one's body during his lifetime has been recognized the world over. *See*, Moore v. Regents of Cal., 793 P.2d 479, 505 (Cal. 1990).

120 In cases where the property has not been disposed in a particular manner, the family of the deceased has the right to do so.

eyes of law, the rights can only be vested in a 'person' and not dead corpses[121], irrespective of the fact that such person is living or artificial.[122]

Could a dead corpse then be included within the definition of 'person'? It seems that in protecting the right to life and human dignity under Article 21, courts have adopted an eclectic approach in granting a limited right to respectful treatment of dead corpse after death.[123]Notably, SC have been very restrictive in interpreting rights of dead person, extending such rights only in cases where undignified treatment of dead corpses is required to be prevented.[124]However, such rights relating to burial or undignified treatment are seemingly insufficient for purpose of cryonics, since (i) the dead corpse is required to be stored by the cryonics institute and (ii) decisions regarding preservation, care, maintenance and even reanimation has to be taken by somebody.[125]Thus, in circumstance where obligations listed above are to be exercised, can the cryonics institute or any other person claim ownership of such corpse?

In India, a dead corpse is not a property of any person, except for religious[126] and burial reasons where the property can be claimed by the next of kin. This *quasi property* approach of dead corpses is in line with United States which recognizes *some* right in dead person with the executor of the deceased.[127] Acknowledging the legal conundrum as it exists, it can only be opined that in absence of a settled law, one can only hope for courts to recognize legal successor's property rights in deceased body. Doing so would be consistent with THOA where organs may be donated by the lawful possessor of body if no objection has been made by deceased during his lifetime.[128] Alternatively, merely recognizing the dead corpse as a property itself would enable deceased to transfer his body akin to testamentary disposition of any other estate, enabling the person to execute his desire to be cryo-preserved. In this regard, it is also essential to make necessary amendments in THOA/Anatomy Act, as has been discussed before, to allow institutes preserving bodies cryonically to obtain ownership of such corpses.

D.2. Ownership of Estate of Suspended individuals

The devolution of property of a deceased in India is mainly governed by Indian

121 Under § 3(42) of General Clauses Act, a person has been defined to include any company or association or body of individuals, whether incorporated or not

122 Salmond, J.W. (1920). *Jurisprudence* (4th ed.) London: Sweet and Maxwell.

123 Ram Sharan Autyanuprasi v. Union of India (AIR 1989 SC 549), PL Parmanand Katara v. Union of India, (1995 (3) SCC 248), S. Sethu Raja v. The Chief Secretary, Government of Tamil Nadu and others W.P.(MD)No.3888 of 2007, Ramji Singh alias Mujeeb Bhai v. State of U.P. and others. Civil Misc. Writ Petition No.38985 of 2004.

124 Such cases involve necrophilia, damage or misuse of corpses etc, http://jurip.org/wp-content/uploads/2017/03/Kritanjali-Sarda.pdf

125 Ugaz, A., Floyd, J., & Wahlen, H. (2016). Freeze a Jolly Good Fellow: Cryonauts and the Law. *Journal of Law and Social Deviance,11*, 54-204.

126 Dilip Kumar Jha v State of Punjab AIR 2015 (NOC 562) 209

127 Ritter v. Couch, 76 S.E. 428, 430 (W. Va. 1912).

128 § 3 (3), THOA.

Succession Act, 1930 ("ISA") when it is a case of testamentary succession[129]. In cases where individual dies intestate (without will[130]), the personal laws would govern succession i.e. when the deceased is a Hindu, Buddhist, Sikh or Jaina, Hindu Succession Act, 1956 ("HSA") would apply[131] and when he is a Mohammedan, the deceased would be governed by customary law of Islam i.e. Sharia law[132]. Further, when a marriage is solemnized under Special Marriage Act, 1954 or in case of intestate succession by persons other than Hindus or Muslims, the testamentary succession is governed by ISA irrespective of the religion of the deceased.[133] For the sake of this article, only devolution of property by way of testamentary succession is considered.

Normally, when an individual dispose off property by way of will, the property vests in his legal successor/heir after his death. Assuming that the individual who has been preserved cryo-genically is successfully reanimated in future, can he reclaim *his* property already devolved? It would seem that there is little scope in this argument- since the legal title of the property has already been passed, no claim to property could vest in such person, much akin to grant of gifts or donations. Fortunately, there are ways through which an individual can govern the rules of disposition of his estate to himself. One of such methods is establishments of private trusts.

The Indian Trust Act, 1882 ("ITA") deals with *inter vivos* establishment of private trusts in India.[134] A private trust must fulfil certain conditions, those being certainty[135], lawfulness[136] and in favour of beneficiaries[137]. Under the ITA, an individual (author) can establish a private trust in favour of the cryonic institute (beneficiary) before his death, who can also act as trustee of the property. Though a deceased person can neither be a trustee nor a beneficiary[138], he can enter into an agreement with cryonic institute for re-transfer of property on reanimation in future. However, one of the foremost considerations in establishment of private trusts is that it should not be perpetual in nature[139], except in cases of charitable

129 § 30, Hindu Succession Act, 1956.

130 § 3(1)(g), Hindu Succession Act, 1956- "intestate"-a person is deemed to die intestate in respect of property of which he or she has not made a testamentary disposition capable of taking effect

131 § 2, Hindu Succession Act, 1956.

132 § 2, The Muslim Personal Law (Sharia) Application Act, Act 26 of 1937, Laws of Parliament, 1937.

133 § 21, Special Marriage Act, 1954, LCI 110th report

134 § 1, Indian Trust Act, 1882. ("ITA") Trusts can also be of public nature, which are mainly governed by Charitable and Religious Trusts Act, 1920. If the private trust us created through will, it will be governed by Indian Succession Act, 1930.

135 § 6, Indian Trust Act, 1882.

136 § 4, ITA, 1882.

137 § 9, ITA, 1882 - Who may be beneficiary- Every person capable of holding property may be a beneficiary.

138 § 9, 10 of ITA, 1882- the trustee or beneficiary must be capable of holding property.

139 § 14 of Transfer of Property Act, 1882. **("TOPA")** "The general rule against perpetuities is also applicable in Trust Act". *See* Income-Tax Officer vs Wanson (India) Ltd. 1983 5 ITD 102 Pune.

trusts[140], irrespective of whether made by will or *inter vivos.*[141]The *rule against perpetuities* says that any person must not endeavour to restrain free alienation of property by its possessor beyond the life in being and for a time unreasonably great with respect of public interest.[142]Broadly, an individual can address this in two ways- (i) he can establish a trust for a certain definite period with hope of revival in that period and (ii) he can institute a personal revival trust (PRT)[143].

It must be noted that in the first instance, the period of perpetuity must not exceed twenty-one years, being the time limit for rule against perpetuity under common law system.[144] It is argued that the rule of perpetuity has been sparingly used by courts and it must be left to the court to determine whether this period can be extended beyond the time limit or not. The other alternative, i.e. a PRT is a type of trust specifically formed to hold assets until the person is revived from cryonic preservation.[145]

While creating trust for a maximum period of twenty-one years seems not enough given the current state of technology[146] and establishment of PRT in India might be considered by courts as violative of rule against perpetuity, there might also be *third* alternative, which entitles cryo-enthusiasts to hold title in trust property until revival. Since Indian courts have consistently held that for the purpose of § 9 of Trust Act, an unborn/conceived person can also be a beneficiary[147],it follows that cryogenically preserved beings not yet been revived are also eligible as beneficiaries.[148] While proponents of this theory have undertaken the view that it may be possible to convince the courts that the same reasoning applies to persons in suspended state[149] (namely that the suspended person is only an 'interim being' not classified as a either 'person' or 'property' because of their potential for human life[150]) as is applicable to conceived child, it is debatable whether Indian courts would accept it. This is due to the fact that under Indian Trust Act, both beneficiary

---

140 § 17, TOPA, 1882. *Se,* Re Bowen [1893] 2 Ch. 491: 62 L.J. Ch. 681

141 *Ibid*

142 Ganendra Mohan Tagore vs. Upendra Mohan Tagore and Ors 4 B.L.R. 1059.

143 Levenberg, I. (2009). Personal Revival Trusts: If You Can't Take It with You, Can You Come Back to Get It. *St. John's Law Review*. 83, 1469, 1500.

144 Derived from English Law in the case of Cooper v. Laroche (1881) 17 Ch. D. 368, the rule against perpetuity is equally applicable in Indian law, *See* Jamshedji Cursetjee Tarachand vs. Soonabai and Ors.1 Ind Cas 834.

145 Levenberg, I. (2009). Personal Revival Trusts: If You Can't Take It with You, Can You Come Back to Get It. *St. John's Law Review*.83, 1469, 1500.

146 Devlin, H. (2016, November 16). Cryonics: does it offer humanity a chance to return from the dead?. *The Guardian.* Retrieved from https://www.theguardian.com/science/2016/nov/18/cryogenics-does-it-offer-humanity-a-chance-to-return-from-the-dead.

147 CIT v. Ram Krishna Gupta [1979] 117 ITR 218.

148 Levenberg, I. (2009). Personal Revival Trusts: If You Can't Take It with You, Can You Come Back to Get It. *St. John's Law Review*. 83, 1469, 1500.

149 *Ibid*

150 David v David 842 S.W.2d 588 (Tenn. 1992),

and trust must be capable of being ascertained.[151] As against conceived child where there is reasonable guarantee of being born, there is no guarantee that a suspended person will ever be reanimated in future (and therefore *also* violative of rule against perpetuity). Nevertheless, changing technologies may as well be a motivating factor for courts to adopt an approach consistent with principles listed above.

E. Issues under Criminal Laws

The central premise of cryonics is to preserve the 'patient' to revive him in future, when the technology makes it possible to undergo reanimation.[152] More interestingly, cryopreservation of brain (called as neuropreservation) is based on the idea that an individual might be reanimated in future by either fitting the brain in some other body or even uploading it in a machine. This has remained no longer the classical sci-fi stuff seen in movies and novels, with ventures such as *Neuralink* already being backed and explored by entrepreneurs.[153] However, it also raises intriguing questions of identity and criminal liability of these animated beings or *cyborgs,* which is essential to this article.

E.1. Identity

Assuming that cryonics is a successful science in future, establishing any connection between the future individual and present individual is a pure challenge to not only law but also the society. Could the future individual bind the past individual? Or could the liability of past individual carry forward to future individual? Does he retain his identity or should he be allowed to live independent of his past?

Two theories exist which shed light on such a possibility. One, where identity is determined by virtue of persisting body and second, where psychological accounts are considered.[154] Although both these theories present their own variations and conclusions in the identity debate, proponents of psychological theory have vehemently put forth the idea that the identity is a product of one's mind and no body.[155] A possible consequence of psychological theory would be that a successful cyron maintains his identity, since the objective of cryonics is to keep neurons intact, which are subsequently responsible for memories, personality and thoughts.[156] However, it is worth noting that there are contrary views which reject psychological theory on the ground that a mind cannot be considered *separate* from body and hence, a reanimated individual without his physical aspect would constitute a new identity.[157]

151 § 6, ITA 1882.

152 *See,* Part I-Process of Cryonics.

153 Ernst, D. (2017, March 28). Cyborg future: Elon Musk's Neuralink Corp. seeks to merge humans and machines. *Washinghton Times*. Retrieved October 13, 2017, from https://www.washingtontimes.com/news/2017/mar/28/elon-musks-neuralink-corp-seeks-to-merge-humans-an/

154 Huxtable, R. (2017). Cryonics in the Courtroom: Which Interests? Whose Interests? *Medical Law Review*, 045. doi:10.1093/medlaw/fwx045.

155 Sinnott-Armstrong, W. & Behnke, S. (2001). Criminal Law and Multiple Personality Disorder: The Vexing Problems of Personhood and Responsibility, *CAL. INTERDISC. L.J.*, 277, 284-85.

156 Moen, O.M. (2015). The Case for Cryonics. *J Med Ethics*. doi:10.1136/medethics-2015-102715, 2

157 Fox, M. & Stein, A. (2015). Dualism and Doctrine, *Indiana L.J.*, 90, 975, 982.

Moving further, one could also argue the classic case of Phineas Gage, who miraculously survived a tragic accident after a three feet iron spike passed through his skull and resulted in a complete changeover of his personality after accident.[158] Would the new Gage be regarded as having the same legal personality? Much akin to an individual who is presumed dead under § 108 of Evidence Act is regarded as a same personality after he re-appears, it might seem that instances like those of Gage when extended to current identity dilemma would produce similar results. Perhaps identification techniques like Turing Test[159] would prove to be beneficial in this regard. However, in case of significant alterations in personality, a separate legal personality is also possible.[160]

E.2. Criminal Liability

If cryonic suspension is merely considered as a mechanism which *pauses* instead of restoring a user from death[161], the criminal liability will remain associated with the identity of the individual. Hence, such an individual will be absolutely responsible for his past actions. However, the same cannot be said for a person shifting identities or those who have undergone substantial alteration, as punishing them would be punishing a person having no association with the former identity.[162] Looking at it from another direction, the reanimated individual having shifted bodies, through neuropreservation or otherwise may raise a defence that though he had *mens rea* for a past act, there was no *actus reus* and hence no liability would arise. Indeed, issues relating to intent, identity, motive, capacity etc. under criminal law would pose complex challenges for legislature and judiciary.

F. Issues under Insurance Laws

One of the most interesting implications of cryonics lies in the area of insurance laws. Broadly, insurance laws in India is spearheaded by Insurance Act of 1938 combined with other legislations such as Life Insurance Corporation of India Act (LIC), Insurance Regulatory and Development Authority Act (IRDA), Marine Insurance Act (MI), etc. along with Indian Contract Act, 1872 (ICA) which acts as a general law governing insurance contracts. Since the cost of cryonics is extremely expensive[163], at least for now, special life insurance policies have been devised to

---

158 Hamilton, J. (2017, May 21). Why Brain Scientists Are Still Obsessed with the Curious Case of Phineas Gage. Retrieved from https://www.npr.org/sections/health-shots/2017/05/21/528966102/why-brain-scientists-are-still-obsessed-with-the-curious-case-of-phineas-gage.

159 Turing, A.M. *Computing Machinery and Intelligence, in* COMKruERS AND THOUGHT 11 (Edward A. Feigenbaum & Julian Feldman eds., 1963). Turing Test is used in determining identity under Artificial Intelligence. It states that in a conversation between a natural person with a computer and another human, if no reliable difference can be made between them, the computer is a person.

160 Ugaz, A., Floyd, J., & Wahlen, H. (2016). Freeze a Jolly Good Fellow: Cryonauts and the Law. *Journal of Law and Social Deviance, 11*, 54-204.

161 Shaw, D. (2009). Cryoethics: Seeking Life After Death. *Bioethics*, 23, 515, 521.

162 *Supra* note at 159.

163 The minimum fee of cryo-suspension is not less than two lacs, with additional costs for neurosuspension being 35-40 lacs and whole-body preservation crossing over one crore. The costs may vary with additional facilities. https://www.theguardian.com/money/2013/sep/20/cryonics-death-insurance-policies.

enable individuals to bear the costs. In this section, we discuss certain consequences that cryonics could have on Insurance laws-

F.1. Death and Legal Claims in Life Insurance

As stated earlier, there are two types of death- (i) clinical i.e. brain stem death and (ii) biological i.e. natural death.[164] After the amendment in THOA, India recognizes brain stem death as a form of death, in line with the UK Approach.[165] This is however subject to necessary approvals by certifying authorities without which no declaration of death can be made.[166]In the context of life insurance contractually agreed between the individual and insurance company, recognition of brain stem death is a major development, especially in cases where accidental deaths leave the victim in a comatose condition. However, certification of brain stem death is often a strenuous procedure and could pose difficulties in insurance claims. It is therefore recommended that terms stating brain stem death and corresponding circumstances be clearly identified in the insurance contract itself.

Furthermore, in circumstances where an individual wishes his body to be cryo-genically preserved before his death, insurance companies can refuse coverage on the ground of assisted suicide. These scenarios are highly prevalent in euthanasia-specific cases where individuals exercising their right to die have been denied insurance coverage.[167]In India, passive euthanasia is legal by virtue of landmark ruling in *Aruna Shanbaug* case.[168] However, there does not exist any right to die[169], which poses an apparent contradiction in law. Only in cases of permanent vegetative state or terminal illness can a patient be allowed to withhold any medical treatment.[170]

Interestingly, a recent debate on legality of Advanced Medical Directives (AMD), more commonly 'living wills' seems relevant to this issue.[171] Under the proposed Medical Treatment of Terminally Ill Patients (Protection of Patients and Medical Practitioners) Bill ("Passive Euthanasia Bill"), an advanced medical

164 See Part III.B-Clinical Death v. Biological Death.

165 Dhanwate, A.D. (2014). Brainstem death: A comprehensive review in Indian perspective. *Indian Journal of Critical Care Medicine,* 18(9), 596–605. Retrieved from https://www.ncbi.nlm.nih.gov/pmc/articles/PMC4166875/

166 For example, Maharashtra has made it mandatory to certify brain death. *See,* Government of Maharashtra, Public Health Department, Government Resolution No. MAP2012/C.R.289/AROGYA 6. Mumbai: Mantralaya. [2012 Sep 13].

167 Richardson, B. (2016, October 20). Assisted-suicide law prompts insurance company to deny coverage to terminally ill California woman. *The Washington Times.* Retrieved from https://www.washingtontimes.com/news/2016/oct/20/assisted-suicide-law-prompts-insurance-company-den/

168 Aruna Ramchandra Shanbaug v. Union of India and Ors. (2011) 4 SCC 454.

169 Gian Kaur vs The State of Punjab 1996 SCC (2) 648.

170 Aruna Ramchandra Shanbaug v. Union of India and Ors. (2011) 4 SCC 454.

171 Staff, F.P. (2017, October 11). What is living will? Supreme Court says 'complex concept', to decide whether people can demand passive euthanasia. *The First Post.* Retrived from http://www.firstpost.com/india/what-is-living-will-supreme-court-says-complex-concept-to-decide-whether-people-can-demand-passive-euthanasia-4131315.html.

directive is defined as "a directive given by the person that he/she hall not be given medical treatment in future when he or she becomes terminally ill.[172] The bill seeks to declare living wills as void and not binding on the medical practitioners.[173] However, courts seem skeptical in declaring living wills as illegal, with a recent constitutional bench ruling on October 10, 2017 opining for 'guidelines for drafting living wills and authenticating them'.[174] The issue that arise here is whether a declaration by an individual in a living will to preserve body for suspension during the period of insurance could enable insurance companies to exclude liability on the grounds that such an act would constitute suicide? Notably in US, a protection from insurance policy avoidance to patients using AMDs is provided and withholding/withdrawal of life sustaining procedures in accordance with law is excluded from the ambit of suicide.[175] However, no such legal protection exists in India and a life insurer could possibly deny claim under suicide clause. The legislature must therefore account for such circumstances. Declaring 'right to die' outside the ambit of suicide for the purpose of insurance laws would be a positive step in this direction.

G. Cryonics and Euthanasia: Is cryonics within the meaning of assisted suicide?

The core difference between Euthanasia and Cryothanasia lies in the end result of these process. While through Euthanasia, the life of a person suffering from unbearable and incurable disease is ended to prevent suffering in future. Cryothanasia is practised to pause the span of life of a person suffering from incurable disease so that he is able to resume a healthy life after the cure of disease is found. There is an element of euthanasia in cryonics but since the intention of practice to health and life, goals of euthanasia and cryonics are contrary to each other.[176] Chances of success are great if the patient is cryo-thanized before the disease results in substantial deterioration of health. Cryopreservation brings an advantage against euthanasia as the factor of death which is a reason for opposition of euthanasia by the law is eliminated.[177] Even if the person is not able to achieve the health status he had before the incurable disease, reduction in certainty of death is certainly an improvement.[178] Administration of palliative care in case of terminal illness is also prescribed instead of permitting euthanasia. In case of cryothanasia, the possibility of such care is not eliminated but kept on hold.

172 § 2(1) of the Medical Treatment of Terminally Ill Patients (Protection of Patients and Medical Practitioners) Bill available at http://www.prsindia.org/uploads/media/draft/Draft%20Passive%20Euthanansia%20Bill.pdf

173 § 11, Medical Treatment of Terminally Ill Patients (Protection of Patients and Medical Practitioners) Bill

174 http://www.thehindu.com/opinion/editorial/the-will-to-die/article19840981.ece

175 ALA. CODE § 22-8A-9(a) (Supp. 1982).

176 Shaw, D. (2009). Cryoethics: Seeking Life After Death. *Bioethics*, 23, 515, 521.

177 Moen, O. M. (2015). The case for cryonics. *Journal of medical ethics* 41(8), 677–681.

178 Ord, T., Hillerbrand, R. & Sandberg, A. (2010). Probing the improbable: methodological challenges for risks with low probabilities and high stakes. *Journal of Risk Research* 13(2), 191–205.

In India, Euthanasia is permissible but only in passive form. There is a reduction of suffering of a person who might have suffer longer if the meaningless treatment would have continued. This is still disadvantageous from the viewpoint of cryonics because suffering can be eliminated in the first place before the disease deteriorates the body to such an extent where it reaches to a permanent vegetative state. Today, the patient may choose to end or continue lifespan as per the option provided by the medical science and law, her eventual state is in many ways more open than dying conventionally.[179]

4. International Practices Concerning Cryonics

There is no legislation in the world that has provisions to govern the practice of Cryonics.[180] The first suspension for Cryonics took place in the United States. Though they are yet to reanimate any human, the Courts across USA have acknowledged patient's right to refuse medical treatment[181] and right to privacy and self-determination.[182] Some states even permitted right to assistance for the purpose of committing suicide.[183] The States which refused to provide such rights acknowledged that there remained a conflict between privacy rights and competing state interests in preserving life, preventing suicide and maintaining medical integrity. Priority was given to competing state interest and accordingly, physician-assisted suicide was prohibited.[184]

In 1988, Dr Thomas K. Donaldson was diagnosed with an astrocytoma, a malignant brain tumour with poor long-term prognosis. He made arrangements that his body gets preserved before a large of his brain gets damaged diminishing chances of future revival of healthy life. In 1990, he sued the Attorney General of the State of California for the right to a pre-mortem cryopreservation, so as to improve his chances of a complete preservation.[185] The court found Donaldson had no constitutional right to an assisted death, and he lost the case.[186] He got cryosuspended when cancer went into remission in year 2006.

But subsequent to this case, a court in Montana delivered a judgment in favour of interests of the individual against the interest of the state and found that right to die exists in Constitution. Oregon and Washington established the right to assisted suicide through state statute.[187] Oregon passed the Death with

179 Glover, J. (1990). Causing death and saving lives: The moral problems of abortion, infanticide, suicide, euthanasia, capital punishment, war and other life or death choices. United Kingdom. Penguin.

180 Perlin A. (2007). To Die In Order To Live: The Need for Legislation Governing Post- Mortem Cryonic Suspension. *SW. U. L. REV.* 36, 33.

181 Cruzan v. Director, Missouri Dept. Health 497 U.S. 261 (1990).

182 *Griswold v. Connecticut* 381 U.S. 479 (1965); *Roe v. Wade* 410 U.S. 113 (1973).

183 Oregon Death with Dignity Act, (2009); Washington Death with Dignity Act, WASH. (2010).

184 *Washington v. Glucksberg* 521 U.S. 702 (1997).

185 Pommer, R. W. (1993). The Thomas Donaldson Case. *Journal for Contemporary Health Law and Policy,* Spring; 9:589.

186 Donaldson v. Lungren 4 Cal. Rptr. 2d 59, 60 (Cal. Ct. App. 1992).

187 Oregon Death with Dignity Act, 1997.

Dignity Act in 1997. In the US, many courts have held that there is a distinction between the right to refuse medical treatment and a right to assisted suicide.[188] The prevailing argument supporting this distinction is that the former is passive, and the latter is an affirmative act to hasten death.[189] But it is pertinent to note that practitioners in the US view cryonics as a process to temporary pause the cellular activities through preservation[190] and not a process to attain death which is permanent cessation of life.[191] Also, the process is not in conflict with the ethical duties of physicians as and this view is developing after the Cruzan judgment.[192]

In the UK, a High Court granted a 14-year-old girl's request to have her body cryogenically frozen upon her untimely death.[193] However, this does not mean that court or law approved the practise of cryonics in the UK. The judgment was taken in light of decay of girl's body from cancer which was incurable at that point of time. Since, the girl was a minor, the mother was given the sole power to make arrangements for the disposal of the body by the court. If the girl was an adult, she could have made a will appointing her mother her executor. The judge concluded by remarking that the case might suggest "the need for proper regulation of cryonic preservation in this country if it is to happen in future".[194] Previous to this, in Airedale NHS Trust v. Bland,[195] the House of Lords unanimously permitted a person in charge a patient in permanent vegetative state to stop his medical treatment so that his suffering can end.

In New Zealand, Human Tissue Act 2008 makes no reference to cryonics.[196] There is no statute or case law on cryonics in New Zealand. As per the provisions of the Burial and Cremation Act 1964, a person having charge of a dead body has to make arrangements for its disposal within a reasonable period but no mode of disposal is specified.[197] Under *Williamss v Williams*, there is no property in a body.[198] This essentially means that a person can wish to get his body preserved through cryonics and a person charged to dispose the body can also give it for preservation. This would be a disposal with dignity and would not be in contravention of Sec 150 of the Crimes Act 1961 which makes it an offence to interfere improperly or indecently with, or offer any indignity to, human remains.[199]

---

188 *Cruzan v. Director, Missouri Dept. Health* 497 U.S. 261 (1990).

189 *Vacco v. Quill* 179 521 U.S. 793 (1997).

190 Sullivan, R. (2010). Pre-Mortem Cryopreservation: Recognizing a Patient's Right to Die in Order to Live. *Quinnipiac Health Law Journal* 14, 49.

191 *Ibid.*

192 *Cruzan v. Director, Missouri Dept. Health* 497 U.S. 261 (1990).

193 Re JS (A Child) (Disposal of Body: Prospective Orders) [2016] EWHC 2859 (Fam).

194 Re JS (A Child) [2017] 4 WLR 1.

195 Airedale NHS Trust v. Bland (1993) All E.R. 82) (H.L.).

196 Human Tissue Act, 2008.

197 § 46 E(1), Burial and Cremation Act, 1964.

198 Williams v Williams (1882) 20 CH. D. 659.c.

199 § 150(b), Crimes Act, 1961.

'Death' is not statutorily defined in New Zealand.[200] Earlier, a person was considered dead when he stopped breathing and his heart stopped beating and medical professional used to declare the death.[201] But advancement of medical technology has made a point that declaration cannot be final as there remains a chance of resuscitation even in the case of cardiac or respiratory arrest.[202] Disposal through cryonics can be done in the same line. Also, practitioners in New Zealand are demanding permission for pre-mortem cryopreservation so as to avoid any damage to brain which can cause information rhetoric death of a person.[203] Thus, some have suggested that there may be a 'right to die in order to live'.[204]

In Australia, practice of organ transplantation and elective ventilations is permissible.[205] Also, assisted suicide can be permitted by the state.[206] In Netherlands, euthanasia and physician-assisted suicide are not punishable if the attending physician acts in accordance with the criteria of due care.[207] Switzerland permit active euthanasia and assisted suicide. Active euthanasia can be committed without the assistance of physician and assistance in suicide is not a crime if done with unselfish motive.[208]

5. Conclusion and Recommendations

When we go through the massive compilation of scientific, biological and medical advancements of the last two centuries, it can be observed that we have come a long way. This exponential growth can be seen from the fact that the disease which appeared to be incurable at one point of time have become curable in the matter of past few decades. So much so that attempts have been made across the globe to achieve immortality through cryobiology. Today, preservation of blood, organs, and even human embryos at low temperature has already become mainstream. Some scientists already believe that by 2040, first human would be reanimated through the process of cryonics[209], making it all the more necessary to give it at least due consideration.

Laws in the many nations across the globe have already taken the first step by granting the right to refuse medical treatment and even physician-assisted

200 Skegg, P. (2015). Death. In Peter Skegg & Ron Paterson (Eds.), Health Law in New Zealand (689). Wellington, New Zealand: Thomson Reuters.

201 Nicola P. (2015). Human Tissue. In Peter Skegg & Ron Paterson (Eds.), Health Law in New Zealand (705). Wellington, New Zealand: Thomson Reuters.

202 *Ibid.*

203 Sullivan, R. (2010). Pre-Mortem Cryopreservation: Recognizing a Patient's Right to Die in Order to Live. *Quinnipiac Health Law Journal* 14, 49.

204 *Ibid.*

205 Australian Organ and Tissue Donation and Transplantation Authority Act, 2009.

206 Bartels, L. & Otlowski, M. (2010). A right to die? Euthanasia and the law in Australia. *J. Law Med.* 17(4), 532-55.

207 Termination of Life on Request and Assisted Suicide (Review Procedures) Act, 2002.

208 Hurst S.A. & Mauron A. (2003). Assited suicide and euthanasia in Switzerland: allowing a role for non-physicians. *BMJ* 326, 7383.

209 A Few Questions and Answers with Robert Freitas, the Author of Nanomedicine [Interview by B. Shock]. (1999). *Cryonics 20*, 23-24.

suicide. This has led to successful preservation of body in some those countries. In the absence of legislation on cryonics anywhere in the world, efforts are now been made to have the right to pre-mortem cryopreservation. Granting this right would subsequently boost the practice of cryonics while also not tarnishing the integrity of the medical professionals, as terminally-ill patients will be eligible to avail cryonic preservation before ailments destroy all hope of reanimation.

In contrast to developed nations across the world, India has not seen the surge on cryo-preservations as yet, primarily due to religious and ethical considerations as discussed above. Nevertheless, as the country gains traction towards its goal of being a superpower, such cases will probably arise. Owing to the extreme complexities that the issue raises, combined with the equivalent inefficiency of our current laws, it is necessary to take positive steps in this direction. Specific and structured policies in this regard would be supportive to persons who seek to exercise their fundamental right to life. Also, this would pave way for development of other fields of law to compliment the practice of extending life span.

Throughout centuries, death has been the basic assumption of our laws. It has consequences on rights, responsibilities, entitlements and obligations of a person. While we have tried to address some of these consequences, this article is merely meant to stimulate more discussion in this direction. In light of this objective, certain recommendations have been proposed as given below-

i) Recognizing and qualifying the practice of cryonics (pre-mortem and post-mortem) as lawful and constitutionally valid and framing comprehensive laws concerning the same.

ii) Amending THOA to include within its scope whole-body donations to cryonic institutions for cryo-preservation purposes.

iii) Granting appropriate powers to registered medical practitioners under § 3, THOA and Authorisation Committee under § 9 (4) to authorise and approve cryonic suspension in a timely and proper manner. In this regard, a specified authorisation body may be set up to deal specifically with such cases.

iv) Providing beforehand requisite regulatory approvals to cryonics institute to make arrangements for suspension in furtherance of the wishes of the individuals. At present, cryonic institutes are not allowed to receive bodies of dead patients without approval of Authorisation Committee which causes undue delay, defeating the purpose of cryonics itself.

v) Solving the inconsistencies in the definition of death under various laws (viz. THOA, IPC, Registration of Births and Deaths Act, 1969 etc.). A major consequence of such inconsistency can be seen when a person is declared brain dead under THOA but not 'legally dead' as per RBD Act, creating problems for cryonics institutes in obtaining necessary approvals (given the extremely time sensitive nature of the preservation process).

vi) Making provisions in criminal, property and other laws to account for situations arising as a result of cryopreservation. Some of these include legalizing establishment of personal revival trusts, enabling granting of property right to dead corpses to cryonic institutes for preservation,

vii) Promoting cooperation between state healthcare systems and cryonic organisations; training and licensing medical practitioners in cryonic processes; establishment of cryonic-friendly healthcare facilities and general positive approach towards cryonics and cryonic processes.

Technology will never stop in presenting newer challenges to legal mandate. The lack of legislative action will only be detrimental to interests of both science and general public welfare. Hence, a pre-emptive step in this regard may as well do wonders for humanity.

Chapter 7

Patenting Life: Genetic Patenting in India

Angela Dsouza
LLM Student of Intellectual Property Law
Queen Mary University of London
Email: angelabdsouza@yahoo.com

Abstract

The past decade has witnessed a significant revolution in the field of science and technology, especially in the arena of biotechnology. Biotechnology has transformed into an extremely dynamic industry, spanning across multiple sectors and touching the lives of millions of people every day. From medical device manufacturing to biofuels, from drugs and pharmaceuticals to agricultural chemicals and feedstock, and research and development activities in medical labs, a multitude of market segments constitute the biotechnology industry and make it a dynamic force for the present and future (The Future of Medicine, 2017).

The primary concern clouding biotechnological development is its immense interplay with intellectual property, more particularly patents. Many believe that the grant of patents to biotechnological inventions has resulted in an exorbitant commercialisation of the same, thus impeding further research and growth. Patents form an integral part of our world today. Every product, right from a safety pin to a space shuttle was once patented before eventually falling into public domain. In fact, no field has been spared from the clutches of patent protection. The rapid development of science and technology is bit of a curate's egg. While it has paved the way for access to better health care, increased production, booming economy and a comfortable lifestyle for man, it has also run into several controversies, particularly with respect to intellectual property.

Introduction

16 June 1980 is a red-letter day in the history of law and science. On this day, Ananda Chakraborty won a US Supreme Court case permitting him to patent a genetically engineered bacterium that could digest oil. The US Supreme Court in a decision of 5:4 held that human made living matter is a patentable subject matter. Chakraborty's oil-eating bacteria opened the floodgates in the United States. Soon the United States Patent and Trademark Office (USPTO) granted patents on genetically modified plants, seeds and plant tissue. By 1987, animal patenting was permitted. Today, almost three decades after the judgment, most

biopharmaceutical products are natural proteins based on the cloning of human genes (Caulfield & Williams – Jones, 1999).

The past decade has witnessed a significant revolution in the field of science and technology, especially in the arena of biotechnology. Biotechnology has transformed into an extremely dynamic industry, spanning across multiple sectors and touching the lives of millions of people every day. From medical device manufacturing to biofuels, from drugs and pharmaceuticals to agricultural chemicals and feedstock, and research and development activities in medical labs, a multitude of market segments constitute the biotechnology industry and make it a dynamic force for the present and future (The Future of Medicine, 2017). Today, genetic engineering techniques are utilised to produce a wide range of new products. While most of these involve plants and animals, emphasis is now being laid on genetically engineered microbes, especially nitrogen fixing bacteria, frost suppressive bacteria and certain microbial soil amendments.

The worldwide market for biotechnology-based products has in fact, seen a spurt from $ 15 billion in 1995 to $38 billion in 2005. With an estimated global industry size of $ 270.5 billion and a growth rate of 12.3%, the biotechnological sector is touted to escalate in the following years (Biotechnology, 2015). Consider the example of the United States of America where the US biotech industry accounted for $ 111.2 billion in annual revenue in 2015. The graph below projects the growth of the US biotechnology industry and its estimated growth until 2020, with contributions of biopharma, bio services, bio agriculture and bio industrial segments (The Future of Medicine, 2017).

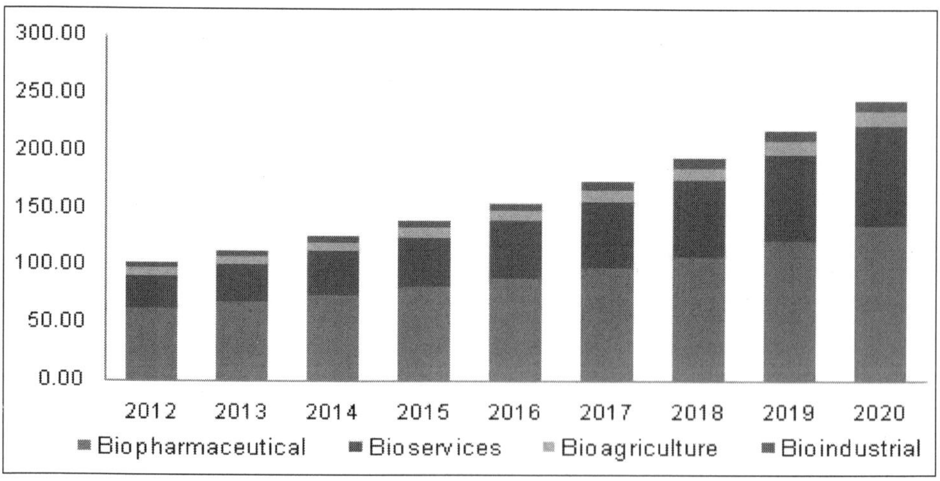

Closer home, the biotechnology sector of India is highly innovative and has seen rapid growth in the past few years. Ranked among the top 12 biotech destinations in the world, the Indian biotech industry holds about 2 percent share of the global biotech industry. With a growth of 57.14 percent in 2016, the industry is projected to be valued at US $ 11.6 billion in 2017 (Biotechnology, 2015).

While biotechnology and its many contributions, especially in the field of health care have proved immensely beneficial, it has also been a victim to controversy and severe criticism. Understanding the biotechnology industry is rather complicated because its scope extends to much more than what's obvious (The Future of Medicine, 2017). As the march for biotechnology results in a furore of research and products globally, the distinction between the products of nature and human-made inventions is increasingly difficult to trace in the chain of living matter (Caulfield & Williams – Jones, 1999).

The primary concern clouding biotechnological development is its immense interplay with intellectual property, more particularly patents. Many believe that the grant of patents to biotechnological inventions has resulted in an exorbitant commercialisation of the same, thus impeding further research and growth.

The patenting of life further opens up a Pandora's box of not only technical and legal issues but also ethical, moral, social and religious concerns. Scientific development in genetic technology has seen such a spurt that their consequences have generated wide ranging apprehensions (Menon, 1999). It is almost as if man has acquired 'superhuman abilities' through his knowledge and control over life at the cellular level.

Genetic technology coupled with the cloning of cells lead to the creation of 'Dolly' the sheep. This was soon followed by mice, calves, pigs, ox, cats and even human beings. Ideas which were once restricted to the realm of science fiction have today transformed into an actuality. Although many are toying with the idea of granting patent protection to such inventions, there are many others who believe that granting a patent to such inventions will not be dangerous but will also deface all social values.

Jurisdictions globally, have divergent views on the permissibility of such biological patents. While countries such as the Canada, Japan, China and a major part of the European Union Union consider biological patents as a valid form of patents, there are many others, such as the United States of America and who have reserved opinions primarily on the grounds of public order and morality.

Closer home, India also shares similar sentiments. However, over the past few years, the Indian Patent Office has granted patents over biological inventions, more particularly genes. While this is considered as a welcome step by many, there are many others who question the validity of such grant. The primary reason for this is that India lacks a well-formulated policy with respect to biological patents. Owing to a lackadaisical approach, corporations and institutions are able to secure a patent protection for those biological inventions which do not satiate even the basic requisites for an invention to be patentable.

In light of this, it becomes imperative to question the grounds on which the Indian Patent Office has been granting these patents. Moreover, it serves as a wake-up call to ascertain whether the Indian Patent Act requires a revamp in light of the evolving sphere of biological inventions.

Defining Patents and Patentability

Patents form an integral part of our world today. Every product, right from a safety pin to a space shuttle was once patented before eventually falling into public domain. In fact, no field has been spared from the clutches of patent protection.

Patents prove to be of immense value to people, especially corporations. While tangible assets do play an important role in the valuation of a company, it is intellectual property, more particularly patents that bolster the company's value. Further, patents provide licensing opportunities with companies within and sometimes outside the company's field. This in turn aids in the generation of revenue through licensing fees. In addition, patents allow individual inventors and small businesses the option of obtaining licenses or selling the rights to those who may be in a better position to produce or utilize the patent.

What is A Patent?

The origins of the word 'patent' lie in the Latin word *patere*, which means 'to lay open' or 'to make available for public inspection'. The word is also a shortened version of the term *letters patent*, an open document issued by the monarch to grant exclusive rights to a person, thus predating the modern patent system.

In modern parlance, however, the term patent refers to the right granted to the inventor of an invention. They are legal rights granted for new inventions employing scientific and technical knowledge (Goel & Parashar, 2013). A patent is a restricted monopoly granted by the government to the inventor in lieu for the technical disclosure of technical information employed in the invention. This in turn excludes others from making, using, selling or importing the patented product or process producing that product. The patent is granted for a limited period to the inventor and upon the expiry of such term, the patent falls into public domain.

The objective of patent law is to promote innovation by furthering their protection and utilization for the development of industries, promotion of technological innovation and transfer and dissemination of technology. Recognition and reward fosters industrial and technical progress thus paving the way for a vibrant socioeconomic structure.

The grant of a patent, however, is subject to certain criteria that need to be met in order to render the invention patentable. In order to be eligible for a patent, an invention must first be novel. In addition, it should include an inventive step and should also possess industrial application. These criteria are like filters arranged in succession and every invention must pass through all these filters in order to be eligible for a patent grant. Therefore, the grant of a patent is the cumulative effect of these criteria; the non-satisfaction of even one of these requirements will render the invention ineligible for a patent grant.

Article 27.1 of the Agreement on Trade Related Aspects of Intellectual Property Rights (TRIPS) reads as follows:

> *'Subject to the provisions of paragraphs 2 and 3, patents shall be available for any inventions, whether products or processes, in all fields of technology, provided that they are new, involve an inventive step and are capable of industrial application.'*

Patentability Requirements

As once stated by Justice Learned Hand, 'the question whether there is a patentable invention is as fugitive, impalpable, wayward, and vague a phantom as exists in the whole paraphernalia of legal concepts' (*Harries v. Air King Prod Co.*, 1950). This is because patent law has to, very often, engage itself in technologies that are yet not fully understood. In addition, the grant of a patent also brings with it complex legal questions entwined with cultural, political and social concerns.

As a consequence, patent legislations, globally, have laid down certain elementary requisites that verify the worthiness of an invention to be granted a patent protection. These requisites are:

Industrial Application

An invention, in order to be patentable, must be of a kind which can be applied for practical purposes and not be purely theoretical. Thus, in order to be patentable, the alleged invention must be capable of industrial application i.e., if the invention is a product, it must be capable of being made or used in an industry; and if it is a process, it must be possible to use or perform it. The need to show industrial applicability reflects the image of the patentable invention as having a concrete and technical character (Bently & Sherman, 2008).

An invention would satisfy this requirement, if it can be made any multiple times and can be made use of in at least one industry (Kankanala, 2013). It should be noted here that the term 'industry' is interpreted in the widest sense and includes activities such as agriculture and even those which do not yield any profit (Bently & Sherman, 2008). One can therefore imply that the invention must have a useful purpose.

In addition to being used or made in any industry, an invention must also possess a useful purpose in order to be industrially applicable. However, it is essential to note that the actual use need not be demonstrated. Ascertainment of the potential use of the invention alone would suffice to deem it to be an industrially applicable invention. Therefore, where a product has been used or put on the market, the commercial success of the product is not a determinant to ascertain the industrial applicability of the invention (*Harvard/OncoMouse*, 2003).

Novelty

An invention will be patentable only if it is novel or new in the light of prior art or is not anticipated by the prior art (Kankanala, 2013). Novelty requires that an invention be quantitatively different from what has been disclosed previously; that is, the technical information disclosed by the patent is not already available to the public (Bently & Sherman, 2008). Where an invention is already disclosed or can be anticipated by the prior art, a patent will not be granted.

The ascertainment of novelty of an alleged invention depends on two yardsticks. First, before being in a position to determine whether an invention is new, it is first necessary to identify what the alleged invention is (Bently & Sherman, 2008). This is crucial because the law of patents (by virtue of Article 27.3) lays down an exhaustive list of inventions that are excluded subject matter. These include *inter alia* scientific theories or mathematical methods, methods of medical and veterinary treatment, immoral inventions and those contrary to *odre public*. Therefore, if an invention falls under any of these heads, it is *prima facie* ineligible to be patented.

The second yardstick is the information that forms a part of prior art. Prior art includes all information and knowledge relating to the invention that was available on the date of patent application (Kankanala, 2013). Therefore, in order to negate novelty of an invention, all elements of an invention must be present in a single prior art reference. There are no geographical limits for where the prior art should be disclosed. Prior art includes information available anywhere in the world. Further, information will be considered prior art irrespective of the manner in which it is disclosed. Information may be part of prior art through written descriptions, past use, exhibitions, sales or even by oral communication. There are no minimum requirements on how widely the information must be published to be disclosed (Bently & Sherman, 2008). Therefore, even a single copy of a document or the sale of a single item will suffice for the information to be a part of prior art (*Fomento Industrial SA and Others v Mentmore Manufacturing Co Ltd*, 1956).

Inventive Step or Non-Obviousness

Inventive step or non-obviousness is the toughest and the most ambiguous requisite to ascertain the patentability of an invention. The non-obviousness doctrine provides that an invention cannot be patented if it does not possess an inventive step. An inventive step is a feature of an invention that involves technical advance as compared to the existing knowledge or economic significance or both and that makes the invention not obvious to a person skilled in the art (Bently & Sherman, 2008). The non-obviousness bar, hence, is a measure of what we, as a society, accept as a valuable discovery (Mojibi, 2010).

The philosophy behind the doctrine of obviousness is that the public should not be prevented from doing anything which was merely an obvious extension or workshop variation of what was already known at the priority date (*PLG Research Ltd and Another v Ardon International Ltd and Others*, 1993). The yardstick of inventive step acts as qualitative threshold and ensures that patent protection is only granted to non-obvious inventions. When applied correctly, the test of inventiveness excludes all results of ordinary innovation from the gamut of patent protection while rewarding those who expend energy and resources to undertake research projects that are highly uncertain and seem unlikely to succeed (Roin, 2009). This also encourages others to undertake further research which would have, otherwise not been undertaken.

Biotechnology and Patents: Global Standards

Intellectual property rights, from their inception, have been predominantly molded by international treaties. These treaties in turn determined the national scene for the protection and regulation of intellectual property rights. This trend was inconspicuous in the field of patent law and it was only after the Agreement on Trade-Related Aspects of Intellectual Property Rights (TRIPS Agreement) was brought into effect that global standards with respect to the grant, scope and use of patents were established.

The TRIPS Agreement came about as an annex to the WTO Agreement (Overwalle, 2008). Articles 27.1 elaborates the international standard for patent protection and states that patents protection shall be available for any invention, whether product or process, in all fields of technology, provided that they are new, involve an inventive step and are capable of industrial application. In addition, the TRIPS Agreement also seeks to address evolving arenas of science and law, more particularly biological patents.

A biological patent is a patent obtained in the field of biology that confers the patent holder with the right to exclude others from making, using, selling or importing the protected invention for a limited period of time. Biological patents include patents in the arena of biotechnology and biotechnological products as well as genetically modified organisms and genetic material.

Article 27.3.2 states in its first sentence that member states may exclude from patentability plants and animals other than microorganisms, and essentially biological processes for the production of plants or animals other than non-biological and microbiological processes (Overwalle, 2008). However, the optional nature of this statement has led to many discrepancies among member states, especially with regard to the patentability of genes.

Some countries such as the United States of America and the European Union opine that patents on biological resources are essential and useful and, therefore, do not opt to implement the exclusionary provisions of the TRIPS Agreement in their national legislations. Usually under such legislations, patent protection is granted to *inter alia* gene sequences, vectors, plant cells and animal cells on the sole condition that they satiate the patentability standards laid down in their respective national legislations.

On the other hand, there are several other countries which seek to categorically exclude biological material from the gamut of patent protection. A typical example is the Andean Pact Community, which has collectively agreed that the entirety or part of living beings as encountered in nature, natural biological processes, biological material existing in nature or which may be isolated, including the genome or germ plasm of any natural living being, shall not be considered inventions (Overwalle, 2008). A similar situation also prevails in Brazil and Argentina.

In this regard, it is essential to consider the patentability of genes. The patentability of genes has been under a continuous dispute owing to its ambiguous nature and the thin line between a natural substance and an artificially procured substance.

Patentability of Genes

A gene patent is a patent on a specific gene which is isolated from a naturally occurring body. It includes its chemical composition, the processes for obtaining or using it, or a combination of such claims. Gene patents are a part of the broader category of biological patents.

Gene patents may claim the isolated natural sequences of genes, the use of a natural sequence for the purposes such as diagnostic testing, or a natural sequence that has been altered by adding a promoter or other changes to make it more useful. The courts have upheld claims on altered sequences, but courts' and lawyers' opinions have been mixed on upholding the use of natural sequences and particularly the sequence itself. Patents on genes have only been granted on isolated gene sequences with known functions, and these patents cannot be applied to the naturally occurring genes in humans or any other naturally occurring organism.

At this juncture, it is also crucial to ascertain whether genes form a patentable subject matter in accordance with the minimum standards laid down by the TRIPS Agreement. As stated previously, Articles 27.1 of the TRIPS Agreement states that patents protection shall be available for any invention, whether product or process, in all fields of technology, provided that they are new, involve an inventive step and are capable of industrial application. These standards have to, therefore, be applied to genes in order to determine their patentability.

While a number of changes have been made to patent law to accommodate biotechnological inventions, for the most part these are treated in a similar manner to other types of invention (Bently & Sherman, 2008). The test of novelty is no different. A biological or biotechnological invention can only be anticipated and will therefore be invalid if an enabling disclosure has been made. Despite this, there are several concerns with respect to biotechnological inventions that rely on natural materials. In this context it is important to note that a natural substance that has been isolated for the first time (such as a polynucleotide sequence) will lack novelty because it was already present in nature (Bently & Sherman, 2008). However here, patent law draws a distinction between the invention i.e. the isolated 'artificial' polynucleotide and the natural nucleotide existing in nature. The artificial nature of the isolated polynucleotide forms the difference between the prior art and novelty, thus fulfilling the requisite for novelty.

The requirement that inventions need to exhibit a useful purpose is also vital in relation to biological research. This is because while researchers have been successful in locating and identifying new gene structures, there has not been much development in ascertaining the functions of these genes. Therefore, unless a useful purpose can be found for these genes, they will not be industrially applicable and, as such, not patentable (Bently & Sherman, 2008).

While dissidents of genetic patents consider this requirement to be of utmost importance, there are others who do not find it satisfactory enough. It is now being suggested that the problem with patents over genes is that, while a patentee only has to disclose one specific use to show industrial applicability (Bently & Sherman, 2008). Once this threshold is satisfied, the patent holder secures control over it as well as all its uses, including those which were, till the grant of the patent, unknown. This in turn creates an imbalance between disclosed and protected matter. Many, therefore, opine that the patent protection should be limited to only what is disclosed in the patent application. Despite its importance, this issue has not been satisfactorily addressed.

Patentability of Genes: A Comparative Analysis

Various countries such as Canada, Europe and Japan are clearly of the view that genes can be patented (Genetic Rights, 2014). However, it is more practicable to focus on the patent legislations of the United States of America and the European Union to gauge the global temperament with respect to the patentability of genes.

These countries are pioneers in genetic technology and have a robust patent legal framework to support the same. Therefore, an understanding of their patent legislations, especially with respect to gene patentability would aid in the appreciation of the global trends in gene patenting.

Gene Patentability in Europe

The basic principles governing gene patents in Europe are summarized in Article 3 of the EC Biotechnology Directive which states that, for the purpose of the Directive, inventions which are new, which involve an inventive step, and which are susceptible to industrial application shall be patentable even if they are products consisting of or containing biological material or a process by means of which a biological material is produced, processed or used.

The basic principles governing gene patents in Europe are summarized in Article 3 of the EC Biotechnology Directive which states that, for the purpose of the Directive, inventions which are new, which involve an inventive step, and which are susceptible to industrial application shall be patentable even if they are products consisting of or containing biological material or a process by means of which a biological material is produced, processed or used (Cook, 2009).

In Europe, it is possible to obtain patent protection for biotechnological inventions by applying for a European patent at the European Patent Office (EPO). On the basis of a single application and examination procedure, it is possible to protect an invention in almost thirty-one European countries, all of which have ratified the European Patent Convention (Overwalle, 2008).

However, the term 'European patent' is a misnomer. A European patent does not connote a single patent that is valid across the whole of Europe; instead, while the application and examination is a single one, the patent is split into a number of different national patents upon grant. These national patents are then subject to the respective national legislations.

While a European patent may be granted for any invention that is new, involves an inventive step and is capable of industrial application, certain inventions are barred from being patented under the European Patent Convention. In light of this, two provisions of the European Patent Convention hold extreme importance. The first is Article 53(1), which prescribes that European patents shall not be issued in respect of inventions either the publication or exploitation of which would be contrary to *ordre public* or morality. The second provision is Article 53(2) of the EPC which states that European patents shall not be granted in respect of plant or animal varieties or essentially biological processes for the production of plant and animals.

Article 53 of the EPC served as the sole guide for the EPO with respect to biotech patenting. It should, however, be noted that the EPC contained no specific provisions for the admissibility of patents on human beings and human body material. Patents were granted solely on the basis of the general requirements outlined in the EPC.

Therefore, in order to resolve these lacunae in the European patent law and to harmonise national legislations with respect to genetic patenting, a Directive (The EU Biotechnology Directive) for the legal protection of biotechnological inventions was adopted by the European Parliament on 6 July 1998.

The EU Biotechnology Directive, vide Article 3(1) stipulates that inventions which are new, possess an inventive step and are capable of industrial application merit a patent even if it relates to a product consisting of or containing any biological material or a process through which the biological material is produced, processed or utilized. This provision categorically states that living matter can also be patented under the European patent law.

Under European patent law, the inventiveness requirement will not be satisfied by an invention involving isolated genetic sequences that have a structure closely related to existing sequences with a known function. The EPO has stated that sequences as well as all other chemical compounds should solve a technical problem in a non-obvious manner to be recognised as inventive.

The EPO will regard a genetic invention as involving an inventive step only if the applicant can demonstrate that obtaining the sequence was in fact a technical achievement or that they have discovered a new or unexpected property associated with the gene.

Gene Patentability in the United States of America

Prequel to the Myriad Genetics Case

The US Patent law states that whoever invents or discovers any new and useful process, machine, manufacture, or composition of matter, or any new and useful improvement thereof, may obtain a patent, subject to other conditions and requirements (35 U.S. Code § 101). In addition, the United States Patent and Trademark Office (USPTO) have issued certain guidelines stipulating the statutory requirements for an invention to be patentable. These guidelines assert that a process, including a process for doing business, must produce a concrete, useful and tangible result to be patentable (*State Street Bank & Trust Co. v. Signature Financial Group, Inc.*, 1998).

The long-standing practice of the USPTO was, however, to refuse claims to living systems as not being patentable subject matter (Rimmer, 2008). Notably, in 1873, Louis Pasteur was granted a patent by the United States Patent and Trademark Office (USPTO), claiming yeast, free form organic germs of disease, as an article of manufacture (Chawla, 2005). A patent attorney, Grubb, noted that "in the USA, in spite of the precedent of the Pasteur patent… it had become the practice of the Patent Office to refuse claims to living systems as not being patentable subject matter" (Grubb, 2004, p. 24).

However, in 1889, the Commissioner of Patents rejected a patent application which lay claim to 'cellular tissues of the Pinus australis' tree separated from the 'silicous, resinous, and pulpy parts of the pine needles and subdivided into long, pliant, filaments adapted to be spun and woven (Rimmer, 2008). The Commissioner of Patents ruled that patents could not be granted in respect of products of nature:

> *"It cannot be said that the applicant in this case has made any discovery, or is entitled to patent the idea, or fact, rather, that fibre can be found in the needle of the Pinus australis, or that it is a longer fibre than can be found in other leaves, or that it possesses more or less strength of fineness, because the mere ascertaining of the character or quality of trees that grow in the forest and the construction of the woody fibre and tissue of which they are composed is not a patentable invention, recognised by the statute, any more than to find a new gem or jewel in the earth would entitle the discoverer to patent all gems which should be subsequently found. The result would be that patents might be obtained upon the trees of the forest and the plants of the earth, which of course would be unreasonable and impossible"* (Rimmer, 2008).

The USPTO was soon faced with its major challenge in 1972 when a microbiologist, Ananda Chakrabarty applied for a patent for genetically-engineered bacteria that could eat all the different components of oil. There were a total of thirty-six claims made and these claims were of three types: first, there were process claims for the mode of producing the bacteria, the second comprised of claims on the inoculum to culture the bacteria and the third comprised of claims to the bacteria itself.

The USPTO allowed the first two claims but rejected the third on the ground that vide 35 U.S. Code § 101, living things are not patentable subject matter. The USPTO opined that an invention be manufactured or a composition of matter and since living matter are neither manufactured nor a composition of matter, they are unpatentable.

Chakrabarty, on the other hand, argued that the genetic engineering impressed on the bacteria was a form of a manufacturing process and was therefore eligible for patent protection. The Court of Customs and Patent Appeals conceded to Chakrabarty's argument and this was subsequently affirmed by the US Supreme Court.

The US Supreme Court noted that the laws of nature, physical phenomena and abstract ideas cannot be patented. This also includes plants and minerals available in the environment, as well as mathematical formulas. However, the Court opined that genetically engineered organisms fall with the gamut of 'manufactured'. The Court held that the bacteria was Chakrabarty's own 'handiwork' and should therefore be granted a patent.

Therefore, biotechnological patents, subject to the exclusion of 'laws of nature' are patentable. US courts have consistently held that as per the exclusion anything that naturally exists or is a 'product of nature' is not patentable (Kankanala, 2007). This, however, resulted in a spurt of applications with the USPTO permitting patenting of genes, more particularly isolated and human genes. It was not until 2009 that this long standing USPTO practice was challenged by a group of medical researchers, advocacy groups, medical doctors and patients in a case relating to patents granted to Myriad Genetics for the BRCA 1 and BRCA 2 genes (NG, 2015).

The Myriad Genetics Case

By 2013, almost 2000 genes of the human body were already patented. As a result, scientific research and genetic testing has been delayed, limited or even shut down due to concerns about gene patents (The Fight, 2013). In such a scenario, the case of *Association for Molecular Pathology v. Myriad Genetics, Inc.* was responsible in questioning the status quo and highlighting the detrimental effects of patenting isolated human genes.

In this case, Myriad Genetics (Myriad) made a medical breakthrough when its scientists discovered the precise location of the BRCA I and BRCA two genes on chromosomes 17 (comprising of approximately 80 million nucleotides) and 13 (comprising around 114 million nucleotides) (NG, 2015). This was an immensely significant contribution towards the development of medical tests for detecting mutations of these two genes in patients thereby enabling an assessment to be made on their risks of developing breast and ovarian cancer.

Upon this discovery, Myriad Genetics sought to and successfully patented the isolated DNA and complementary DNA (cDNA) that encodes for the genes BRCA 1 and BRCA 2. Assuming that these patents were held valid, Myriad Genetics would be conferred with the exclusive right to isolate these genes as well as to artificially create the BRCA cDNA.

Since isolation is an essential step in conducting genetic and diagnostic testing, Myriad tried to enforce its patents against entities that were performing the BRCA testing (NG, 2015). However, in a unanimous decision, the Supreme Court invalidated Myriad's claims to isolated genes stating that naturally occurring DNA sequences, even when isolated from the body, cannot be patented, but artificially created DNA is patent eligible because it does not occur naturally.

The court focused on the 'product of nature' exclusion and re-affirmed the implicit exception to 35 U.S. Code § 101 that laws nature, natural phenomena and abstract ideas are not patentable. The Court reiterated that these were the primary tools of scientific and technological research and therefore lie out of the gamut of patentability. Without this exception, there would be considerable danger that the grant of patents would tie-up the use of such tools and thereby inhibit future innovation premised upon them (*Association for Molecular Pathology v. Myriad Genetics, Inc.*, 2013).

The Court, however, also held that a blanket prohibition on the patentability of naturally occurring things is not viable. This is because every invention, at some level entails the use of or applies the laws of nature, natural phenomena or abstract ideas. A broad interpretation of this exclusionary clause, would therefore, vitiate the very purpose of patent law. Therefore, there ought to be a fine balance between incentives that bolster creation and invention and impending the flow of information that might spur invention.

Genetic Patents: The Indian Landscape

The Indian Patents Act 1970 is the governing legislation for patents in India. The Act, vide Section 2(1)(m), provides that a patent may be granted for an 'invention', which is further defined as a new product or process involving an inventive step and capable of industrial application.

The three terms 'new', 'inventive step' and 'industrial application', provide the three main criteria for patentability (Matthew, 2011). According to the Act a new invention is any invention or technology which has not been anticipated by publication in any document or used in the country or elsewhere in the world before the date of filing of the patent application i.e. such matter should not have fallen into public domain or formed a part of prior art. In addition, the invention seeking patent protection should include an inventive step i.e. such invention must possess a technical advancement or economic significance or both that makes the invention non-obvious to a person who is skilled in the art at the time the invention was made. In addition, the alleged invention must be capable of industrial application.

In addition to these elementary requisites, the Patent Act, vide Section 3 provides an exhaustive list of inventions that are barred from being patented. Such non-patentable inventions include *inter alia*:

Any invention that claims to be contrary to the established laws of nature.

- Any invention whose use or commercial exploitation would prove detrimental to public order, morality or would result in serious prejudice to human, animal or plant life, health or the environment.
- Any discovery of a scientific principle or discovery of any biotic or abiotic substance occurring in nature.
- The discovery of a new form of a known substance which does not result in the enhancement of the known efficacy of that substance.
- Any substance obtained by an admixture.
- Any arrangement, rearrangement or duplication of devices.
- Any agricultural or horticultural method.
- Any medicinal, surgical, curative, diagnostic, therapeutic or prophylactic treatment for humans or animals.
- Any mathematical or business method or a computer program or algorithm.
- Plants and animals in whole or in part thereof other than microorganisms but including seeds, varieties and species and essential biological processes for production and propagation of plants and animals.

Patentability of Genes Under the Indian Patent Act 1970

At the outset, it is essential to recall that the Patent Act 1970 bars the patenting of plants and animals in whole or in part thereof other than microorganisms but including seeds, varieties and species and essential biological processes for production and propagation of plants and animals.

As a consequence, prior to 2000, the Indian Patent Office (IPO) did not grant patents to inventions that entailed living entities of natural or artificial origin, biological materials or other materials having replicating properties, substance derived from such materials or any processes for the production of living substances/entities including nucleic acids (Kalyan, 2007).

However, in 2002, in the case of *Dimminaco AG v. Controller of Patents & Designs*, the High Court of Calcutta granted patents for the processes involved in the preparation of the Bursitis vaccine where the final product of that process contained living organisms. Though the grant was opposed by the IPO on the ground that the process for the preparation of the said vaccine could not be considered as a mode of manufacture since its end product contained a living entity, the Calcutta High Court, led by Justice Asok Kumar Ganguly held that there was no statutory bar to the patentability of living organisms (Basheer, 2005).

Statutory changes soon followed with the Patents Act being amended in 2002 to specifically permit, *inter alia*, the patenting of biotechnological and microbiological processes (NG, 2015). The definition of the term 'invention' was amended to contain 'new product or process involving an inventive stp and capable of industrial application.' Subsequently, a 2005 amendment rendered the grant of patents in any field of technology as permissible.

The Patents Act, vide Section 3(c) stipulates that the mere discovery of a scientific principle or the formulation of an abstract theory, discovery of any living or non-living substance occurring in nature would not be patentable. Further Section 3(j) of the Act states that any plant or animal, in whole or any part thereof, except microorganisms but including seeds, varieties and species and essentially biological processes for production or propagation of plants and animals are not patentable.

A gene occurs in nature and can therefore not be patented. However, it must be noted that there is considerable skill involved in identifying its function, location and isolation (Ravi, 2013). With regard to Section 3(j), while plants and animals in whole or part are unpatentable, it is imperative to ascertain whether genes would form a 'part' of such plant or animal and would therefore be unpatentable. Further, it is also essential to determine whether genes can be patented at all under the Patents Act. These concerns are, unfortunately, unanswered by the Act.

As a consequence, reliance must be placed on the Manual of Patent Practice and Procedure issued by the Indian Patent Office over a period of time to understand their approach towards the grant of patents. While the 2005 draft manual of the Manual had an annexure dedicated to biotechnological and pharmaceutical inventions, it was deleted in the 2008 draft. The 2005 draft categorically provided for the patenting of recombinant DNA and plasmids in the event of substantial human intervention. However, in the 2008 draft, the explanations under Section 3(j) only elucidate the manner in which microorganisms can be patented in the light of the *Dimminaco* case. However, under the description of unity of an invention, the Manual provides an example:

> *When a genetically modified gene sequence/amino acid sequence is novel, involves an inventive step and has industrial application, the following can be claimed:*
>
> *a. Gene sequence/amino acid sequence.*
>
> *b. A method of expressing the above sequence*

c. *An antibody against the protein/sequence.*

d. *A kit made from the antibody/sequence.* (Draft Manual, 2008)

This gives an impression that a gene may be patented if it is a recombinant gene involving an inventive step and possessing industrial application.

However, the final Manual that was released by the Indian Patent Office in 2011 provides no further explanation on the subject matter. The only provisions that were retained were the ones pertaining to sequence listing that had to be provided by the patentee and the aforementioned claims under the unity of invention. The requirement of human intervention did not find a place in the manual (Ravi, 2013).

Subsequent to this, there were several grants made by the Indian Patent Office, patenting genes. However, in almost every case, the Patent Office has failed to stipulate the legislative framework that they were relying on to grant such patents. Consider the example where the Universiti Sains Malaysia applied for a patent grant on a vector or cloning vector encoding a filarial parasite polypeptide. The abstract of the invention stipulated that the alleged invention was a cDNA sequence or any functional equivalent, fragment, analogue, mutant or variant thereof. While the original claim sought to cover the entire cDNA, the claim was subsequently narrowed to cover only an expression vector containing the particular nucleotide sequence for the polypeptide (Universiti Sains Malaysia, 2011).

In the first examination report, the patent office had objected to multiple claims on the ground that since the cDNA was obtained from what was already existing in nature, it cannot be patented. Subsequent claims based on the RNA and the polypeptides were also objected on similar grounds. However, all these claims were ultimately withdrawn with the patent being granted for the expression vector containing the particular sequence for the polynucleotide alone. While the claims made definitely fall outside the purview of Section 3(c), it is unclear if they are entirely non-obvious as ultimately, the particular nucleotide sequence is inserted is put inside a vector which is known recombinant DNA technology with no enhanced utility as compared to the prior art (Ravi, 2013).

Another example is when the University of Copenhagen sought a patent on an Isolated Nucleic Acid Molecule Comprising an Allele of a Genetic Polymorphism Linked to Resistance to Enterotoxigenic Escherichia Coli (ETEC) (University of Copenhagen, 2010). Here the subject matter in consideration was a nucleic acid sequence resistance to a particular type of E.coli in pigs. The invention covered methods to identify this sequence using probes and primers crafted for this purpose. The application comprised of several claims, the first one being a claim on the particular sequence that results in the trait of resistance in pigs (which is a naturally occurring substance). The patent application covered both, the original sequence as well as the man made probes/primes for identifying the trait (Ravi, 2013). Surprisingly, the examination report raised no objection to the fact that the application sought to patent an isolated gene derived from an animal. This in turn goes to prove that animal genes are patentable in India.

Both these examples reflect a complete ignorance or rather a lackadaisical attitude of the Indian Patent Office in granting genetic patents. The fact that the Indian patent law makes no mention of genetic patents is completely disregarded while accepting such applications. This in turn reveals the several lacunae and unresolved areas with respect to genetic patents within the Indian law. As the arena of biotechnology continues to escalate both in terms of development and costs, it becomes extremely imperative for India to devise a clear-cut policy on genetic patents in order to prevent grants to undeserving or frivolous claims and subsequently avoid incertitude in the future.

Conclusion and Suggestions

The rapid development of science and technology is bit of a curate's egg. While it has paved the way for access to better health care, increased production, booming economy and a comfortable lifestyle for man, it has also run into several controversies, particularly with respect to intellectual property.

Intellectual property is one of the fastest growing integrant of both global economy as well as government policy decisions. The sheer value imputed to it has resulted in a expansive framework of both international and domestic legislations regulating it.

The spurt in the development of science and technology has also contributed to bolster the value of intellectual property rights, particularly patents. Inventions coupled with continual development has not only fuelled people to take up uncertain research but also seek for protection upon success. This in turn incentivises others to enter this ever-evolving field of science and technology.

The sphere of biotechnology is no different. Though a relatively new field, biotechnological development has seen unprecedented growth. Today, biotechnological inventions and processes are used to produce a wide number of products including food and medicines. This has paved the way for people to seek patent protections on their inventions in the field of biotechnology.

However, being a developing field, its nuances are still not fully understood, thus leaving the patent protection framework within a lurch. The very nature biotechnological inventions render it difficult to ascertain standard criteria for the grant of patents. Several countries, however, have modified their patent legislations to accommodate patents on biotechnological inventions, more particularly patents on genetic material. They opine that this would further bolster research and development in the field of genetics and biotechnology. On the other hand, there are others who believe that this would make people owners of nature and life while also resulting in the debasement of social value.

While the European has opted for a more liberal view by permitting patents on genetic material, the United States of America, through the course of several judicial decisions have arrived at a policy of restrictive patenting for genetic material and biotechnological inventions. Irrespective of which side they stand on, many countries have a crystal-clear take on their policy for genetic patenting.

India, to the contrary, appears to be sitting on the fence. Despite the Indian patent law making no express provision for the patenting of genes, the Indian Patent Office has gone ahead and granted patent protection to several claims of genes both, naturally occurring as well as artificially produced. Such grants not only highlight the insouciant attitude of the patent office but also bring to the forefront the glaring lacunae in the Indian patent law. Despite the meteoric development of biotechnology in India, the Indian law has failed to take cognizance of the same. Today, India ranks as one of the top 12 biotech nations in the world with a market share of approximately 2 percent. Gaining a strong foothold in the biotech industry is only possible with further development. However, such development should be complemented by an equally robust legislative mechanism. Lack of a clear policy and laws for the same will only prove detrimental to the body of patents in India. Irrespective of what the policy ought to be, it is imperative that a policy be primarily formed to prevent grants to ill-considered claims and incertitude in patent grants that defeat the very purpose of patent law.

References

Association for Molecular Pathology v. Myriad Genetics, Inc. 569 U. S. ___ (2013).

Basheer, Shamnaad (2005). 'Policy Style' Reasoning at the Indian Patent Office. *Intellectual Property Quarterly, 3,* 309-323.

Bently, L. & Sherman, B. (2008). *Intellectual Property Law.* New York: Oxford University Press.

Biotechnology. (2015). New Delhi, India, India Brand Equity Foundation.

Chawla, H.S. (2005). Patenting of Biological Material and Biotechnology. *Journal of Intellectual Property Rights, 10,* 44-51.

Cook, Trevor. (2009). *Pharmaceuticals, Biotechnology and the Law.* Reed Elsevier, United Kingdom: Lexis Nexis.

Draft Manual of Patent Practice and Procedure (2008). Retrieved from http://www.ipindia.nic.in/ipr/patent/DraftPatent_Manual_2008.pdf

Fomento Industrial SA and Others v. Mentmore Manufacturing Co Ltd 1956 RPC 87.

Genetic Rights and Wrongs. (2014, September). Retrieved from http://www.nature.com/news/genetic-rights-and-wrongs-1.15877

Goel, D. & Parashar S. (2013). *IPR, Biosafety and Bioethics.* Delhi, India: Pearson.

Grubb, Philip W. (2004). *Patents for Chemicals, Pharmaceuticals and Biotechnology.* New York: Oxford University Press.

Harries v. Air King Prod. Co., 183 F.2d 158, 162 (2d Cir. 1950).

Harvard/OncoMouse [2003] OJ EPO 473, 494.

Kankanala, Kalyan C. (2007). *Genetic Patent Law and Strategy.* Noida, India: Manupatra.

Kankanala, Kalyan C. (2013). *Fun IP: Fundamentals of Intellectual Property.* Bangalore, India: Brain League IP Services.

Knoppers, Bartha Maria. (1999). Biotechnology: Sovereignty and Sharing. In T.A. Caulfield & B. William-Jones (Eds.), The Commercialization of Genetic Research: Ethical, Legal, and Policy Issues (pp. 1-12). New York: Kluwer Academic/Plenum Publishers.

Matthew, R. (2011). *Patentability Requirements in India.* Retrieved from https://www.lakshmisri.com/Uploads/MediaTypes/Documents/L&SWebsite_IPR_Featured_Ranjan.pdf

Menon, M.G.K. (1999). *Human Genome Research: Emerging Ethical, Legal, Social, and Economic Issues.* Mumbai, India: Allied Publishers.

Mojibi, A. (2010). An Empirical Study of the Effect Of Ksr v. Teleflex on the Federal Circuit's Patent Validity Jurisprudence. *Albany Law Journal of Science and Technology, 20*(3), 559-596.

NG, Elizabeth Siew-Kuan (2015). Patenting Human Genes: Wherein lies the balance between Private Rights and Public Access in India and the United States. *The Indian Journal of Law and Technology, 11,* 3-51.

Overwalle, Geertrui van. (2008). Biotechnology and Patents: Global Standards, European Approaches and National Accents. In D. Wüger & T. Cottier (Eds.), Genetic Engineering and the World Trade System (pp. 77-108). Cambridge, United Kingdom: Cambridge University Press.

PLG Research Ltd and Another v Ardon International Ltd and Others [1993] FSR 197.

Ravi, Bhavishyavani (2013). Gene Patents in India: Gauging Policy by an Analysis of the Grants made by the Indian Patent Office. *Journal of Intellectual Property Rights, 18,* 323-329.

Rimmer, Matthew. (2008). *Intellectual Property and Biotechnology: Biological Inventions.* Cheltenham, United Kingdom: Edward Elgar Publishing Limited.

Roin, B.N. (2009), Unpatentable Drugs and the Standards of Patentability. *Texas Law Review, 87*(3), 503-570.

State Street Bank & Trust Co. v. Signature Financial Group, Inc. 149 F.3d 1368 (Fed. Cir. Jul. 23, 1998).

The Fight to take back Our Genes: Challenging Patents on Cancer Genes. (2013, June). Retrieved from https://www.aclu.org/cases/association-molecular-pathology-v-myriad-genetics?redirect=free-speech-womens-rights/aclu-challenges-patents-breast-cancer-genes-0

The Future of Medicine is Biotechnology: An Industry Rundown. (2017, January). Retrieved from http://www.portfoliowealthglobal.com/the-future-of-medicine-is-biotechnology-an-industry-rundown/

Universiti Sains Malaysia, (2011), Indian Patent Application No. 953/MUM/2000. Retrieved from http://www.allindianpatents.com/patents/246865-an-expression-vector-or-cloning-vector-encoding-a-filarial-parasite-polypeptide

University of Copenhagen, (2010), Indian Patent Application No. 2286/DELNP/2005. Retrieved from http://www.allindianpatents.com/patents/244118-an-isolated-nucleic-acid-na-molecule-comprising-an-allele-of-a-genetic-polymorphism-linked-to-resistance-to-enterotoxigenic-escher-ichia-coli-etec

Chapter 8

The Effects of Chemotherapy Treatment on Male Reproductive Functions

Khaled Habas, Martin. H. Brinkworth and Diana Anderson

Faculty of Life Sciences, University of Bradford, Bradford, Richmond Road, West Yorkshire, BD7 1DP, UK.

Email: d.anderson1@bradford.ac.uk

Abstract

There is increasing concern about paternal exposure to environmental and chemotherapeutic agents which may have adverse effects on offspring. However, a long-term effect of most chemotherapy drugs is disruption of germ cells and a large reduction in sperm count and quality. Germ cells are unique cells in the body that transfer genetic information between generations. The chance of recovery of germ cells following cytotoxic insult, and also the extent and speed of recovery, are associated with the type of agents used and the dose received. Treatment with cytotoxic chemotherapy is associated with significant gonadal damage in men, causing adverse effects in the reproductive system and stress in germ cell development. Many studies have shown that men especially young patients receiving chemotherapy regimens for the treatment of different types of cancers are associated with infertility. However, the impact of different therapies on fertility with patients prior to treatment and a consideration of fertility-preserving measures before and during treatment should be discussed.

Male subfertility and infertility can be caused by somatic or psychosocial factors. This study mainly will discuss the phase specificity of the susceptibility of germ cells to genetic damage induced by chemotherapy agents.

Keywords: DNA damage; male germ cells; infertility; chemotherapy; spermatogenesis.

Introduction

Reproductive toxicity has been an area of increasing interest and concern over the past decade, as human exposure to a substantial number of possible toxicants like environmental pollutants, industrial products, and drugs (Pasqualotto, Lucon, Sobreiro, Pasqualotto, & Arap, 2004). Thus, the effect that these drugs and toxic agents can have on the male reproductive system, in young patients exposed to chemotherapy drugs is of concern whether these anticancer agents can induce male germ cell mutations which lead to transmissible genetic damage in posttreatment progeny (Signorello *et al.*, 2012). Infertility is a particular focus among all reproductive toxic effects [2]. Onco-infertility is identified as an important issue in cancer survivors in the reproductive age range (Surampudi *et al.,* 2015). Epidemiological studies have reported that approximately 50 % of infertility cases have found to be due to male-related factors (Baysal *et al.,* 2017). Drugs are considered one of the main factors that could lead to infertility in men by a reduction in the quality of semen (Liu, Bao, Liu, Zhang, & Shen, 2012). Treatment and preservation of chemotherapy induced onco-infertility has become increasingly important and is a dynamic research area in reproductive biology (Duffy, Allen, Dube, & Dickersin, 2012). This issue may become more important in young man where sperm banks are not available (Dohle, 2010; Loren *et al.,* 2013; Trost & Brannigan, 2012). There is concern that males of young age exposed to chemotherapy drugs and toxicants, mainly for the treatment of testicular and blood cancers, could have adverse effects on testicular function and the reproductive system and development (Dere, Anderson, Hwang, & Boekelheide, 2013). Preconceptional exposure to chemotherapy drugs and chemicals results in disruption of spermatogenesis, embryo loss, birth defects, and a reduction in sperm count and quality (Brinkworth, 2000; Dere *et al.,* 2013). In addition, exposure to chemotherapy drugs to males prior to conception may affect the outcome of subsequent progeny due to a drug induced fault in the spermatozoa itself, including an effect on the DNA and chromosomal proteins. There are different mechanisms by which chemotherapeutic agents influence male reproduction including non-genetic effects such as the presence of a drug in the seminal fluid, genetic effects such as gene mutation or chromosomal abnormalities, and epigenetic effects such as altered gene expression and DNA methylation (Trasler & Doerksen, 1999). The genetic consequences of paternal exposure to chemotherapy drugs may cause abnormalities in sperm, thus contributing to infertility and adverse maternal and offspring outcomes (Codrington, Hales, & Chen, 2004). Studies have been reported that show significant associations among sperm DNA damage and effects on fertilization in addition to pregnancy rates (Brachtchenko *et al.,* 2015; Jiang, He, Wang, & Zhu, 2011). Screening for sperm DNA damage can offer valuable evidence in cases of male idiopathic infertility and males following assisted reproduction (Agarwal & Said, 2003).

The molecular mechanisms by which these chemotherapeutic agents induce damage and activate apoptosis in each germ cell type are not fully developed. The current chapter will discuss the present knowledge of the effects of cytotoxic chemotherapy agents as induces of DNA damage in the germ cells, and outline the molecular mechanisms by which these compounds target phase specificity in germ cells. We shall also discuss the different vulnerabilities in response to DNA damage among the different germ cell phases to various chemotherapeutic agents. Unravelling the molecular mechanisms involved due to chemotherapy in both somatic and germ cells could lead to new targets for treatment, thereby improving the quality of sperm and reproductive organs in patients suffering from infertility.

Damage in male germ cells after exposure to chemotherapeutic agents

Evidence accumulated from several human epidemiological studies and animal studies have indicated that environmental agents can interact with the male genome, causing specific types of genetic alteration in spermatozoa that affect fertility (Olsen, Lindeman, Wiger, Duale, & Brunborg, 2005). Spermatogenesis is a highly ordered and regulated differentiating system. The spermatogenic stem cells differentiate during division of spermatogonia to form spermatocytes that undergo two meiotic divisions to give rise to spermatids that mature into functional spermatozoa (L. D. Russell, Chiarini-Garcia, Korsmeyer, & Knudson, 2002). Germ cells proliferate via a series of mitotic and meiotic complex divisions in which genetic stability is maintained by the accurately controlled DNA duplication and repair, and different mechanisms of the cell cycle (Ruwanpura, McLachlan, & Meachem, 2010).

Germ cell development involves not only mitotic and meiotic divisions but a balance between differentiation or dying and requiring master regulators and a variety of hormones including, follicle-stimulating hormone (FSH) and testosterone. The stability of the germ cell is regulated by the balance between death and division, which are affected by many biochemical factors. The highly synchronized nature of germ cells requires accurate functional and junctional links between the Sertoli and germ cells (Kierszenbaum & Tres, 2004). Any alterations at the fine regulation in any of these processes may lead to testicular diseases (Giampietri *et al.*, 2005). Exposure to reproductive cytotoxic agents can induce damage in somatic testicular and germ cells at different phases of differentiation, resulting in a temporary or permanent damage to fertility (Fossa & Magelssen, 2004; Zhang, Shao, & Meistrich, 2007). Exposure of germ cells to mutagens can induce DNA damage, resulting to fetal abnormalities, heritable mutations and genetic disorders in the offspring (L. Russell, Selby, Von Halle, Sheridan, & Valcovic, 1981). Germ cells phases have different unique properties in DNA synthesis, chromosome-related proteins, and DNA repair capability. The susceptibility of cells to induced mutation could be affected by such factors due to the accessibility of DNA to carcinogenic/mutagenic insults, the intermission between DNA damage and the next round of DNA synthesis, and the ability of cells to repair DNA damage (Cordelli *et al.*, 2003). Damage in germ cells is associated with the type and dose of chemotherapy drugs and the period of treatment. Male germ cells are susceptible to environmental gentoxicant and chemotherapy drugs at different phases of spermatogenesis. Unrepaired DNA damage during spermatogonial division processes could be fixed as mutations through replication giving rise to clones of mutated spermatozoa. The last stage of the spermatogenic phase is unable to replicate, and fixation of premutagenic DNA damage as mutations rely on replication-independent DNA synthesis related to DNA repair (Olsen *et al.*, 2005). Studies have reported that the levels of DNA damage and DNA repair related genes in response to DNA damage are dependent on the type of germ cells and the gentoxicant *in vitro* (Habas, Anderson, & Brinkworth, 2016b; Habas, Brinkworth, & Anderson, 2017b). Thus, the most susceptible germ cells to chemotherapeutic drugs are cells those undergoing continuous mitotic activities, which are the rapidly dividing differentiating spermatogonia (Kangasniemi *et al.*, 1990; Meistrich, 2013). Studies have shown that the initiation phase of germ cells is highly susceptible to chemotherapy drugs such as doxorubicin (Habas, Anderson, & Brinkworth, 2017; Hou *et al.*, 2005). The damage to spermatogonial cells can lead to a alterations of later phases of germ cells and a reduction of sperm counts (Drumond *et al.*, 2011).

Cytotoxic chemotherapy agents target phase specificity of germ cell

Germ cells are unique cells that transfer genetic information from generation to generation. Damage in spermatogenesis as a primary morphological events a common indicator after administration of cytotoxic chemicals (Vidal & Whitney, 2014). Following exposure to cytotoxic chemotherapy agents, histopathological changes occur in the testis, which are dependent on drugs used and cell types. In the testicular cells, different target cells for reproductive cytotoxic agents are somatic cells (Leydig and Sertoli cells) and germ cells (spermatogonia, spermatocytes and spermatids). A previous study has shown that each spermatogenic cells isolated from rodent animals *in vitro* can selectively be targeted by specific reproductive cytotoxic agents (Figure 1). Treatment with cytotoxic chemotherapy has been found to be associated with significant gonadal damage in males. Among the commonly used chemotherapy drugs, alkylating agents have been associated most often with infertility. In males receiving procarbazine-containing regimens for the treatment of lymphomas are most of patients become infertile (Howell & Shalet, 2005). In most male patients receiving treatment with other cytotoxic chemotherapy drugs such as doxorubicin hydrochloride (adriamycin), bleomycin and dacarbazine there seems to be a significant benefit, with a return to normal fertility in the vast majority of patients (Howell & Shalet, 2005). Ethane-1, 2-dimethanesulfonate is a cytotoxic alkylating agent that targets Leydig cells and causes ablation, a rapid decrease in testosterone levels, and a typical pattern of spermatogenesis loss (Bartlett, kerr, & sharpe, 1986). Cisplatin is one of the most important chemotherapeutic agents that is reported for its activity against testicular germ cell cancer (Boekelheide, 2005). It has been reported that exposure to cisplatin caused the dilatation of the endoplasmic reticulum, changes the structure of mitochondria and an increase in the numbers of inclusion bodies in Leydig and Sertoli cells (Aydiner, Aytekin, & Topuz, 1997). Cisplatin induces cross-links, including DNA cross-links resulting in its antineoplastic influence (Malina, Novakova, Vojtiskova, Natile, & Brabec, 2007).

Doxorubicin is commonly used drug employed in the treatment of solid or soft cancers. Doxorubicin induces DNA damage and apoptosis in male germ cells (Habas, Anderson, & Brinkworth, 2017; Jia *et al.*, 2015). Doxorubicin can intercalate into germ cell DNA through division and causes cellular death in the seminiferous epithelium as well as affecting the number of germ cells located in the vicinity of the basement membrane of the testis (Vendramini, Sasso-Cerri, & Miraglia, 2010). It can also intercalate with DNA and results in the inhibition of topoisomerase II (Topo II) activity, leading to replication-dependent, site-selective double-strand breaks in DNA (Quiles, Huertas, Battino, Mataix, & Ramirez-Tortosa, 2002). A study has shown that spermatogonia and spermatocytes are highly susceptible target cells (Habas, Anderson, *et al.*, 2017). Phthalates, such as di-(2-ethylhexyl) phthalate, are universal environmental toxicants able to induce testicular atrophy. Sertoli cell exposure to mono-(2-ethylhexyl) phthalate (MEHP) has shown it causes dysfunction, due its active metabolite and results in a rapid depletion of germ cell apoptosis (Boekelheide, 2005). Alkylating agents are electrophilic chemicals which have the ability to attack the nucleophilic centres of DNA, resulting in base mismatch during DNA replication (Friedberg, Walker, Siede, & Wood, 2005). Alkylating agents which are monofunctional and bifunctional include single or double-reactive groups (Jenkins *et al.*, 2005). N-ethyl-n-nitrosourea (ENU) and N- methyl-n-nitrosourea (MNU) cause mutations that affect spermatogonial stem cells (L. B. Russell, Hunsicker, & Russell, 2007). A recent studies in rodents have also shown that germ cells treated with ENU and MNU have the greatest response in spermatogonial stem cells (Habas, Anderson, & Brinkworth, 2016a; Habas, Brinkworth, & Anderson, 2017a). Cytotoxic nucleoside analogues including 6-mercaptopurine (6-MP) and 5-bromo-2'-deoxyuridine (5-BrdU) have been found to be associated with DNA damage and apoptosis. 6-MP is metabolized by the thiopurine methyltransferase (TPMT) enzyme, resulting in the depletion of cytotoxicity as a result of its incorporation into DNA synthesis (Kanemitsu *et al.*, 2009). 5-BrdU is a thymidine analogue that is combined into replicating DNA, resulting in specific-locus mutations (Kagawa, Noge, Higashigawa, & Komada, 2008). Germ cell exposure to 6-MP showed the greatest response in DNA damage and apoptosis in early meiotic spermatocytes (Habas *et al.*, 2016a). Methyl methanesulphonate (MMS) and ethyl methanesulphonate (EMS) are the common species of anticancer drugs that employed to treat different types of cancer (Kondo, Takahashi, Ono, & Ohnishi, 2010). Germ cell exposure to MMS and EMS causes a high incidence of DNA damage and apoptosis in spermatids in rodents (Habas, Brinkworth, *et al.*, 2017a).

Defects or delay at all stages of the spermatogenesis process lead to infertility. Targeted cytotoxic chemotherapy agents in rodents provide great tools to study these phases, and examine the impact of gene function on specific phases and thus have provided new insights into the origins of male infertility (Yauk *et al.*, 2015).

Evaluation of male germ cell cytotoxic chemotherapy agents

Sperm DNA integrity is essential for the accurate transmission of genetic information and maintaining the reproductive function in males, development of embryos and fertilization (Spano *et al.*, 2000). Any changes of chromatin structural abnormalities and DNA damage could lead to male infertility. There are several methods used to evaluate the integrity of DNA in male germ cells induce by cytotoxic chemotherapy agents, which are considered an independent measure of DNA quality that may yield better diagnostic and prognostic methods. The mechanisms of cytotoxic chemotherapy damage on specific target cells in spermatogenesis and the molecular mechanism of drug action by which these cytotoxic chemotherapy agents induce DNA damage in germ cells are not well known. Understanding the molecular mechanisms of chemotherapeutic drug action and DNA damage in each cell type in germ cells is an important step toward the understanding of novel therapeutic treatment to regulator accelerated DNA damage or apoptosis during abnormal germ cell development. A molecular biological study of chemotherapy agent mechanisms in germ cells requires the isolation and enrichment of these different cell types. Isolation of germ cell types using STA-PUT velocity sedimentation has recently shown that a number of chemotherapy agents can be tested in different cell types of germ cells. This high yield method during short a time frame at a reasonable cost according to the principles of the 3Rs, replacement, refinement and reduction is now available (Habas *et al.*, 2016a).

Chemotherapeutic targets in rapidly dividing cancer cells by directly or indirectly inducing different types of DNA damage are required (Woods & Turchi, 2013). Personalized medicine should be modified to individual patients utilizing genetic or other information (Ogino, Fuchs, & Giovannucci, 2012). Predicting clinical responses to chemotherapeutics drugs is a main concern in treatment of cancers (Tofilon, Basic, & Milas, 1985). There are a number of methods available to predict chemotherapy responses. Methods relying on polymerase chain reaction (PCR) can display genes for enzymes that disturb metabolism of these drugs (Denkert *et al.*, 2013). Reliable and rapid results are urgently needed. The influence of a chemotherapeutic drug cannot always be predicted by assessing gene expression (Borst & Wessels, 2010). The single cell gel electrophoresis also known as the Comet assay is a rapid and highly sensitive test and allows the detection of both single strand and double strand DNA damage (ASSAY(OECD 489), 2014; Tice *et al.*, 2000). *In vivo* test systems, carcinogens and non-carcinogens have been assessed by several methods but the micronucleus assay also provides the sound data to estimate the carcinogenic potential of compounds (ASSAY(OECD 487), 2012; Ashby, 1985). Chromatin condensation and internucleosomal DNA fragmentation as well as cell shrinkage and shedding of apoptotic bodies are commonly identifying hallmarks of programmed cell death (Nagata, Nagase, Kawane, Mukae, & Fukuyama, 2003). These features can be detected by terminal deoxyncleotidyl transferase (TdT) – mediated deoxyuridine triphosphate (dUTP) nick end-labelling (TUNEL) assay (Gavrieli, Sherman, & Ben-Sasson, 1992). Chemotherapy agents can induce oxidative stress in organ systems. Oxidative stress during cancer chemotherapy induces lipid peroxidation and generates many electrophilic aldehydes that can attack numerous cellular targets (Conklin, 2004). A combination of the STAPUT method and theses methods can provide better understanding of molecular mechanisms of cancer chemotherapy and their side effects in each cell type in spermatogenic cells that may cause to idiopathic subfertility.

Concluding remarks

Men undergoing chemotherapy treatment for cancer are susceptible to the toxic and enduring reproductive effects of these cytotoxic chemotherapy agents. These concerns are particularly significant for couples considering having children. This is because gonadotoxic effects may not only impact their progeny, but also their generation. Long term after effects of chemotherapy for cancer during childhood has been found to be related to increased risk of psychosocial problems often associated with infertility issues. However, oncologists should be prepared to discuss the negative impact of cancer chemotherapy on the reproductive system with their patients, including both the children and their parents where/when necessary.

Table 1: Different responses and properties of DNA-damaging in germ cells compounds used in cancer chemotherapies

Drug	Mode of Action	Target cells	References
EDS	Hormone insufficiency response	Leydig cells	(Sadate-Ngatchou, Pouchnik, & Griswold, 2004)
MEHP	Metabolite in these cells	Sertoli cells	(Richburg, Nanez, Williams, Embree, & Boekelheide, 2000)
Doxorubicin	Topoisomerase II poison	Spermatogonia	(Habas, Anderson, & Brinkworth, 2017a)
ENU	Induced mutation	Spermatogonia	(Habas *et al.*, 2017a)
MNU	Induced mutation	Spermatogonia	(Habas, Anderson, & Brinkwor, 2016a)
6-MP	Interferes with nucleic acid synthesis by inhibiting purine metabolism	Spermatocytes	(Habas *et al.*, 2016a)
5 BrdU	Incorporated into synthesized DNA of replicating cells	Spermatocytes	(Habas *et al.*, 2016a)
MMS	Methylates DNA predominantly on N7 -deoxyguanosine	Spermatids	(Habas *et al.*, 2016a)
EMS	Reacts with guanine in DNA, forming the abnormal base O6-ethylguanine	Spermatids	(Habas *et al.*, 2016a)

EDS:Ethane 1,2-dimethane sulphonate

MEHP:Mono(2-ethylhexyl) phthalate

Doxorubicin

ENU: N-ethyl-N-nitrosourea

MNU: N-methyl-N-nitrosourea

MMS: Methyl methanesulfonate

EMS: Ethyl methanesulfonate

6-MP: Mercaptopurine

5-BrdU: 5-Bromo-2′-deoxyuridine

Figure legends

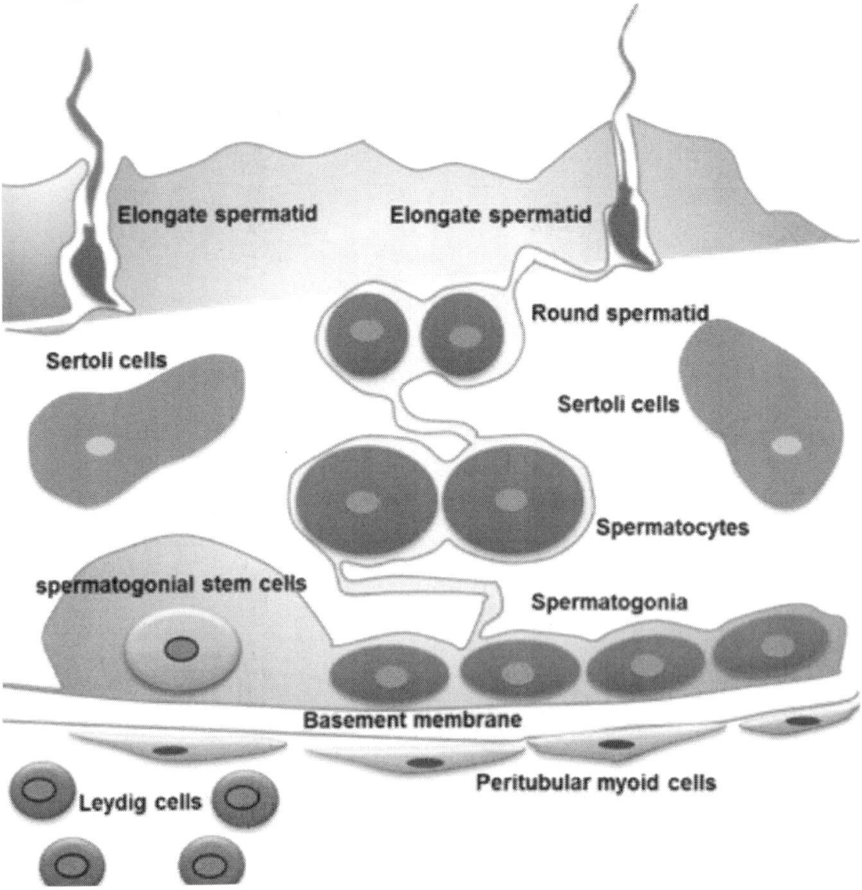

Fig. 1: Spermatogenesis is the process in which rodents produce spermatozoa from spermatogonial stem cells by way of mitosis and meiosis. The initial cells in this process are diploid spermatogonia, producing primary spermatocytes by mitosis. The primary spermatocytes divide meiotically (meiosis I) into two secondary spermatocytes; each secondary spermatocyte divides into two spermatids by meiosis II, making a total of four haploid spermatids. These develop into mature spermatozoa.

References

Agarwal, A., & Said, T. M. (2003). Role of sperm chromatin abnormalities and DNA damage in male infertility. *Human Reproduction Update, 9*(4), 331-345. doi:10.1093/humupd/dmg027

Ashby, J. (1985). Evaluation of short-term tests for carcinogens: report of the International Programme on Chemical Safety's collaborative study on in vitro assays. In *Progress in mutation research* (Vol. 5): Elsevier.

ASSAY, I. V. M. A. C. (2014). OECD Guideline for the Testing of Chemicals.

No, O. T. (2010). 487: in vitro mammalian cell micronucleus test. OECD Guidelines for the Testing of Chemicals, Section, 4.

Aydiner, A., Aytekin, Y., & Topuz, E. (1997). Effects of cisplatin on testicular tissue and the Leydig cell-pituitary axis. *Oncology, 54*(1), 74-78.

BARTLETT, J., KERR, J. B., & SHARPE, R. M. (1986). The effect of selective destruction and regeneration of rat Leydig cells on the intratesticular distribution of testosterone and morphology of the seminiferous epithelium. *Journal of Andrology, 7*(4), 240-253.

Baysal, M., Ilgin, S., Kilic, G., Kilic, V., Ucarcan, S., & Atli, O. (2017). Reproductive toxicity after levetiracetam administration in male rats: Evidence for role of hormonal status and oxidative stress. *Plos One, 12*(4), e0175990.

Boekelheide, K. (2005). Mechanisms of toxic damage to spermatogenesis. *J Natl Cancer Inst Monogr*(34), 6-8. doi:10.1093/jncimonographs/lgi006

Borst, P., & Wessels, L. (2010). Do predictive signatures really predict response to cancer chemotherapy? *Cell Cycle, 9*(24), 4836-4840.

Brachtchenko, J., Moskovstev, S., Swanson, S., Shlush, E., Kan-Ool, L., Sharma, P., . . . Librach, C. L. (2015). Significant Correlation between Sperm DNA Damage and Achieving a Pregnancy in 1847 Non-Ivf Fertility Treatment Cycles. *Fertility and Sterility, 104*(3), E297-E297.

Brinkworth, M. H. (2000). Paternal transmission of genetic damage: findings in animals and humans. *International Journal of Andrology, 23*(3), 123-135. doi:DOI 10.1046/j.1365-2605.2000.00222.x

Codrington, A. M., Hales, B. F., & Chen, C. C. (2004). Spermiogenic germ cell phase-specific DNA damage following cyclophosphamide exposure. (vol 25, pg 354, 2004). *Journal of Andrology, 25*(4), 657-657.

Conklin, K. A. (2004). Chemotherapy-associated oxidative stress: impact on chemotherapeutic effectiveness. *Integr Cancer Ther, 3*(4), 294-300. doi:10.1177/1534735404270335

Cordelli, E., Fresegna, A. M., Leter, G., Eleuteri, P., Spano, M., & Villani, P. (2003). Evaluation of DNA damage in different stages of mouse spermatogenesis after testicular X irradiation. *Radiation Research, 160*(4), 443-451. doi:Doi 10.1667/Rr3053

Denkert, C., Loibl, S., Kronenwett, R., Budczies, J., von Torne, C., Nekljudova, V., . . . von Minckwitz, G. (2013). RNA-based determination of ESR1 and HER2 expression and response to neoadjuvant chemotherapy. *Annals of Oncology, 24*(3), 632-639. doi:10.1093/annonc/mds339

Dere, E., Anderson, L. M., Hwang, K., & Boekelheide, K. (2013). Biomarkers of chemotherapy-induced testicular damage. *Fertility and Sterility, 100*(5), 1192-1202. doi:10.1016/j.fertnstert.2013.09.017

Dohle, G. R. (2010). Male infertility in cancer patients: Review of the literature. *International Journal of Urology, 17*(4), 327-331. doi:10.1111/j.1442-2042.2010.02484.x

Drumond, A. L., Weng, C. C., Wang, G. S., Chiarini-Garcia, H., Eras-Garcia, L., & Meistrich, M. L. (2011). Effects of multiple doses of cyclophosphamide on mouse testes: Accessing the germ cells lost, and the functional damage of stem cells. *Reproductive Toxicology, 32*(4), 395-406. doi:10.1016/j.reprotox.2011.09.010

Duffy, C., Allen, S. M., Dube, C., & Dickersin, K. (2012). Oncologists' Confidence in Knowledge of Fertility Issues for Young Women with Cancer. *Journal of Cancer Education, 27*(2), 369-376. doi:10.1007/s13187-011-0304-1

Fossa, S. D., & Magelssen, H. (2004). Fertility and reproduction after chemotherapy of adult cancer patients: malignant lymphoma and testicular cancer. *Annals of Oncology, 15,* 259-265. doi:10.1093/annonc/mdh936

Friedberg, E. C., Walker, G. C., Siede, W., & Wood, R. D. (2005). *DNA repair and mutagenesis*: American Society for Microbiology Press.

Gavrieli, Y., Sherman, Y., & Ben-Sasson, S. A. (1992). Identification of programmed cell death in situ via specific labeling of nuclear DNA fragmentation. *The Journal of cell biology, 119*(3), 493-501.

Giampietri, C., Petrungaro, S., Coluccia, P., D'Alessio, A., Starace, D., Riccioli, A., . . . De Cesaris, P. (2005). Germ cell apoptosis control during spermatogenesis. *Contraception, 72*(4), 298-302. doi:10.1016/j.contraception.2005.04.011

Habas, K., Anderson, D., & Brinkworth, M. (2016a). Detection of phase specificity of in vivo germ cell mutagens in an in vitro germ cell system. *Toxicology, 353,* 1-10. doi:10.1016/j.tox.2016.04.001

Habas, K., Anderson, D., & Brinkworth, M. (2016b). Detection of phase specificity of in vivo germ cell mutagens in an in vitro germ cell system. *Toxicology, 353-354,* 1-10. doi:10.1016/j.tox.2016.04.001

Habas, K., Anderson, D., & Brinkworth, M. H. (2017). Germ cell responses to doxorubicin exposure in vitro. *Toxicol Lett, 265,* 70-76. doi:10.1016/j.toxlet.2016.11.016

Habas, K., Brinkworth, M. H., & Anderson, D. (2017a). In Vitro Responses to Known in Vivo Genotoxic Agents in Mouse Germ Cells. *Environmental and Molecular Mutagenesis, 58*(2), 99-107. doi:10.1002/em.22075

Habas, K., Brinkworth, M. H., & Anderson, D. (2017b). In vitro responses to known in vivo genotoxic agents in mouse germ cells. *Environmental and Molecular Mutagenesis, 58*(2), 99-107. doi:10.1002/em.22075

Hou, M., Chrysis, D., Nurmio, M., Parvinen, M., Eksborg, S., Soder, O., & Jahnukainen, K. (2005). Doxorubicin induces apoptosis in germ line stem cells in the immature rat testis and amifostine cannot protect against this cytotoxicity. *Cancer Research, 65*(21), 9999-10005. doi:10.1158/0008-5472.CAN-05-2004

Howell, S. J., & Shalet, S. M. (2005). Spermatogenesis after cancer treatment: damage and recovery. *JNCi Monographs, 2005*(34), 12-17.

Jenkins, G., Doak, S., Johnson, G., Quick, E., Waters, E., & Parry, J. (2005). Do dose response thresholds exist for genotoxic alkylating agents? *Mutagenesis, 20*(6), 389-398.

Jia, Y., Ohanyan, A., Lue, Y. H., Swerdloff, R. S., Liu, P. Y., Cohen, P., & Wang, C. (2015). The effects of humanin and its analogues on male germ cell apoptosis induced by chemotherapeutic drugs. *Apoptosis, 20*(4), 551-561. doi:10.1007/s10495-015-1105-5

Jiang, H., He, R. B., Wang, C. L., & Zhu, J. (2011). The relationship of sperm DNA fragmentation index with the outcomes of in-vitro fertilisation-embryo transfer and intracytoplasmic sperm injection. *Journal of Obstetrics and Gynaecology, 31*(7), 636-639. doi:10.3109/01443615.2011.590910

Kagawa, Y., Noge, I., Higashigawa, M., & Komada, Y. (2008). Combined antitumor effect of cyclophosphamide and bromodeoxyuridine in BDF1 mice bearing L1210 ascites tumors. *Biological & Pharmaceutical Bulletin, 31*(1), 57-61. doi:Doi 10.1248/Bpb.31.57

Kanemitsu, H., Yamauchi, H., Komatsu, M., Yamamoto, S., Okazaki, S., & Nakayama, H. (2009). Time-course changes in neural cell apoptosis in the rat fetal brain from dams treated with 6-mercaptopurine (6-MP). *Histology and Histopathology, 24*(3), 317-324.

Kangasniemi, M., Veromaa, T., Kulmala, J., Kaipia, A., Parvinen, M., & Toppari, J. (1990). DNA-Flow Cytometry of Defined Stages of Rat Seminiferous Epithelium - Effects of 3 Gy of High-Energy X-Irradiation. *Journal of Andrology, 11*(3), 312-317.

Kierszenbaum, A. L., & Tres, L. L. (2004). The acrosome-acroplaxome-manchette complex and the shaping of the spermatid head. *Archives of Histology and Cytology, 67*(4), 271-284. doi:Doi 10.1679/Aohc.67.271

Kondo, N., Takahashi, A., Ono, K., & Ohnishi, T. (2010). DNA damage induced by alkylating agents and repair pathways. *J Nucleic Acids, 2010.*

Liu, L., Bao, H., Liu, F., Zhang, J., & Shen, H. (2012). Phthalates exposure of Chinese reproductive age couples and its effect on male semen quality, a primary study. *Environment international, 42*, 78-83

Loren, A. W., Mangu, P. B., Beck, L. N., Brennan, L., Magdalinski, A. J., Partridge, A. H., . . . Oktay, K. (2013). Fertility Preservation for Patients With Cancer: American Society of Clinical Oncology Clinical Practice Guideline Update. *Journal of Clinical Oncology, 31*(19), 2500-+. doi:10.1200/Jco.2013.49.2678

Malina, J., Novakova, O., Vojtiskova, M., Natile, G., & Brabec, V. (2007). Conformation of DNA GG intrastrand cross-link of antitumor oxaliplatin and its enantiomeric analog. *Biophysical Journal, 93*(11), 3950-3962. doi:10.1529/biophysj.107.116996

Meistrich, M. L. (2013). Effects of chemotherapy and radiotherapy on spermatogenesis in humans. *Fertility and Sterility, 100*(5), 1180-1186.

Nagata, S., Nagase, H., Kawane, K., Mukae, N., & Fukuyama, H. (2003). Degradation of chromosomal DNA during apoptosis. *Cell Death and Differentiation, 10*(1), 108-116. doi:10.1038/sj.cdd.4401161

Ogino, S., Fuchs, C. S., & Giovannucci, E. (2012). How many molecular subtypes? Implications of the unique tumor principle in personalized medicine. *Expert review of molecular diagnostics, 12*(6), 621-628.

Olsen, A.-K., Lindeman, B., Wiger, R., Duale, N., & Brunborg, G. (2005). How do male germ cells handle DNA damage? *Toxicol Appl Pharmacol, 207*(2), 521-531.

Pasqualotto, F. F., Lucon, A. M., Sobreiro, B. P., Pasqualotto, E. B., & Arap, S. (2004). Effects of medical therapy, alcohol, smoking, and endocrine disruptors on male infertility. *Revista do Hospital das Clínicas, 59*(6), 375-382.

Quiles, J. L., Huertas, J. R., Battino, M., Mataix, J., & Ramirez-Tortosa, M. C. (2002). Antioxidant nutrients and adriamycin toxicity. *Toxicology, 180*(1), 79-95. doi:Pii S0300-483x(02)00383-9

Doi 10.1016/S0300-483x(02)00383-9

Russell, L., Selby, P., Von Halle, E., Sheridan, W., & Valcovic, L. (1981). The mouse specific-locus test with agents other than radiations: interpretation of data and recommendations for future work. *Mutation Research/Reviews in Genetic Toxicology, 86*(3), 329-354.

Russell, L. B., Hunsicker, P. R., & Russell, W. L. (2007). Comparison of the genetic effects of equimolar doses of ENU and MNU: While the chemicals differ dramatically in their mutagenicity in stem-cell spermatogonia, both elicit very high mutation rates in differentiating spermatogonia. *Mutation Research-Fundamental and Molecular Mechanisms of Mutagenesis, 616*(1-2), 181-195. doi:10.1016/j.mrfmmm.2006.11.003

Russell, L. D., Chiarini-Garcia, H., Korsmeyer, S. J., & Knudson, C. M. (2002). Bax-dependent spermatogonia apoptosis is required for testicular development and spermatogenesis. *Biology of Reproduction, 66*(4), 950-958. doi:DOI 10.1095/biolreprod66.4.950

Ruwanpura, S. M., McLachlan, R. I., & Meachem, S. J. (2010). Hormonal regulation of male germ cell development. *Journal of Endocrinology, 205*(2), 117-131. doi:10.1677/Joe-10-0025

Signorello, L. B., Mulvihill, J. J., Green, D. M., Munro, H. M., Stovall, M., Weathers, R. E., . . . Boice, J. D. (2012). Congenital Anomalies in the Children of Cancer Survivors: A Report From the Childhood Cancer Survivor Study. *Journal of Clinical Oncology, 30*(3), 239-245. doi:10.1200/Jco.2011.37.2938

Spano, M., Bonde, J. P., Hjollund, H. I., Kolstad, H. A., Cordelli, E., Leter, G., & Stu, D. F. P. P. (2000). Sperm chromatin damage impairs human fertility. *Fertility and Sterility, 73*(1), 43-50. doi:Doi 10.1016/S0015-0282(99)00462-8

Surampudi, P., Chang, I., Lue, Y., Doumit, T., Jia, Y., Atienza, V., . . . Wang, C. (2015). Humanin protects against chemotherapy-induced stage-specific male germ cell apoptosis in rats. *Andrology, 3*(3), 582-589. doi:10.1111/andr.12036

Tice, R. R., Agurell, E., Anderson, D., Burlinson, B., Hartmann, A., Kobayashi, H., . . . Sasaki, Y. F. (2000). Single cell gel/comet assay: Guidelines for in vitro and in vivo genetic toxicology testing. *Environmental and Molecular Mutagenesis, 35*(3), 206-221. doi:Doi 10.1002/(Sici)1098-2280(2000)35:3<206::Aid-Em8>3.0.Co;2-J

Tofilon, P. J., Basic, I., & Milas, L. (1985). Prediction of in vivo tumor response to chemotherapeutic agents by the in vitro sister chromatid exchange assay. *Cancer Research, 45*(5), 2025-2030.

Trasler, J. M., & Doerksen, T. (1999). Teratogen update: paternal exposures—reproductive risks. *Teratology, 60*(3), 161-172.

Trost, L. W., & Brannigan, R. E. (2012). Oncofertility and the Male Cancer Patient. *Current Treatment Options in Oncology, 13*(2), 146-160. doi:10.1007/s11864-012-0191-7

Vendramini, V., Sasso-Cerri, E., & Miraglia, S. M. (2010). Amifostine reduces the seminiferous epithelium damage in doxorubicin-treated prepubertal rats without improving the fertility status. *Reproductive Biology and Endocrinology, 8*. doi:Artn 3

10.1186/1477-7827-8-3

Vidal, J. D., & Whitney, K. M. (2014). Morphologic manifestations of testicular and epididymal toxicity. *Spermatogenesis, 4*(2), e979099. doi:10.4161/21565562.2014.979099

Woods, D., & Turchi, J. J. (2013). Chemotherapy induced DNA damage response: convergence of drugs and pathways. *Cancer Biol Ther, 14*(5), 379-389. doi:10.4161/cbt.23761

Yauk, C. L., Aardema, M. J., van Benthem, J., Bishop, J. B., Dearfield, K. L., DeMarini, D. M., . . . Douglas, G. R. (2015). Approaches for identifying germ cell mutagens: Report of the 2013 IWGT workshop on germ cell assays. *Mutation Research-Genetic Toxicology and Environmental Mutagenesis, 783*, 36-54. doi:10.1016/j.mrgentox.2015.01.008

Zhang, Z., Shao, S., & Meistrich, M. L. (2007). The radiation-induced block in spermatogonial differentiation is due to damage to the somatic environment, not the germ cells. *Journal of Cellular Physiology, 211*(1), 149-158. doi:10.1002/jcp.20910

Chapter 9

Molecular Diagnostics-Nucleic Acid based Techniques for Modern Diagnostic Tools

Yachana Jha

Assistant Professor Biotechnology, N. V. Patel College of Pure & Applied Sciences, S. P. University, V.V. Nagar, Anand (Gujarat), India.

Email: yachanajha@ymail.com

Abstract

Molecular diagnostics is a dynamic and transformative area of diagnostics, leading to insights in research and treatment in many disease states that are revolutionizing health care. There are many progresses made in human genomics, which have changed the approach towards diagnosis and therapeutic diseases. There are many ways discovered for curing inherited genetic diseases as well as settling crucial diagnostic troubles. Nucleic acid-based diagnostics are widely used in centralized laboratory settings to diagnose both infectious and non-infectious conditions. Nucleic acid-based diagnostics are used to diagnose a wide range of conditions, including cancer, genetic markers associated with a high risk of cancer, and genetic diseases (e.g. cystic fibrosis). The basic application is to determine changes in sequence or expression levels in crucial genes involved in disease. The scope of molecular diagnostics in molecular medicine could be expanded well beyond current nucleic acid testing. It plays an important role in practice of medicine, public health, pharmaceutical industry, forensics and biological warfare and drug discovery. The molecular diagnostic marketplace offers a growth opportunity given the interest in utilizing molecular tools to precisely target therapeutics. Molecular diagnostics detect and measure the presence of genetic material or proteins associated with a specific health condition or disease, helping to uncover the underlying mechanisms of disease and enabling clinicians to tailor care at an individual level – facilitating the practice.

1. Introduction

A successful healthcare system includes prefect and precise diagnostic tests, to acquire the best information for doctors to make right decisions about the individual. Health care basically dependents on detecting, diagnosing, treating and preventing for managing health conditions of human beings. In which diagnostics are an integral and critical part of our health care system, as the results of these tests inform a wide range of medical decision making i.e. from the genetic tests that inform personalized physiological treatment to the microbial culture that identifies the right antibiotic to fight an infection. Diagnostic tests broadly classified into two primary areas of health care diagnostics, that are "in vivo" imaging and "in vitro" diagnostics. The main categories of diagnostics are clinical chemistry, immunology, hematology, microbiology and molecular diagnostics.

Traditional methods of diagnosis basically depend on blood screening for the presence of antibodies or antigens. Due to the delay in production of antibodies (seroconversion) or the generation of significant amount of antigens, the window period, the time between disease and ability to diagnose disease, was significantly longer for serology methods. So to overcome the limitation of serology based diagnosis, molecular diagnostics now become a growing part of the clinical laboratory. Molecular diagnostics is a subset of in vitro diagnostics techniques. The diagnostics industry continues to innovate in all of these important areas, and molecular diagnostics has captured particular attention in recent years because of the deep insights these types of tests bring to diagnosis and treatment. Molecular diagnostics is one of the most dynamic and transformative areas of diagnostics, leading to advances in research and treatment that are revolutionizing health care across a wide range of diseases and health conditions.

At every stage of healthcare depends on preventing, detecting, diagnosing, treating and managing health conditions of human beings. Molecular diagnostics are transformative and diagnostic areas leading towards research and development by specialist scientists/doctors. Scientists also make it a point to consider these molecular findings for getting best measurements. Molecular diagnosis are defined as analysis of genetic material that helps to establish diagnosis, choice of treatment, long term follow-up of a patient and family counseling. The report provides the view for molecular diagnostics in consideration to the major technologies related to molecular diversities. There are several complexities related to molecular diagnostics and these are meant to be researched even more to get appropriate results for different chronic diseases, such as cancer or tumor. It is reshaping the approach of medicines for best diagnostic and curing options. Most of the findings have DNA or RNA analysis as their base.

Human diseases are mainly caused by problems in regulation and functioning of internal body parts due to genetic impact or problems caused during their lifetime. There are many complex biological processes occurring in the body cells and there are many interactions between proteins and other elements carried out as molecular interactions. Molecular diagnostics also helps in measuring the protein material measurements or genetic associations of any disease.

There are many diseases spreading like fire in today's generation and they can be cured with tailored care for the patients. Expert doctors can facilitate the practice of personalized medicine concepts with the use of best technology and science. Continuity in technology innovation has led the scientists to produce high performance of molecular diagnostics and the future of gene-driven medications. There are increasing ways to save human life by efforts of scientists. There are diagnostics available all over the world and research institutes are responsible for holding these molecular tests. There are regular studies based on gene expression and these practices enable the large scale gene analysis for knowing about tumor cell in humans. The expression of genes is monitored well through these tumor samples. Transcriptomics and genetic studies have revealed the concept of molecular medication from many years and there are studies based on proteomics approach. There is information flowing through extra and intra-cellular molecular protein circuits with interactions of organs with circulatory systems of the body.

The benefit of identification of new biomarkers for diseases has increased through posttranslational modifications and RNA splicing. The concept of molecular medication has become very important in the development of cancer therapeutics. Cancer is included in the list of genetic diseases based on genetic mutations helping in modification of protein functioning. It has generation of proteomic patterns and it has been observed from the samples of patients being monitored for these diseases. There are integrated proteomic and genomic information defining diseases and their related therapies. There are many molecular techniques available for proteomic and genomic profiling of patients. This is done so for the major reason of development of bio markings and bio sensors for diagnosis, therapeutics and responsiveness for any new diseases. These molecule-based techniques are becoming useful in providing best tools for curing patient diseases by generating specific patient tailored therapeutics.

The healthcare centers try to make personalized approach for all kinds of diseases and craft specific medications for different people. Molecular medication mechanisms have been introduced into trend with the aim of providing safe and effective ways of diagnosing the disease and work out for its prognosis. There are many ways to allow the development of diseases by therapeutic strategies done through molecular medication process. There are many ways discovered by scientists for personalizing the medications in the best way to eliminate even chronic diseases in human beings.

Nowadays, these tests are an integral part of medicine, available for a large number of human disorders, including single gene diseases, polygenic diseases and chromosomal syndromes. Molecular theory in medicines has made it feasible to treat many chronic diseases having genetic base or non-genetic character. There is revolution made in medicines at present and insights of research have made scientists know about the effects of medications on chronic diseases. It includes all tests and methods to identify a disease and understand the predisposition for a disease analyzing DNA or RNA of an organism. Rapid advances in molecular diagnostics enable basic research and results in practical diagnostic tests.

2. Various Methods for Analysis

Molecular diagnostics is growing rapidly. Molecular diagnostic tests detect specific sequences in DNA or RNA that may or may not be associated with disease, including single nucleotide polymorphism (SNP), deletions, rearrangements, insertions and others. Clinical applications can be found in at least six general areas: infectious diseases; oncology; pharmacogenomics; genetic disease screening; human leukocyte antigen typing; and coagulation. (Grody *et al.*, 2010). Each molecular assay requires three basic steps:

i) **The extraction and purification of nucleic acid-** Many different methods of DNA analysis have been described and applied. In every laboratory, a method is chosen based on the required sensitivity, necessary equipment, number of samples and economic capacity (Khoury *et al.*, 2003). Genomic DNA is required for genetic analysis, but quantity and quality of DNA preparation may vary, depending on the requirements of the assay. Majority of laboratories routinely purify DNA for the analysis, using either the manual methods or commercial methods. The source of DNA could be any tissue with nucleated cells: usually, it is blood or bucal swab; in prenatal diagnosis these are chorionic villi samples, cells from amniotic fluid etc (Turnpenny and Ellard, 2005).

ia) Isolation of genomic DNA from blood sample

About 5 ml of blood was taken in a fresh tube, to this equal volume of solution I was added. (Solution 1 contains 1M Tris, 1 M Potassium chloride and 1M magnesium chloride), Tris helps in maintaining pH while KCl and Mgcl2 maintains the ionic balance and thus prevents the cells from bursting. The samples were mixed properly and about 72 µl of Nonidet P-40 was added, NP-40 is a detergent that ruptures the cell membrane (Salazar et al. 1998). The tube was then centrifuged at 3500 rpm for 10 minutes at 4ºC temperature. The supernatant was discarded and the pellet was dislodged from the sidewall by vortexing, add 2 ml of solution II (1M Tris, 1M KCl, 1M MgC12, 5M Nacl, 10%SDS and 0.5M EDTA), SDS is a detergent aid the process of nucleus rupture by removing lipid molecules and thereby causing disruption of nuclear membrane. EDTA on the other hand chelates magnesium ion which are essential for preserving the overall structure of the cell envelop and also inhibits cellular enzymes that could degrade DNA. The tube was mixed properly by inverting up and down and was incubated at 37 ºC for an hour. The DNA was then purified by extracting once with phenol, phenol-chloroform (1:1 v/v) and chloroform-isoamyl alcohol (24:1). These organic solvents precipitate proteins but leave the nucleic acid in aqueous solution. The cell extract is mixed gently and the layers then separated by centrifugation, precipitated protein molecules are left as a white coagulant mass at the interface between the aqueous and organic layers. The aqueous solution of the nucleic acid is then removed with a pipette. The DNA is then concentrated by the addition of 1/10th volume of 3M sodium acetate and double volume of absolute ethanol. The precipitated DNA was then taken in a fresh sterilized 1.5 ml microfuge tube and pelleted by centrifugation at 12000 rpm for about 15 minutes. The pelleted precipitate was then washed with 70% ethanol to remove the excess of salt and pellet air dried. Finally about 50 µl of TE buffer was added to dissolve DNA.

ib) Quantitative and purity analysis of isolated DNA by UV spectrophotometer

Prepare the dilution of isolated sample in TE buffer, for example if 1 ml of liquid is pipette into 9 ml of diluents, the original liquid is said to be diluted to 1/10 or 10-1. After preparation of dilution take the optical density of the solution at 260 nm and 280 nm wavelengths against the reference TE buffer (Sambrook & Russell, 2001).

Calculation:

1 OD = 50μgm/ml (Standard)

Quantity of DNA = O.D. at λ260nm × 50 × Dilution factor μgm/ml

Purity of DNA = O.D. at λ260nm / O.D. at λ280nm

Values 1.8 = Pure DNA, <1.8 =Protein contamination, > 1.8 RNA

ii) **The amplification or making copies of the nucleic acid of interest (target)-** Most of the methods of molecular analysis are based on amplification of the DNA region of interest by the polymerase chain reaction (PCR), using synthetic oligonucleotide primers and the enzyme Taq polymerase. PCR with a number of its modifications has been the golden standard in molecular genetic testing for more than 20 years (10). The PCR makes it possible to perform selective amplification from complex genomes. This technique is based on the process of denaturing a double-stranded genomic DNA template using heat. Next, the temperature is lowered to ensure that primers can anneal to their complementary sequences into the template. Thus, the elongated DNA template follows in both directions from the primer site by means of enzymatic catalysis with a thermostable DNA polymerase, generating double-stranded products (Gasser, 2006). PCR-based techniques have revolutionized many areas of study because the enzymatic amplification of DNA can be performed *in vitro* from small amounts of material.

iia) **Real time PCR-** An important and innovative modification of standard PCR is Real Time PCR, which provides elegant and effective quantification or genotyping of the tested material. Detection of the amplification range in real time is enabled by the measurement of increasing fluorescence from dye linked to DNA. This is used to measure the quantity of a target sequence (commonly in real-time). It quantitatively measures starting amounts of DNA, cDNA, or RNA. Quantitative PCR is commonly used to determine whether a DNA sequence is present in a sample and the number of its copies in the sample. *Quantitative PCR* has a very high degree of precision. Quantitative PCR methods use fluorescent dyes, such as Sybr Green, Eva Green or fluorophore-containing DNA probes, such as TaqMan, to measure the amount of amplified product in real time. It is also sometimes abbreviated to RT-PCR (*real-time* PCR). qPCR is the appropriate contractions for quantitative PCR (real-time PCR). Amplified DNA are analysed by agarose gel electrophoresis (Shokoples *et al.*, 2009).

iib) **Agarose gel electrophoresis-** Electrophoresis is rapid and relatively inexpensive method and can be easily set up in any laboratory. DNA can be checked for size and intactness, homogeneity and purity by this technique importantly, this technique is central to molecular diagnosis to check target gene amplification. Agarose forms gel and the gel pore size depends on the agarose concentration. The DNA molecules are separated by electrophoresis on the basis of their size, shape and magnitude of the net charge on the molecules. The dye ethidium bromide intercalates between the bases of RNA and DNA and fluorescence orange when irradiated with U.V.Light. Low concentration agarose gel with large pores permits fractionation of high mol. Wt. molecules and vice versa. Under an U.V. transilluminator, bands of DNA are appeared which were fluorescent orange in colour (Aaji & Borst. 1972).

iii) The detection of the amplified target or end product detection-

iiia) Recently, the MLPA (multiplex ligation-dependent probe amplification) method has been developed as rapid and effective for detection of gene deletions/duplications as well as targeted substitutions. Since 2003, several hundred commercial MLPA assays have been available for routine usage. It consists of multiple primer sets within a single PCR mixture to produce amplicons of varying sizes that are specific to different DNA sequences. By targeting multiple genes at once, additional information may be gained from a single test-run that otherwise would require several times the reagents and more time to perform. Annealing temperatures for each of the primer sets must be optimized to work correctly within a single reaction, and amplicon sizes. That is, their base pair length should be different enough to form distinct bands when visualized by gel electrophoresis.

iiib) Direct DNA sequencing-

This is an extremely sophisticated method of analysis, gives exact data about the primary structure of a particular DNA segment. Classic, famous and well established method Sanger's method of sequencing, but in the last few years several new platforms of "next generation sequencing" (NGS) have been developed, in order to provide faster and cheaper sequencing analyses (Harris et al.2013). The available personal whole genome/exome sequencing is one of the NGS goals, likely to be achieved in the next few years.

Pyrosequencing is the first alternative to the conventional Sanger method for de novo DNA sequencing. Pyrosequencing is a DNA sequencing technology based on the sequencingbysynthesis principle. It employs a series of four enzymes to accurately detect nucleic acid sequences during the synthesis. Pyrosequencing has the potential advantages of accuracy, flexibility, parallel processing, and can be easily automated. Furthermore, the technique dispenses with the need for labeled primers, labeled nucleotides, and gelelectrophoresis. Pyrosequencing has opened up new possibilities for performing sequencebased DNA analysis. The method has been proven highly suitable for single nucleotide polymorphism analysis and sequencing of short stretches of DNA. Pyrosequencing has been successful for both confirmatory sequencing and de novo sequencing. By increasing the read length to higher scores and by shortening the sequence reaction time per base calling, pyrosequencing may take over many broad areas of DNA sequencing applications as the trend is directed to analysis of fewer amounts of specimens and largescale settings, with higher throughput and lower cost. This article considers key features regarding different aspects of pyrosequencing technology, including the general principles, enzyme properties, sequencing modes, instrumentation, limitations, potential and future application.

Ion Torrent™ technology directly translates chemically encoded information (A, C, G, T) into digital information (0, 1) on a semiconductor chip. This approach marries simple chemistry to proprietary semiconductor technology; it's Watson meets Moore. The result is a sequencing technology that is simpler, faster, more cost effective and scalable than any other technology available. The semiconductor has transformed every industry it's touched. Just as the microprocessor enabled desktop computing to displace the mainframe, semiconductor technology will inevitably democratize sequencing, putting it within the reach of any lab or clinic. In nature, when a nucleotide is incorporated into a strand of DNA by a polymerase, a hydrogen ion is released as a byproduct. If there are two identical bases on the DNA strand, the voltage will be double, and the chip will record two identical bases. Because this is direct detection—no scanning, no cameras, no light—each nucleotide incorporation is recorded in seconds. The semiconductor will inevitably transform the life sciences, just as it has transformed every other industry it has touched. By creating a direct connection between chemical and digital information, Ion Torrent technology will democratize research, providing a fast, simple, scalable sequencing solution that every lab can afford. Eventually, Ion Torrent technology will also be able to provide diagnostics that are less expensive and more reliable, improving human health a Here's how the technology is used to call a base: If a nucleotide, for example a C, is added to a DNA template and is then incorporated into a strand of DNA, a hydrogen ion will be released. The charge from that ion will change the pH of the solution, which can be detected by our proprietary ion sensor. Our sequencer—essentially the world's smallest solid-state pH meter—will call the base, going directly from chemical information to digital information round the world.

iiic) Microarray analysis has emerged in the last few years as a flexible method for analyzing large numbers of nucleic acid fragments in parallel. Its origins can be traced to several different disciplines and techniques. Microarrays can be seen as a continued development of molecular biology hybridization methods, as an extension of the use of fluorescence microscopy in cell biology, as well as a diagnostic assay using capture to solid surface as a way to reduce the amount of analytes needed. The convergence of ideas and principles utilized in these fields, together with technological advancements in preparing miniaturized collections of nucleic acids on solid supports, have all contributed to the emergence of microarray and microchip technologies. Microarray format of DNA testing is also technically sophisticated, modern and has perspective, allowing more than 100.000 simultaneous microhybridization tests in one assay. Gene chips created for molecular genetic testing of some groups of diseases are based on this method (Templeton *et al.*, 2004).

iiid) Flow cytometry is a technique of quantitative single cell analysis. The flow cytometer was developed in the 1970's and rapidly became an essential instrument for the biologic sciences. Spurred by the HIV pandemic and a plethora of discoveries in hematology, specialized flow cytometers for use in the clinical laboratory were developed by several manufacturers. The major clinical application of flow cytometry is diagnosis of hematologic malignancy, but a wide variety of other applications exist, such as reticulocyte enumeration and cell function analysis. The technique of analyzing individual cells in a fluidic channel was first described by Wallace Coulter in the 1950s, and applied to automated blood cell counting. Subsequent developments in the fields of computer science, laser technology, monoclonal antibody production, cytochemistry, and fluorochrome chemistry led to the development of the flow cytometer two decades later. Because the first commercial flows cytometers were large, complex, expensive, and difficult to operate and maintain, they were primarily used in the research laboratory (Davis, 2001). However, the enormous value of the flow cytometer in the medical and biologic sciences was quickly appreciated, and its cost and complexity gradually decreased as its analytic capability increased.

iv) Southern blot- In some cases, however, time consuming classic tests of hybridization (Southern blotting, dot blot) are still the methods of choice. **Southern blot** is a method used in molecular biology for detection of a specific DNA sequence in DNA samples. Southern blotting combines transfer of electrophoresis-separated DNA fragments to a filter membrane and subsequent fragment detection by probe hybridization. Southern transfer may be used for homology-based cloning on the basis of amino acid sequence of the protein product of the target gene. Oligonucleotides are designed that are similar to the target sequence. The oligonucleotides are chemically synthesized, radio labeled, and used to screen a DNA library, or other collections of cloned DNA fragments. Sequences that hybridize with the hybridization probe are further analyzed, for example, to obtain the full length sequence of the targeted gene. Southern blotting can also be used to identify methylated sites in particular genes. Particularly useful are the restriction nucleases *MspI* and *HpaII*, both of which recognize and cleave within the same sequence.

A dot blot is a technique in molecular biology used to detect biomolecules, and for detecting, analyzing, and identifying proteins. It represents a simplification of the northern blot, Southern blot, or western blot methods. In a dot blot the biomolecules to be detected are not first separated by electrophoresis. Instead, a mixture containing the molecule to be detected is applied directly on a membrane as a dot, and then is spotted through circular templates directly onto the membrane or paper substrate. This differs from the western blot because protein samples are not separated electrophoretically. This is then followed by detection by either nucleotide probes (for a northern blot and southern blot) or antibodies (for a western blot). The technique offers significant savings in time, as chromatography or gel electrophoresis, and the complex blotting procedures for the gel are not required. However, it offers no information on the size of the target biomolecule. Furthermore, if two molecules of different sizes are detected, they will still appear as a single dot. Dot blots therefore can only confirm the presence or absence of a biomolecule or biomolecules which can be detected by the DNA probes or the antibody. Because dot blot does not require complicated instrument to operate, lots of dot blot assays are developed using antibodies with high specificity to detect different protein targets. Dot blot is also used to evaluate or screen the effectiveness of the antibodies.

Common nucleic-acid based diagnostic techniques used to diagnose infectious diseases (Weile & Knabbe, 2009) are summarized in the table below-

	Description	**Strengths**	**Weaknesses**
PCR/RT-PCR	DNA (or RNA reverse transcribed to cDNA) is amplified to detect the presence of a pathogen or host gene of interest	DNA is amplified which allows for sensitive detection	Requires highly skilled technician and laboratory equipment, amplified material can contaminate subsequent samples
Isothermal amplification	Similar to PCR, but uses simplified amplification techniques that operate at a single temperature	DNA is amplified which allows for sensitive detection, simplified isothermal amplification is more amenable to point-of-care devices/low-resource settings	Newer technology that has not been extensively clinically validated, amplified material can contaminate subsequent samples
Hybridization	DNA probes bind directly to DNA of pathogen or host gene of interest	No risk of contamination of new samples with amplified material	Because the target DNA is not amplified, technique can be less sensitive, requires highly skilled technician and laboratory equipment
Sequencing	The specific genetic code is determined for an amplified piece of DNA or the full genome of an organism	Beyond confirming the presence of a pathogen, sequencing can provide detailed information about the original and unique characteristics of the pathogen in a specific patient, not practical for low-resource settings	Sequencing techniques are expensive, time consuming, and require both a highly skilled technician and expensive laboratory equipment

3. Different types of disease diagnosed in detail

There are approximately five to six areas of molecular diagnostics carried out by hospital, reference laboratories and research institutes worldwide. Not every laboratory will perform all of them as different laboratories have their own expertise and interest. In general, they all use the same molecular tools and technologies, and they can be classified as

3a. Infectious diseases molecular testing

This involves the design of DNA probes that are directed against the specific sequences of viruses, bacteria, or parasites.

3b. Molecular oncology testing

This looks at individual cancer markers and involves detecting any derangements or alterations in either in the DNA sequence or gene expression that could be found in a tumor and nowhere else in the body.

3c. Inherited diseases molecular testing

This looks at inherited disease (genetic diseases) where one should be able to locate mutations in the cell inherited from the parents (parent).

3d. Identity testing — DNA fingerprinting

This looks at benign variations in DNA sequences that exist between people in a population and has many applications, such as, forensic testing to solve crimes, paternity testing, monitoring bone marrow transplants as it can be used to distinguish donor from recipient cells.

3e. Tissue type testing — HLA (Human Leukocyte Antigen) typing or histocompatibility testing

This is a blood test that measures substances called **antigens** on the worldwide. Not every laboratory will perform all of them as different laboratories have their own expertise and interest. In general, they all use the same molecular tools and technologies, and they can be classified as: surface of body cells and tissues. Checking the antigens can tell if donor tissue is safe (compatible) for transplant to another person. In some cases, a tissue type test may be done to see whether a person has a chance for developing certain diseases that cause the body to attack its own cells, such autoimmune diseases.

3f. Pharmacogenetics testing

This is probably the newest area which looks at benign variants in the human genome in genes that are involved in drug metabolism and alter subtly how a drug is metabolised. Such tests will be useful prior to initiation of therapy in order to choose the best or most appropriate therapy for the patient. This is a key **technologies popularly referred as "personalized medicine".**

Examples of disease diagnosed by molecular technology-

Nucleic acid-based diagnostics are used to diagnose a wide range of neglected diseases including leishmaniasis, tuberculosis, and HIV (Muldrew, 2009). FDA approved molecular tests for neglected diseases are summarized in the table below-

Disease	Manufacturer	Test Name	Method
Leishmaniasis	Cepheid - Sunnyvale, CA	Smart Leish PCR assay	RT-PCR
Tuberculosis	Gen-Probe, Inc. - San Diego, CA	AMPLIFIED™ Mycobacterium tuberculosis Direct Test (MTD)	Transcription mediated amplification (TMA)
HIV	Abbott Molecular, Inc. - Des Plaines, IL	Abbott Real-time HIV-1	Real-time RT-PCR
	Roche Molecular Diagnostics - Pleasanton, CA	AMPLICOR HIV-1 MONITOR™ Test, v1.5 COBAS AMPLICOR HIV-1 MONITOR™ Test, v1.5 COBAS® AmpliPrep/ COBAS® TaqMan HIV-1 Test	Real-time RT-PCR
	Siemens Healthcare Diagnostics - Deerfield, IL	VERSANT® HIV-1 RNA 3.0 Assay (bDNA)	Branched Chain DNA Signal Amplification

1. Screening Test Example: HPV

The fight against cervical cancer is largely a success story in the developed countries, where the introduction in the 1940s of the Papanicolaou (Pap) smear test to look for abnormal/precancerous cervical cells has driven down death rates from cervical cancer by as much as 70 per cent. The cervical is the second leading cancer of women worldwide, due to poorer access to health care in developing countries. Globally, cervical cancer affects about 500,000 women and kills about 250,000 patients. About 20 years ago, researchers discovered a link between the human papilloma virus (HPV) and cervical cancer. It is now known that, of the 100 or so genetically distinct types of HPV, about fourteen are associated with a high risk of cervical cancer, and just eight of those are responsible for almost all cases. Because HPV types are genetically identifiable, it has been possible to develop molecular diagnostic tests to screen women for the high risk types. Identifying women with these high risk types enables those women to schedule more frequent exams and can guide a physician to follow up more aggressively when a Pap test yields abnormal or inconclusive results. In this way, molecular diagnostics are driving the next advances in early detection and prevention of cervical cancer after the historical success of the Pap test. The most successful treatment of cervical cancer is delivered as a result of early detection. The use of HPV tests to identify women most likely to develop cervical cancer has the potential to revolutionize treatment of this disease.

2. Screening/Diagnostic Test Example: Cystic Fibrosis

The cystic fibrosis test is an example of a molecular diagnostic test that can be classified as a screening test or a diagnostic test, depending on when it is used.

Cystic fibrosis (CF) is an inherited chronic disease that mainly affects the lungs and digestive system and currently afflicts about 70,000 people worldwide. CF is caused by an abnormality in the CF transmembrane regulator (CFTR) gene that prevents the normal movement of chloride ions across membranes. The disease is characterized by a buildup of mucus in the lungs, pancreas, and other organs of the body. Over time, this results in patients having serious breathing and digestive difficulties and an average life expectancy that is less than 40 years. CF is seen in patients with two altered CFTR genes, one from each parent. Those that only have one copy of the altered gene are considered "carriers", and while they do not have symptoms of CF, they can pass the gene to their children. Therefore, "carrier screening" of parents-to-be or pregnant women determines their CFTR gene status and helps families adequately prepare for the results. Testing is also done on amniocentesis samples to directly assess CF status in the unborn child. Newborns are screened in all 50 states to assess CF status. One of the most common mutations causing CF is the delta F508 deletion mutation which can be detected using a number of molecular techniques.

These tests use DNA amplification methods to amplify key portions of the CFTR gene and look for the mutations that cause CF. This helps in identify carriers and thereby informs their reproductive planning. Testing can also be done on the newborn or later in childhood to diagnose CF.

3. Therapeutic Decision-Making Example: KRAS

An example of a molecular diagnostic that improves therapeutic decision-making is K-Ras testing. K-Ras is a protein, encoded by the KRAS gene, that plays a critical role in cell division, cell differentiation, and the self-destruction of cells. KRAS mutations that produce an abnormal, overactive K-Ras protein are found in pancreatic, colorectal, lung and other cancers. Detecting a KRAS mutation is used to determine patient suitability for certain therapies in colorectal and lung cancer. Anti-EG FR (epidermal growth factor receptor) drugs (Erbitux (cetuximab) and Vectibix (panitumumab)) are key therapies for those cancers, but patients whose cancers contain KRAS typically fail to respond to these anti-EG FR therapies. Therefore, Erbitux and Vectibix labels recommend against prescribing the drugs for patients with certain KRAS mutations. KRAS mutation testing is typically performed for patients with metastatic colorectal cancer or metastatic lung cancer via direct DNA sequencing or PCR and other amplification-based methods. KRAS mutation testing is just one of a growing number of examples of molecular diagnostics that help a physician's in decision making regarding appropriate treatment.

4. Therapeutic Monitoring Example: HIV

Finally, many molecular diagnostics improve monitoring and management of disease. Some of the most common monitoring molecular tests are tests for HIV viral load in patients affected with HIV. HIV viral load tests are amplification-based tests that measure the amount of HIV RNA to determine how many copies of the virus are present (measured in copies per milliliter of blood). Keeping viral levels as low as possible is key to staying healthy with HIV. Because researchers and physicians have made great strides in the care of HIV patients in the three decades since HIV was first detected, essentially transitioning it into a chronic disease in many developed countries, the HIV viral load test has become an essential tool as patients cycle through different antiretroviral therapies and develop resistance to certain therapies. Periodic HIV viral load tests indicate whether or not the disease is progressing, either because an untreated patient's immune system can no longer suppress replication of the virus, or because the therapy for a patient in treatment is no longer working. The HIV viral load test is not used for initial diagnosis (this is often done with antibody tests), but typically also is used upon initial diagnosis as a staging diagnostic, to get a first report on the progression of the disease prior to treatment.

5. Screening/Diagnostic Test Example: Oncology

The fundamental premise of cancer genomics is that cancer is caused by somatically acquired mutations, and consequently it is a disease of the genome. With the advent of NGS, cancer genomes can now be systemically studied in their entirety, an endeavour ongoing via several large scale cancer genome projects around the world, including a dedicated paediatric cancer genome project. For the child suffering from cancer this may provide many benefits including a more precise diagnosis and classification of the disease, more accurate prognosis, and potentially the identification of 'drug-able' causal mutations. Individual cancer sequencing may, therefore, provide the basis of personalised cancer management. Currently pilot projects are underway using NGS of cancer genomes in clinical practice, mainly aiming to identify mutations in tumors that can be targeted by mutation-specific drugs. his has seen NGS employed for very sensitive investigations such as interrogating foetal DNA from maternal blood or tracking the levels of tumor cells from the circulation of cancer patients (Dawson *et al.,* 2013). There are few example of molecular diagnostic being used in each of these stages are as bellow-

	Risk Assessment	**Screening**	**Diagnosis**	**Staging & Prognosis**	**Therapy Selection**	**Monitoring**
Description	Diagnostic tests to complement traditional risk factors	Applied to high-risk patient to identify disease early	Use for definitive diagnosis and general cancer typing	Assess severity and/or risk of recurrence Inform adjuvant chemo decision	Used to predict efficacy or safety response to specific treatments	Recurrence monitoring Monitoring for treatment efficacy
Example of Molecular Diagnosis	CF carrier testing BRCA1 testing	MRSA HPV	TB CT/NG	OncoType Dx MammaPrint	BRAF KRAS Her2	BCR-ABL HIV viral load

4. Future application

There are hundreds of examples in which the latest molecular technology is being used for rapid diagnosis and to aid physicians in improving clinical outcomes for their patients. Since it is in the early stages of understanding about the complex fields of genomic and proteomics, however, the diagnostic technologies are evolving rapidly, it seems fair to say that much of the promise of molecular diagnostics is still ahead. As our understanding enhance about the complexity of diseases, there is increasing number of molecular biomarkers that must be identified to fully characterize many subsets of populations that have highly variable symptoms. New technologies are making it possible to gather more information to fully characterize the disease state, the best treatment alternatives for a patient, or in the case of infectious disease, for rapidly identify a specific pathogen out of many that could be responsible for a particular infection (e.g., respiratory viruses). Approaches that may address this need for increasing amounts of data include multiple marker or multiplexed approaches (methods that can test for multiple biomarkers in a single assay) and gene sequencing that can detect multiple defects associated with a particular subset of patients with a disease. Practical application of these methods can be challenging, due to complexity of the assays involved, but these challenges are being met by integration of molecular methods with advanced information technology (IT) and data analysis methods. New technologies also will bring greater efficiency to current methods. There has been a great deal of excitement about the promise of nanotechnology to support in the development of molecular diagnostics. Companies have commercialized technology based on gold nanoparticles that allow increased sensitivity and specificity for molecular diagnostics assays and that also enable multiplexing of assays. Other nanotechnology-enabled approaches include innovative ways to sequence DNA in which a single DNA strand is extruded through a nanopore and the sequence is "read" base pair by base pair. Finally, molecular diagnostics at the point of care is making great strides. Advancements have focused on ease of use, producing tests that can be performed in less specialized laboratories, rapid turn-around time, and appropriately small size and simplicity for resource-constrained settings. Molecular diagnostics are truly transformative technologies. Yet excitement about the future of this field must be tempered by recognition of the challenges of continuing innovation and timely patient access. The challenges include regulatory hurdles, coverage and reimbursement issues, and practical and ethical (privacy) issues associated with generating and storing large volumes of highly detailed and personal health information.

a) The fast pace of technological development in molecular diagnostics, and the rapidly growing research regarding biomarkers, challenge regulatory bodies to stay current. Clear understanding of regulatory expectations for multiplex tests, companion diagnostics and next generation sequencing as well as the increasing investments necessary to generate the clinical evidence required for approval or clearance will be integral.

b) The patenting of gene sequences currently working their way through the courts.

c) Insurance coverage and payment for diagnostics is under constant downward pressure as payers try to keep down escalating health care costs.

d) The ability and capacity to capture, store and analyze the tremendous and rapidly increasing amount of diagnostics data, particularly with gene sequencing tests, is an ongoing challenge. IT systems must have enough power to process and analyze these huge volumes of information.

e) In addition, another key challenge is the need for data standards that would speed interpretation of these complex genomic data sets and make the results relevant for specific patients.

f) This task is further complicated by the fact that the patient's medical record is often in many unconnected places, whether in multiple out-patient offices, multiple hospitals, or multiple pharmacy systems.

g) Finally, ethical questions are also being raised about the disclosure and use of genetic information. Genetic markers are being identified that can signal the propensity of a patient to develop a disease over their lifetime and the question has been raised of how, if at all, such information should be disclosed, particularly in cases where prevention or treatments are not yet available. Policy makers continue to grapple with these challenges.

References

Aaji, C. & Borst, P. The gel electrophoresis of DNA. Biochim. Biophys. Acta. 1972; 269: 192-200.

Burke W. Genetic testing. N Engl J Med 2003; 347: 1867–75.

Davis BH. Diagnostic advances in defining erythropoietic abnormalities and red blood cell diseases. Semin Hematol. 2001; 38:148-59.

Dawson SJ, Tsui DW, Murtaza M, et al. Analysis of circulating tumor DNA to monitor metastatic breast cancer. N Engl J Med 2013; 368:1199–209

Gasser RB. Molecular tools – advances, opportunities and prospects. Vet Parasitol. 2006; 136(2): 69-89.

Gibbs JN. Regulatory pathways for molecular diagnosis. Detailing the various options available and what each requires. Genetic Eng Biotech News 2008; 28(14).

Grody WW, Nakamura RM, Strom CM, Kiechle FL (eds). Molecular Diagnostics: Techniques and Applications for the Clinical Laboratory. Academic Press, Inc.; Boston, MA. 2010.

Harris SR, Cartwright EJ, Török ME, et al. Whole-genome sequencing for analysis of an outbreak of meticillin-resistant Staphylococcus aureus: a descriptive study. Lancet Infect Dis 2013; 13:130–6.

Khoury M, McCabe L, McCabe E. Population screening in the age of genomic medicine. N Engl J Med 2003; 348: 50–8.

Muldrew KL. "Molecular diagnostics of infectious diseases". Curr Opin Pediatr 2009; 21: 102-111.

Salazar LA, Hirata MH, Cavalli SA, Machado MO, Hirata RDC. Optimized Procedure for DNA Isolation from Fresh and Cryopreserved Clotted Human Blood Useful in Clinical Molecular Testing. Clinical Chemistry 1998; 44 (8): 1748-1750.

Sambrook, J. & Russell, D.W. Molecular Cloning, 3rd edition (2001).

Shokoples SE, Ndao M, Kowalewska-Grochowska K, Yanow SK. Multiplexed real-time PCR assay for discrimination of *Plasmodium* species with improved sensitivity for mixed infections. J Clin Microbiol. 2009;47(4):975-80.

Templeton KE, Scheltinga SA, Beersma MF, Kroes AC, Claas EC. Rapid and sensitive method using multiplex real-time PCR for diagnosis of infections by influenza A and influenza B viruses, respiratory syncytial virus, and parainfluenza viruses 1, 2, 3 and 4. J Clin Microbiol 2004; 42: 1564-9.

Turnpenny P, Ellard S. Emery's Elements of Medical Genetics, 12th ed. Elsevier, 2005. pp 59–72.

Weile J and Knabbe C. "Current application and future trends of molecular diagnostics in clinical bacteriology". Anal Bioanal Chem 2009; 394: 731-742.

Chapter 10

Exploring Social, Economic and Emotional aspects of Surrogacy Practice- A Retrospective Analysis of 106 Surrogate Mothers in a Single Centre in Anand

Nayana H. Patel*, Niket H. Patel, Molina Patel, Harsha K. Bhadarka, Yuvraj D. Jadeja and Nilofar R. Sodagar

Akanksha Hospital and Research Institute, A Unit of Sat Kaival Hospital Pvt. Ltd., Lambhvel- 387310. Dist: Anand Gujarat, India.

Email: nayana@ivf-surrogate.com

Abstract

Aim: Surrogacy practice in India has been discussed extensively. When the practice is considered to be extremely fulfilling for patients who are unable by themselves to have a baby, its benefits to surrogate mothers were frequently questioned in past. The present study was undertaken to explore the impact of surrogacy practice on life of surrogate mothers from different perspective.

Materials and Methods: The study was conducted from December 2016 to February 2017 and included 106 past surrogates who had delivered surrogate babies at least 6 months before. Consent was obtained from them before asking them to fill up/answer the questionnaire.

Results: The mean age of surrogate mother while practicing surrogacy was found to be 28.5 years (SD- 3.4 years). Construction of house and education of children were emerged out as the main motives of surrogates for undertaking the practice. It has been found that 57.1% surrogate have had two children while 26.7% had single child before surrogacy. Contradictory to popular belief of unemployment of surrogate's husband, in 99.1% cases, husbands of surrogates were found working at time of her being surrogate mother. Before practicing surrogacy, the highest numbers of surrogates were found to be a housewife (38.8%) while 27.7% were doing labour work. Average compensation received by surrogates was found ₹ 4,48,053/- and all surrogates were able to fulfil their motives, post surrogacy.

Conclusion: This was the first study of its kind which explores impact of surrogacy practice on various aspects of life of surrogate mothers. Rightly practiced compensated surrogacy is mutually beneficial to couple and surrogate mother.

Clinical Significance: When commercial surrogacy practice is at verge of its ban in India, the study divulges various aspects of this form of surrogacy practice in context of surrogate mothers.

Keywords: surrogacy, surrogate mother, Surrogacy (Regulation) Bill 2016

Introduction

After legalization of commercial surrogacy in the year 2002, India emerged as a new surrogacy hub. Many foreign nationals including OCIs and PIOs were choosing India as destination for surrogacy treatment over other countries due to good medical facilities, well-constructed infrastructure, and relatively lower finance for the treatment.

Though being symbiotic arrangement for both, couple and surrogate, the arrangement had gathered many controversies in past. There are numerous stories, articles and researches available on internet and print media which claim the practice to be exploitative for surrogate mothers. Also, compensation given to surrogate mothers considered as commodification of motherhood and offensive to Indian traditional value. Undesirable impact of the practice on relationship of surrogates with their husband and children were also reported in past.[1]

Surrogacy has been depicted controversial practice by thinking that only poor and illiterate women chose obligatory to opt for surrogacy to improve their economic condition and they are being treated as child producing machines so far by the unscrupulous medical fraternity and commission agents.[2]

Though surrogacy is an important fertility treatment that particularly benefits women with medical condition that makes pregnancy unsafe or impossible; it has proved to be the only source for men in same sex couple and sometimes a single parent, Indian government is stepping towards the ban to curb exploitation of poor Indian surrogate mothers by Surrogacy (Regulation) Bill, 2016. The impact of surrogacy on life of surrogate mothers has not been studied extensively yet. When the commercial surrogacy is at the verge of ban, the present study was undertaken to find out the information impact of surrogacy on life of surrogates and to know their experience with process of surrogacy and their viewpoint on the ban.

Materials and Methods

The study population included 106 past surrogates who had delivered surrogate babies at least 6 months before. The study period was spread around a time span of 3 months, from December 2016 to February 2017.

Data collection Methodology

Printed questionnaires were given to the participants. Complete privacy was ensured while filling up the details. For females who were not educated at all, help from a couple of female volunteer was taken and interview sessions were organised to help them understand the questionnaire and so as to let them answer according to their will without having an influence on the participant's answers and opinions. To avoid any biased or influence on surrogate mothers, the questionnaires filling was conducted by NGO representatives not associated with hospitals ensuring the surrogates about confidentiality of their identity. Consent was obtained from surrogates before asking them to fill up/answer the questionnaire.

Result

The present study was carried out at private infertility clinic, by contacting past surrogates to visit the hospital for the interview based study. The aim of our study was to identify the motives of surrogates behind surrogacy, to know the impact of this practice on lives of surrogates, and to know opinion of surrogate mothers on proposed ban.

The mean age of surrogate mother was found to be 28.5 years (Min-21 years, Max-35 years, SD- 3.4 years). It was found that in 76% cases, surrogate and her husband mutually decided on the decision of her becoming surrogate mother, followed by 19% cases where whole family was involved in decision making while in only 5% cases surrogate was the sole decision maker mostly because of her widow status with no adult family members. Only in 0.9% case, surrogate's husband was found to be unemployed at the time of her becoming surrogate mother.

Study showed that before practicing surrogacy, the highest number of surrogates were housewives (30.8%) while 27.7% were doing labour work, 18.5% were domestic helper, 13.8% were doing various jobs and 9.2% were self-employed as well (Figure 1).

Before surrogacy, the mean annual income of surrogate was found to be ₹ 34,188/- (Minimum: ₹ 10,000, Maximum: ₹ 1,80,000) (Table 1). Figure-2 depicts the numbers of children surrogate had before surrogacy, which revealed that highest 57.1% surrogate had two children followed by 26.7% with single baby. The study shows that most of the surrogates (72%) choose to be a surrogate mother once in their life while 27% became surrogate twice and only 1% did it thrice when it was allowed as per ART guideline.

Study also helps in finding the motives of surrogate mothers behind practicing surrogacy. Among other, construction of house and education of children were the main reasons (Figure 3).

The average of compensation surrogate received was found to be ₹ 4,48,053/- (Standard deviation: ₹ 1,29,448/-) for practicing surrogacy(Table 1). All surrogates had confirmed that they got amount as per their contract and no money from their compensation went to any agent. The study even showed that only 11% surrogate kept secrecy about being surrogate from their relatives and friend due to reason of unawareness of scientific facts behind surrogacy procedure in village population. Also, all surrogates had denied being exploited during process of surrogacy by doctor or couple and were of the opinion that surrogacy actually helped all of them in establishment of better life than before.

Furthermore, results of present study confirm that in 97.1% case surrogate did not face any trouble in relationship with their husband during and post surrogacy and this practice does not trouble her relationship. In studied population, 99% of surrogates, 6 months post surrogacy did not have any major health issue, the only health issue came to light was backache, which was in a very minor study population of 1%. When asked about opinion on ban on commercial form of surrogacy, all surrogate mothers conveyed that it would be a loss of one choice from them which had helped them immensely for betterment of life and the practice should be continued in regulated form.

Discussion

Since the legalisation of commercial surrogacy in 2002 in India, due to variety of reasons, the practice gathered controversies at regular interval. Recently, Surrogacy (Regulation) Bill, 2016 came up with ban on commercial surrogacy.

The present study was undertaken to find out the factual information of surrogacy practice, from surrogates themselves and to bring light on issues warped over the practice.

Surrogacy is an arrangement done when any female; incompetent to carry baby in her womb due to any medical condition, and so embryo developed from her/donor's egg and her husband's/donor sperm (any one gamete must belong to the couple), is implanted in another female (Surrogate). In turn, compensation is given to surrogate mother to reimburse her loss of job allowances for nine months while she nurtures the baby in her womb. However, the idea of providing compensation to surrogate mothers seems problematic to many people who wish the female to be reproductive gift-giver with only altruistic arrangements. Many a times, surrogacy practice has been compared with prostitution and act of baby selling due to its incorporation of the monetary exchanges. However, it should be considered that some sort of pressure; social or emotional, only can be the driving force behind altruistic arrangement for surrogacy which would beat the purpose of the Bill.

Many developed countries like New zeal land, Canada and recently New York, are supporting the compensation given to surrogate mothers.[3] Altruistic models have already been failed in a developed country like UK. In present study, we tried to find out motives which encourage a lady to be a surrogate mother. We found that though monetary compensation was a major factor for a lady to be a surrogate mother, but the core motives for getting money were diverse from case to case and were noble. We found that the surrogates do surrogacy not because they want money for getting luxuries; but they pursued in the "hope of better life" for their children and family. Present study revealed that the main motives for which surrogates did surrogacy was either construction of their house or buying the house and education of their children, while other being treatment of a family member, payment of loan and to keep money as deposit in bank for secure future. We also found that all surrogates, at the end of surrogacy, had a feeling of gratification as they were able to gift motherhood to a lady who herself could not be a mother. We also found that surrogates pursue surrogacy as they think it is a nobel cause and simultaneously they get good compensation for 10 months, that they cannot earn doing any other work with their qualifications. Considering surrogacy as a form of medical treatment and arrangement of compensation should be encouraged as it brings happiness in two families with arrival of new life.

In present study, the rate of unemployment, among husbands of surrogate mothers, were found to be 09%, which was not found in concordance with past study with conclusion that surrogate mothers do surrogacy out of choice as to augment the family income because of their unemployed husbands in most of the cases. However, we found that most of the surrogates were either housewives or doing labour work. The mean salary of surrogate mothers before surrogacy was found to be ₹ 34,188/- (Maximum: ₹ 1,80,000/-, Minimum: ₹ 10,000/-)

The present study revealed that majority of surrogates came to know about surrogacy by past surrogates who been either relative or friend and not an agent. As per popular belief in media and other literature, majority of part of surrogate's compensation goes to the agent. But fact differed in this centre which gives ₹ 20,000/- to the person, who brings willing surrogate and her husband to hospital, only after surrogate delivers the baby. Thus, negating the popular notion mentioned before that agents get money from compensation of surrogates. Also the study revealed that surrogacy has always been a combined decision of surrogate and her husband, except for 5% cases where the surrogate was either divorced or widow.

We found that before doing surrogacy, 57.1% surrogates had two children of her their own while 25.7% had only one kid before surrogacy while at the higher edge 16.2% had 3 kids and 1% had 4 kids before doing surrogacy. We also found that 72% surrogates prefer to be a surrogate mother only once in their life while 27% had did is twice and only 1% did it three times. The current data are not in agreement with claims stating surrogates are being treated as baby producing machine/object and surrogates repeat the practice in hope of more and more money.[5]

Also in this study we tried to light the issues related to stay of surrogates in a hostel during the pregnancy. We found that surrogates were allowed to be in contact with their families on phone, also their kids and family were allowed visit them during the stay and surrogates were also allowed to go to home for short stay up to a week or so. As per their opinion, surrogates find the arrangement of stay in surrogacy hostel/house in favour of themselves as they get complete rest during this stay and they have benefit of everyday medical check-up which reduces chances of any pregnancy associated risk. This results are opposite than published in article as research by CSR.[5]

According to one study, though the husbands do not mind their wives to act as surrogate mothers, the spouse and her children distance themselves from her after she returns home following the birth of the baby,[3] but we found completely altered trend. In contrast, we found that 99% of surrogates felt their husband became more supportive and helpful during and after surrogacy. The same study also concluded that many surrogate mothers (100 per cent in Jamnagar, 83 per cent in Surat and 40 per cent in Anand) revealed that they lost contact with friends and members of the family after opting for surrogacy. While in present study revealed different scenario in which all surrogates were in contact with their family and 89% of surrogates did not hide the fact of practicing surrogacy from any one while only 11% kept it secret from others. This data shows a kind of acceptance of practice of surrogacy amongst surrogates themselves and society. This might be because now there is more awareness of science behind surrogacy and lesser stigma allied to surrogacy process.

As 100% of surrogate mothers were able to fulfil their motive/s for which they had opted the practice of being a surrogate mother, the arrangement was found to be more positive for them rather than exploitative. None of the surrogate had felt that her rights were being exploited during the entire period and they had an opinion that this practice had provided them a choice, by which they had been able do something for their better future along with helping a couple. In their opinion, the practice of surrogacy should be continued so more needy women and couples can have synergetic outcomes.

As the present study was undertaken in single centre, it does not give wider view on situation of surrogates in other places. However, with results of this study we can conclude that the arrangement work so positively for surrogates and change their life for better by providing home and supporting the education of children, which certainly make difference in their social wellbeing.

Conclusion

Surrogacy practice is highly misunderstood. This is a first study of its kind which looks into the social economic arm of surrogacy practices in India. This study strongly highlights the fact that if rightly practiced; it could prove beneficial to both the surrogate mother who is compensated in the process which augments for family finance and the intended couple for whom this was the only hope of completing their family.

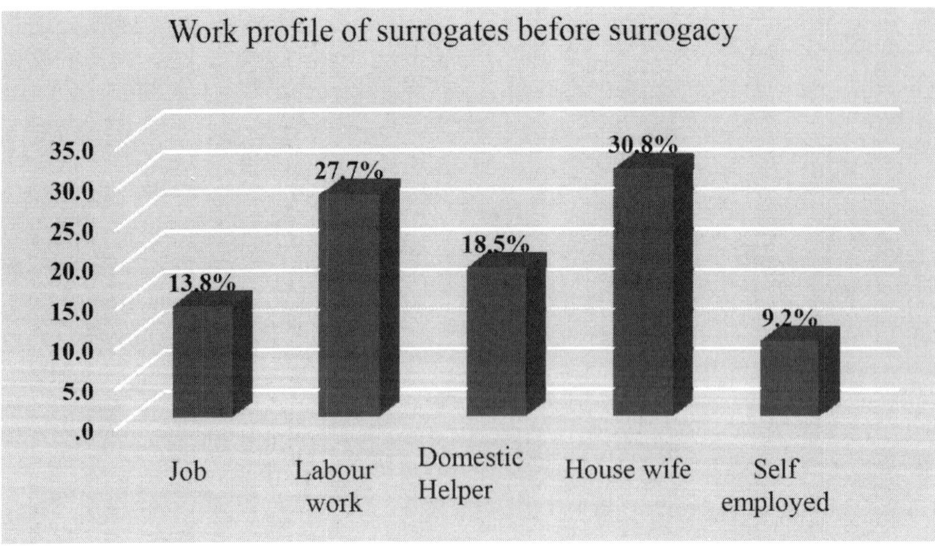

Fig. 1: Work profile of Surrogate mothers before surrogacy

In response to the current movement for ban on commercial surrogacy in India, we feel that government should take the opinion of surrogates as they are one of the most vital stakeholders in this practice and also shall consider potential of compensated surrogacy practice which made positive difference in lives of many surrogate mothers.

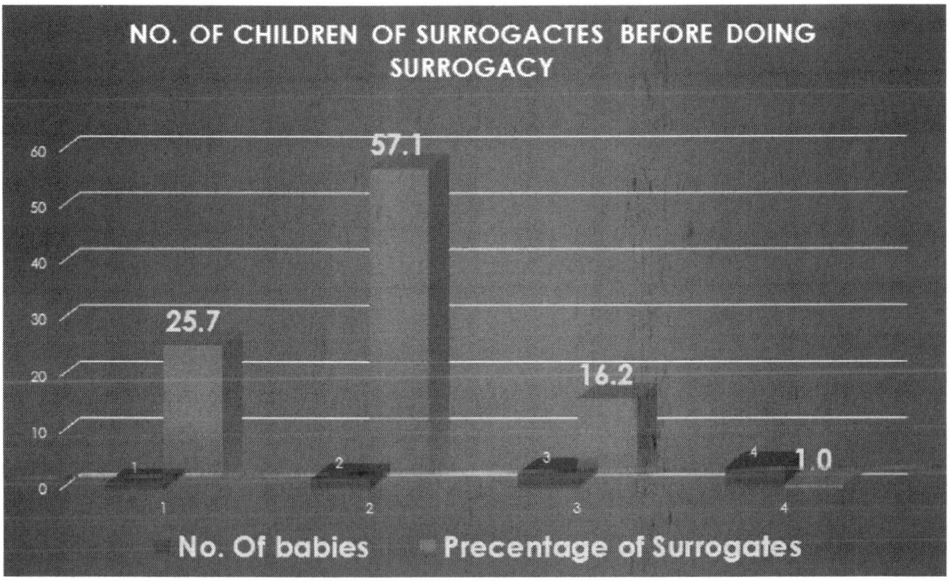

Fig. 2: Numbers of live birth surrogate have before surrogacy

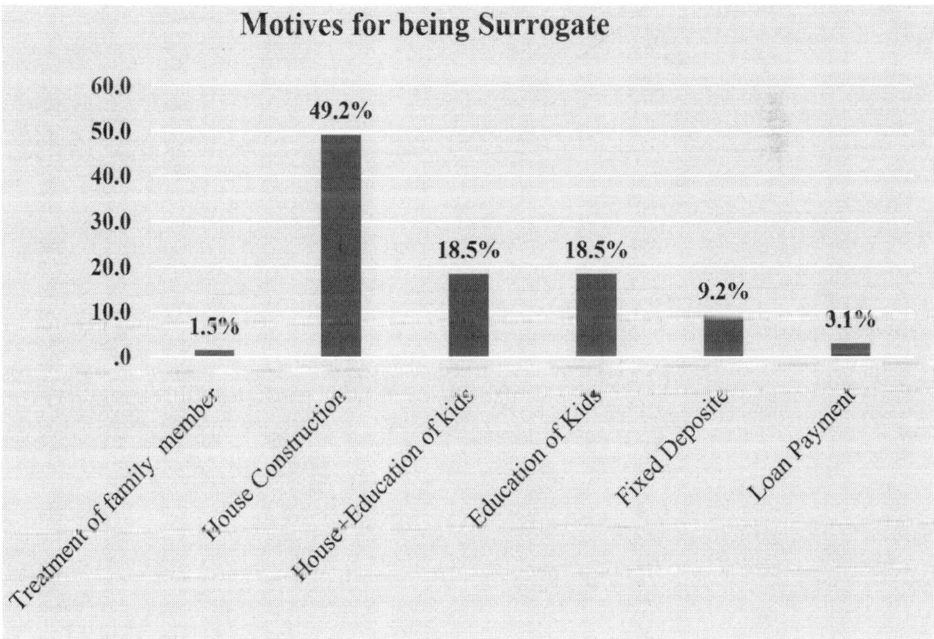

Fig. 3: Motives of surrogate mothers behind practicing surrogacy

Table 1: Compensation of surrogate mothers before and for surrogacy

Annual Income of Surrogate mothers before Surrogacy	
Mean	₹ 34,188/-
Minimum	₹ 10,000/-
maximum	₹ 1,80,000/-
Compensation Given to surrogate mothers for surrogacy	
Mean	₹ 4,48,053/-
Std. Deviation	1,29,448/-

Acknowledgement

The author heartily thanks Ms. Vinita D' Silva, the NGO member and her team of volunteers for conducting interviews of surrogate mothers which was mandatory for the study to get unbiased and non-influential answers from surrogate mothers.

Reference

Verma S. Surrogate mothers face nightmares of surrogacy. India Today. New Delhi, Mar 5, 2012. Available from:http://indiatoday.intoday.in/story/surrogate-mothers-face-nightmares-of-surrogacy/1/176504.html

Singh J, Khanna PK, Khanna A. Consensual Violence against Surrogate Mothers in Kishwar Desai's The Origins of Love. *Paripex - Ind J Res* 2015; 4(2): 90-92

Mahapatra D. Baby Manji's case throws up need for law on surrogacy. The Times of India. Aug 25, 2008. Available from: http://timesofindia.indiatimes.com/india/Baby-Manjis-case-throws-up-need-for-law-on-surrogacy/articleshow/3400842.cms

Zyl LV and Walker R. The future of surrogacy in New Zealand – Beyond the adoption model *Women's Studies Journal* 2015;29 (1): 34-55.

Verma T. What are the surrogacy laws in India: Here is everything you need to know. The Indian express. March 6, 2017. Available from: http://indianexpress.com/article/research/karan-johar-surrogate-children-yash-roohi-what-are-the-surrogacy-in-laws-in-india-here-is-everything-you-need-to-know-4555077/

Chapter 11

Genetic Testing and Privacy

Sejal Pal, Nidhi Patel and Preeti Sharma*

Assistant Professor, Department of Biotechnology, Veer Narmad South Gujarat University, Surat, Gujarat India.
Email: preetisharma26@yahoo.com*, sejalpal15@gmail.com

Abstract

Genetic testing is a type of medical test that identifies any type of changes in chromosomes, genes or proteins which gives us a basic idea about every detail in a person or his/her differential characters. One of the significant dangers of genetic technology lies in its ability to provide substantial and sensitive information about individuals to government and other organizations. There is also a persisting danger that too much reliance on genetic "discoveries" can lead to injustice by labelling individuals. Hence considering all the aspects of genetic testing, privacy laws are designed where confidentially and privacy are essential to all trusting relationship, such as that between patients and doctors, moreover in a healthcare context, patient confidentially and the protection of privacy is the foundation of the doctor–patient relationship. This concept applicable in every field associated with genetics.

There are some of the laws followed in India for Genetic testing and Privacy, still privacy problems are going on, new laws are to be made and amended. While there are no arguments with the overall bills objectives like law, enforcement, identification of missing person, dead bodies in disaster and accidents for identification, for consent use of DNA samples but the problem of developing and maintaining a Data Bank, religious aspects and other such problems are reason for critics

Introduction

Genetic testing is a type of medical test that identifies any type of changes in chromosomes, genes or proteins which gives us a basic idea about every detail in a person or his/her differential characters. Today more than 1000 genetic tests are currently in use, and more are currently being developed (1). Several methods are used for genetic testing like:

- Molecular genetic tests,
- Chromosomal genetic tests,
- Biochemical genetic tests.

Where, molecular tests mostly involve study of single gene of short lengths of DNA. Chromosomal test mainly analyses whole chromosomes or long lengths of DNA. Biochemical test involves the study of the amount and activity of proteins.

Applying genetic information can upgrade public health but at the same time as more connections are uncovered between genes, personality, future health risks and other vital information, there are chances that an individual may suffer from discrimination or other harms associated (2). In addition, genetic technology in criminal investigations have proven a powerful tool to help convict offends and to show the innocence for wrongly convicted serious crime.

One of the significant dangers of genetic technology lies in its ability to provide substantial and sensitive information about individuals to government and other organizations. There is also a persisting danger that too much reliance on genetic "discoveries" can lead to injustice by labelling individuals according to their genetically determined traits (2), for example a supposed genetic tendency for anti-social behaviour, the potential to use genetic information against any individual may discourage them from perusing information that are important for their own health benefits.

Personalized medicine is receiving importance, where patients may receive individually adapted health treatment, based on their unique genetic makeup, this conduct promises to reshape healthcare. Among all genetic testing's the most commonly opted tests among patients are as follows:

1. New-born screening
2. Diagnostic testing
3. Carrier testing
4. Forensic testing
5. Prenatal testing
6. Predictive testing

Newborn screening: Newborn screening is used just after the birth to identify genetic disorders that can be treated early in life.

Diagnostic testing: Diagnostic testing is used to identify or rule out a specific genetic or chromosomal condition.

Carrier testing: Carrier testing is used to identify people who carry one copy of a gene mutation that, when present in two copies, causes a genetic disorder.

Prenatal testing: Prenatal testing is used to detect changes in a foetus gene or chromosome.

Forensic testing: It uses DNA sequences to determine an individual for legal purposes.

Predictive and pre-symptomatic testing: This type of testing is used to detect genetic mutation related with disorders that may appear after birth, or later in life (1).

Hence considering all the aspects of genetic testing, privacy laws are designed where confidentially and privacy are essential to all trusting relationship, such as that between patients and doctors, moreover in a healthcare context, patient confidentially and the protection of privacy is the foundation of the doctor–patient relationship. This concept applicable in every field associated with genetics.

Genetic testing

Genetic tests are performed on samples such as hair, skin, blood, amniotic fluid, or other types of tissues, smear prepared from buccal cavity or tissues collected from the samples like skin, ulcer, wounds, clots on skin or blood etc. can be taken. These samples are forwarded to a laboratory where specialists look for specific changes in shape, size, specific behaviour of cells, chromosomes, DNA or proteins which depends on the suspected case and test performed accordingly (1). Newborn screening tests are done on either amniotic fluid or from skin or blood samples taken from heels or other parts of the body. If the test results are positive than only parents are given the result for further processing or testing consent which makes this testing unique from others. The additional testing would be for further confirmation for the related genetic problem.

The Nature of Genetic Information

The Assessment of Risk for Colorectal Tumours in Canada (ARCTIC) reports the key features of genetic information as follows (3):

Identifying: Genetic information is identified not only on an individual level but also at family level.

Ubiquitous: Identify genetic status and gather small amount of material rather than transitory information

Longevity: Allows for an infinite access to use and reuse technology and scientific samples.

Predictive: The predictive value of genes tends to be inherited, in the form of single gene disorder or any changes in amino acid which can lead to a genetic disorder or mutation only among few people that hold the chances of developing related disease in future.

Individual and Familial nature: Most genetic information flows between generations giving an idea of any heritable disorders or uniqueness.

Shared data: Particularly in the clinical setting hereditary data as shared data influences that might be viewed as the patient or members or individual from the family.

Instructive dangers: Hereditary data may put people, families and groups in danger of separation and defamation particularly with regards to employment and insurance, since it can remarkably uncover the individuals who are asymptomatic or inclined to disease; as well as who are not and may never turn out to be sick. These qualities of hereditary data can prompt conclusions that one's hereditary data is in some way or another unique, and this warrants special principles for administering, gathering, utilizing and revealing data (personalized).

Genetic testing also covers various mutations, genetic variation, hereditary testing, cancer and other genetically associated diseases. Once a person has decided to proceed with genetic testing, a medical geneticist or a primary healthcare doctor can order the test. Genetic testing is often done as a part of a genetic consultation where it is important that a person has/her genetic test done, it is important that he or she understands the testing procedures and benefits and limitation of the test, and the possible consequences of the test results. This process of educating a person about the test and obtaining permission is called informed consent (1). Along with informed consent direct–to–consumer is also included as consent for genetic testing. If the person has enough information to take decision about testing it is called as "informed", and a person's voluntary agreement to have the test done is considered as "consent". Informed consent can only be given by adults, for children and other who are unable to make their own medical decision informed consent can be given by guardian or other person legally responsible for making decision (1).

Several factors are commonly included on an informed consent form like (4):

1. General description of the test.
2. How the test will be carried out.
3. Any physical or emotional risk.
4. Whether the result can be used for research purposes.
5. How and to whom the test result will be reported.
6. Whether the result will provide any information about family members' health or any risk of any disease.

What is direct-to-consumer?

Direct-to-consumer genetic testing refers to genetic tests that are marketed directly to consumers via television, print advertisements or through the internet. This form of testing is known as direct-to-customer or as at-home genetic testing. A consumer chooses to purchase a genetic test directly; the test kit is mailed to the customer instead of being ordered by doctor. Consumers are notified of their results directly (pregnancy kit, malarial kit.etc.) or by mail or telephone (1). At home genetic test, however have noteworthy dangers and recorded constraints. Purchasers are powerless of being deluded by the after effects of invalid tests. Customers may likewise encounter an intrusion of genetic security if testing organizations utilize their data in an unauthorised way. More research is expected to completely comprehend the advantages and limitation of direct to consumer genetic testing.

There are various issues related to personalize medicine concept but considering the benefits of genetic testing, it can direct a person towards available options, as well it may involve emotional, social or financial consequences hence governing all matters privacy loss are undertaking.

Privacy Laws

Genetic privacy laws affect the scattering of personalized medicine, using data based on genetic testing for cancer risk and other genetically associated problems. Genetic privacy laws take three alternative approaches for protecting patient's privacy (5):

1. Requiring informed consent on the part of individual.
2. Restricting discriminatory uses of genetic data by employees.
3. Health care providers limiting re disclosure without the consent of individual.

Finding empirical approaches for genetic health privacy which give users control over re disclosure and to encourage the spread of genetic testing, laws are to be emended.

State associated genetic laws mainly focused on major three points (5):

1. Contribution in building an existing academic literature on genetic testing and relate it to privacy regulation.
2. Literature on genetic testing aims to disentangle its inherent implications for asymmetric information out comes. Hence, these approaches restrict sensitive genetic information flows.
3. Empirical evidence for genetic exceptionalism.

Substantial policy debate has been there on whether genetic health data are distinct from regular health data or not therefore needs a special class of protection (5). These concerns which are specific to genetic information can complicate the legal and ethical issues surrounding disclosure of personal information and are the reasons for new targeted laws which provides empirical evidence on how an individual responds to regulation that protect the privacy of genetic information rather than general health data. This supports the need for separate legislative action.

It also helps policymakers in determining the best approach for regulation of genetic privacy, giving the perceived desirability for personalized medicine (6). This perceived desirability roots both the fact that the personal genetic information can be used by an individual to anticipate the risk of their disease, in selecting investment in preventive care and while facing illness selecting most effective treatment but that are potentially large system gains from analyzing personal genetic data on a large scale.

General well being and consumer advocates have contended for string genetic security assurances however life coverage industry agents have contended that all genetic data from candidates ought to be made accessible to them and that data protection may be a practical solution.

By measuring the effects of genetic privacy on availability of genetic testing and its rate, can provide effective policy for diffusion of genetic medicine. Genetic tests are extremely valuable for an individual as well a sub population or population. Genetic variations can be identified predicting the increased risk of ovarian cancer, breast cancer, cystic fibrosis, colon cancer etc. among other diseases. Always a negative result implies for a normal cancer risk or no cancer, while a positive result would be an elevated cancer (1). For example, someone who has been tested positive for BRCA or BRCA2 mutation elevates the risk of breast cancer or ovarian cancer and that they should be offered enhanced screening for further confirmation and curing of cancer at an early stage. It also suggests that they should be offered prophylactic surgery, double mastectomy or removal of either ovaries or fallopian tubes.

Medical research and health care is rapidly expanding. Most medical research is not complete, unless experimentation on human subjects, including children is undertaken, experimentation on human being is subjected to ethical standards that promote respect for all and protect their health and rights, but these are included in both genetic testing and gene associated laws. Though medical evidence of an early stage is effective but is not always a permanent treatment towards disease. Steps to safe guard genetic information's where laws can be divided into 3 categories:

First category of law relates for collecting and storing genetic information reassuring patients by providing clear information on cost and benefits of testing. Second category includes laws that are explicit anti–discriminative laws which prevent any type of discrimination while using genetic data. These laws can target employers, long term care, and health insurers. This law limit how genetic information is used by certain types of organizations that received it, but not whether or not they received the information, so such laws may provide less privacy assurance to consumers. The third category consist of laws that gives the individual explicit ownership rights over there data by either requiring their consent for data disclosure to any third party, or by giving them actual ownership rights over the data (7). The capacity of a person to seek after a genetic test is restricted by the supply side accessibility of genetic testing. Privacy controls may likewise bring down the supply cost of genetic testing, by forcing extra consistence costs on medicinal services suppliers that make interest on genetic testing (2, 7).

Will health insurance cover the costs of genetic testing?

In many cases, health insurance plans will cover the costs of genetic testing when it is recommended by a person's doctor. Health insurance providers have different policies about which tests are to be covered. A person interested in submitting costs of the testing would contact his/her insurance company to pay for testing or for some coverage. Most of the people choose not to use their insurance to pay for testing because of companies own laws and the fear for test results may affect their insurance coverage , instead they opt to pay out of pocket for such tests (8).

Ethical Guidelines for genetic testing and privacy (In India):

An ethical guideline for biomedical research on human subject by the council in 2000 was revised followed by a number of developments in science and technology. These have lead to further widening of health care between the developed and developing countries. The advances in the area of genetics, genomic and molecular biology have grown by leaps resulting into need of sufficient safe guards to protect the rights and welfare of human participant subjected to biomedical research (5). International agencies have been bringing out guidelines for researchers among which WHO and UNESCO are striving to bring a universal consensus to these guidelines in an attempt to reduce disparity across the world.

Separate guidelines have been brought out by the Indian Council of Medical Research (ICMR) as "National Guidelines for Accreditation, Supervision and

Regulation of ART Clinics in India", which was involved solely in clinical trials but as genetic testing evolved, the ICMR brought out the 'Policy Statement on Ethical Considerations involved in Research on Human Subjects' in 1980 and revised these guidelines in 2000 as the 'Ethical guidelines for Biomedical Research on Human Subjects'. Main two important statements are made by Ethical Guidelines for Biochemical Research for human participants shall be known as the ICMR code and they are as follows (5):

1. Statement of General principles on Research using Human participants in biochemical research.
2. Statement of Specific principles on Research using Human participants in specific areas of biochemical research.

'Policy Statement on Ethical Considerations involved in Research on Human Subjects' for the benefit of all those involved in clinical research in India. In 1982, the World Health Organisation (WHO) and the Council for International Organizations of Medical Sciences (CIOMS) issued the 'Proposed International Guidelines for Biomedical Research involving Human Subjects' (5). Subsequently the CIOMS brought out the 'International Guidelines for Ethical Review in "Epidemiological studies' in 1991 and 'International Ethical Guidelines for Biomedical Research involving Human Subjects" in 1993. Over the years, various bioethical advisory bodies in national jurisdictions like Nuffield Council of Bioethics and European Commission on Ethics have also laid down general and specific principles in specific areas of scientific research involving human beings as subjects in medical research in India (5).

Medical and related research using human as research participants must necessarily ensure that (8):

1. The PURPOSE of such research should be directed towards the increase of knowledge about the human condition in relation to its surrounding and changes.
2. Research is CONDUCTED under conditions in which no person or person's dignity or well beings are harmed.
3. Research of EVALUATION at all stages of the process, that is research design, experimentation, declaration of results and use of the results should ensure safety.

Statement of General principles (6, 8)

1. Essentiality principles: The research entailing the use of human participants is considered to be absolutely after considering all alternatives only.
2. Voluntariness, informed consent and community agreement: The participants/patients involved are fully apprised of the research, impact and risk involved and other such important facts. The participants are under complete right to retain or abstain from participating or from in-between of the procedure. This law is currently applicable on the research involving *mutatis mutandis*.

3. Non exploitation principle: Research participants are remunerated for their involvement in the research or experiment, irrespective of their social, economical and literacy conditions they are to be kept fully apprised of all the dangers arising in/out of the research. Participants should be selected irrespective of their arbitrariness, discrimination or caprice. They should have recompense and rehabilitation rights if they need one.
4. Privacy and confidentiality principles: The identity and records of the human participants in the research or experiment should be kept confidential and no details about identity of the participants must be disclosed without valid scientific and legal reasons like therapeutic purposes on specific consent signed by the participant for the disclosure, ensuring that the human participant does not suffer from any form of hardship, discrimination or stigmatisation.
5. Precautions and risk minimalization principles: Care and caution should be taken at all stages of resource or experiment to ensure that the participant are not affected by any kind of irreversible adverse effect and permanent damage, requisite steps should be taken for the well being of the participants.
6. Professional competent principle: Research or experiment should be conducted all times by competent and qualified person who will act with total integrity and impartiality and who is totally aware of ethical consideration in respect to research or experiment.
7. Accountability and transparency principle: Research or experiment should be conducted in a fair, honest, impartial and transparent manner. Where by subject of principles including privacy and confidentiality and the rights should be incomplete record before the onset of research including all data and notes maintain during the experiment and research.
8. Maximization of public interest and distributive justice principle: Research or experiment are conducted and used for benefit of human kind and not for those who are socially better but also for least advanced people.
9. Institutional agreement principle: It is the duty of all persons connected with the research or experiment to ensure that all the procedure are compiled with institutional agreement required for the use and application of any resource in a bonafide and transparent manner.
10. Public domain principle: It is necessary or experiment are brought into public domain so that its result are generally made known through scientific and other publication or those associated with the research or experiment under the law in force at that time.
11. Totality of responsibility principle: It is a moral responsibility to follow all the principle and guidelines laid down generally in respect of research or experiments including the institution where the research is conducted sponsor or the family members paying for the test result and effect of the result should be monitored by all the above mentioned people involved.

12. Compliance principle: It is necessary to ensure that the participant have both letter and the guidelines as well as other norms, directions and guidelines specifically laid down and which are applicable for that area of research or experiment duly compiled with.

Informed consent process in India

Biomedical research involving human participants must obtain informed consent. Informed consent protects that individual's freedom of choice and respect for autonomy and is given voluntarily a part in research. Adequate information about the research is given in a simple and easily understandable language under the INFORMED CONSENT FORM WITH PARTICIPANTS. Following components are applicable (5):

A) Purpose and nature of study.
B) No of participants and duration of participation.
C) Followed procedure.
D) Any investigation to be performed in the pre or post part of the experiment.
E) Discomforts or foreseeable risk related to project.
F) Benefits for participants, community or medical professionals.
G) Compensation policy.
H) Medical treatments available for any kind of injury or damage during the experimentation.
I) Any substitute treatments available.
J) Ensuring confidentiality.
K) No loss of benefits on withdrawal.
L) Benefits involved on the commercialization of the event.
M) Local PI or PI detail contacts and studies asking for more information related to the experiment.
N) Details of the chairman of Institutional Ethics Committee (IEC) for appeal against any violation of rights.
O) Voluntary participation.
P) Test for genetics and HIV is to be done by counselling for consent.
Q) Storage period of biological sample and related data.

Patients or participant information sheets copy must be maintained. The consent should have in brief highlighted important points including risk and benefit and loss of benefits on withdrawal. Assurance should be given for confidentiality and should be maintained. Written consent should have signature or thumb impression (due to more sensitive nature of the research). Verbal consent can be taken for witness and double assurity. Ombudsman a third party can also take accountability or consent by approval of EC. In drug trials, volunteers can give thumb impression otherwise legal custodian cannot be taken or accepted.

Reconsent can be taken but under following conditions (6):

a) Deviation in the protocol.

b) Study extension

c) Change in treatment, procedures etc.

d) If possibility arises for disclosure of identity through any form like in data, presentation or photographs.

Special rules are there for selection of groups or participants for research they are as follows:

1. Pregnant women: Such women's should in no circumstances be the participants of any research unless there is no more or minimal risk involved for foetus, lactation or on pregnancy. They can only participate in such trials on conditions where the research is to protect or advance the health of women, foetus or nursing infants. In such case women with no pregnancy cannot be involved.
2. Children: If the research can be ensued on an adult than a child cannot be involved. They can only participate if the research focuses on health and brain improvement of children, guardians consent (proxy) should be taken. If child refuses to participate no one can force him/her in any condition or personal interests such type of act is strictly punishable.
3. Vulnerable groups: Racial inequalities should not be there in genetic research. Economically or socially disadvantaged people should not be used for the benefit of those who are better than them. Mentally challenged or mentally differently able person who are unable to give their informed consent should not be harassed in anyway, special care for their rights and welfare should be taken. For participants such as students, prisoners, subordinates or employees requiring adequate justification as they have reduce autonomy as research participants

Privacy and confidentiality are essential for any relationship here we mean between doctor and patients. In context of health care privacy and protection is its foundation. Patients must be comfortable in asking and sharing any kind of information this same follows for doctors.

Medical privacy involves secrecy, data security and modesty. And there are certain situations where health information disclosure is permitted they are as follows (8):

1. While referral.
2. When demanded by police or court.
3. Under Insurance act demanded by insurance companies.
4. Under consumer protection cases, workmen's compensation cases or for income tax authorities demand.
5. For registration of disease.
6. Study of vaccination.

7. Reporting drug adversary effect
8. For investigation of communicable diseases.

Legislation

Epidemic diseases act, 1897 (revised in 2002) (7):

This act was brought under force for the purpose of preventing epidemic diseases, which later on was revised in the case of infectious diseases including the right of accountability, openness, quality verification, security, liability and privacy. Because of the act access and correction, choice and notice could not be applied for this act. Even after being revised in 2002 there were still some principle points missing they are as follows:

1. Notice.
2. Openness.
3. Limitation of collection.
4. Penalty.
5. Verification.

Mental health act, 1987 (revised in 1994) (9)

Under National Human Rights Commission (NHRC) New Delhi which carried out a survey of 37 mental hospitals in country and proposed this law which involves patient's rights with respect to privacy and dignity this law also governs treatments and researches related to mental health and associated diseases.

Preconception and prenatal diagnostic techniques act 1994 was also included under this act the declining sex ratio in India was alarming and to prevent this strength was undertaken where it prohibited the determination of sex and sex selection before and after conception and was prescribed as criminal act and included punishments. However, this test can be followed under following condition:

a) Conception has occurred over the age 35.
b) Two or more spontaneous abortion has already occurred.
c) Exposure to teratogenic agent such as drugs, radiation, infection or any chemical.
d) Family history of retardation or physical deformities.

In order to follow above mention criteria mother has to give informed consent.

Even after being revised following are the missing aspects:

a) Accountability
b) Quality.
c) Consent and choice.
d) Disclosure.
e) Security.
f) Openness.

Medical Termination of Pregnancy Act, 1971 (revised in 2006) (10)

There are legal grounds under which a women can seek and abortion which includes choice and consent (Mother should be aware of risk involved and other options available and of she's below 18 years guardians would be responsible for a informed consent under Indian lunacy act 1912). Disclosure (It is necessary for the chief medical officer to know any kind of termination of pregnancy being performed and the reasons involved).

Termination of pregnancy is granted under following conditions:

1. Failure of contraceptive device.
2. Pregnancy is result of rape.
3. There is fatal result involved for mother.
4. The foetus has certain disability.
5. The baby has some genetic disorder.
6. Any family history involved.

Following are the missing principles in the act:

1. Purpose limitations.
2. Access and correction.
3. Oversight.

The above mention 3 laws are also included in genetic testing and privacy as biomedical procedures are involved in these fields.

Ethical Guidelines for Biomedical Research on Human Subject

Council of Medical Research Published these Guidelines in 2006. Following are the principles (3, 8):

1. Choice and consent. Principle of informed consent forms is available which are responsible for the confidentiality of records in future and present.
2. Collection limitation
   a) Research records: Record should be maintained and retainable when needed.

      Confidentiality of identity: It is mandatory to protect the privacy of a particular community, person or anyone involved in testing.
   b) Collection for surveillance studies: Studies required systematic collection, analysis, interpretation of data related to the research and methodologies.
   c) Collection of disaster management studies requires cope up methods for disaster or emergency situation along with maintaining privacy.
   d) Collection of epidemiological studies: This maintains the confidentiality of epidemiological data which involves national and public safety.
   e) Collection of pedigree studies: Sometimes it is necessary to conduct genetic family studies in order to study heredity disease and privacy laws are applicable for the members of the family involve.

f) Collection for cultural sensitivity in pedigree studies: It maintains privacy for the cultural background of India. This may also involve disease associated to sex chromosome.

g) Collection for DNA banking: Cell line and bio bank maintain different types of cells and tissues hence the source form where they have been collected must be kept private and mostly u identified to large group of people involved.

h) Records keeping of Institutional Ethics Committee: IEC maintains documentation of all data file and preserved accordingly.

3. Disclosure

a) Disclosure of participant information: No hardship or discrimination must occur on enclosure of identity a record personal involved.

b) Identity disclosure: Identity can be only disclosed under specific laws that are prioraly described above.

c) Scrutinization for disclosure: For Scrutiny by legal or administrative authority record should be there.

d) Anonymization: Any information placed in the public domain should use anonymization.

4. Security: Records must be safely maintained before and after completion of the study.

These are some of the laws followed in India for Genetic testing and Privacy, still privacy problems are going on, new laws are to be made and amended. While there are no arguments with the overall bills objectives like law, enforcement, identification of missing person, dead bodies in disaster and accidents for identification, for consent use of DNA samples but the problem of developing and maintaining a Data Bank, religious aspects and other such problems are reason for critics.

References

Genetic Home Reference, retrieved from https://ghr.nlm.nih.gov/.

Miller, A.R. and Tucker, C (2015). Privacy Protection, Personalized Medicine and Genetic Testing, *SSRN Electronic Journal.*

Goldfarb, A. and Tucker, C (2011). Privacy regulation and online advertising. Management of Science, 57(1), 57-71, *SSRN Electronic Journal.*

Patangia Venkata Ganesh vs. state of Andhra Pradesh, 2003 crlj 4508(AP).

Ethical Guidelines for Biomedical Research on Human Participants (ICMR) (2006), New Delhi

Guidelines for Gene Therapy (1996). Department of Biotechnology, New Delhi.

The IRDA, 2011, Health Insurance Portability Guidelines.

Statement of General Principles, Principle 7, (2006). Ethical Guidelines for Biomedical Research on Human Subjects.

The Mental Health Act, 1987, S.3 (2).

Medical Termination of Pregnancy Regulations, 2003, Regulation 4(2).

Chapter 12

Antibiotic Resistance

Dr Gurudas Khilnani[1] and Dr Ajeet Kumar Khilnani[2]

[1]MD (Gen Med), MD (Pharmacology), DHRM, FISC, FIPS,
Dean Gujarat Adani Institute of Medical Sciences, Bhuj-370001, Gujarat, India.

[2]MS (Otorhinolaryngology), ACME, Associate Professor Department of Otorhinolaryngology,
Gujarat Adani Institute of Medical Sciences, Bhuj-370001, Gujarat, India.

Email: drgurudas@gmail.com, ajeetkhilnani@gmail.com

Abstract

Microbes are known to exist since antiquity. Many antibiotics are obtained from soil microbes (fungi and bacteria) and have been present in the environment long before humans started using them in clinical settings. Microorganisms have been naturally exposed to these bioactive products during evolution. Given the billions of years of co-evolution of antibiotic producing and antibiotic resistant organisms. Paul Ehrlich hypothesized "Magic Bullets" against microbes in 1900 and Salvarsan was the first antimicrobial agent used against syphilis in 1906 (Heynick, 2009). Domagk (1933) used prontosil and its metabolite sulphanilamide in infections (Otten, 1986). The Penicillin was discovered in 1928 and put to clinical use in 1940. Therefore, problem of antibiotic resistance (AR) is an ever-increasing menace to mankind (Petri, 2011).

Antibiotic Resistance is an ever increasing public health problem which has evolved from environmental mixing of genes and is further aggravated by unrestricted use of antibiotics in livestock husbandry and poultry farming. Inappropriate use of antibiotics at all levels of health care delivery; poor sanitation and lack of awareness of seriousness of the AR are increasingly realized as modifiable factors.

1. Introduction

Paul Ehrlich hypothesized "Magic Bullets" against microbes in 1900 and Salvarsan was the first antimicrobial agent used against syphilis in 1906 (Heynick, 2009). Domagk (1933) used prontosil and its metabolite sulphanilamide in infections (Otten, 1986). The Penicillin was discovered in 1928 and put to clinical use in 1940. The use of these agents was soon associated with emergence of bacterial resistance against them. Subsequently, it was realized that with introduction of every new antibiotic, bacteria showed insensitivity and resistance to them. Therefore, problem of antibiotic resistance (AR) is an ever-increasing menace to mankind (Petri, 2011).

AR is a global threat today. This has increased the need for newer and newer antibiotics. However, the pace with which development of new antibiotics has occurred has lagged behind the ever-increasing need of newer antibiotics. Thus, a state of "Antibiotic famine" is created in the world. As per a recent WHO report (WHO, 2017) only 51 new antibiotics and biologicals are in clinical development to treat priority antibiotic-resistant pathogens, Mycobacteria and Clostridium difficile. Among all these candidates, only 8 are classified by WHO as true inventions that will add to the current antibiotic battery. This has necessitated steps to be taken to prevent development of AR against existing antibiotics. Development of treatment guidelines, for the responsible use of antibiotics in the humans, animals and agricultural sectors, is the priority area of work for WHO and its constituent member countries. The economic burden of AR is huge with resultant increased morbidity and mortality, loss of man-days and earnings. Other consequences are failure of therapy, prolonged hospitalization, extra expenditure on newer expensive antibiotics and harm due to Adverse Drug Reactions to newer antibiotics. Unfortunately, poor communities have infections due to multidrug resistant (MDR) bacteria such as MDR tuberculosis (TB) for which very few drugs are available today.

This chapter discusses evolution, environmental and human related factors leading to AR, mechanisms of development of AR, and strategies taken at international and national levels to curb the menace of AR in humans.

2. Evolution of Antibiotic Resistance

Microbes are known to exist since antiquity. Many antibiotics are obtained from soil microbes (fungi and bacteria) and have been present in the environment long before humans started using them in clinical settings. Microorganisms have been naturally exposed to these bioactive products during evolution. Given the billions of years of co-evolution of antibiotic producing and antibiotic resistant organisms, many bacteria have developed mechanisms to become intrinsically resistant to antibiotics. Once antibiotics were used to treat bacterial infections it did not take long for the first highly sensitive strains to convert to resistant ones. Strains resistant to the first generation of antibiotics, including Penicillin-G and Streptomycin, were isolated before or shortly after the drugs were introduced to the market (Wright GD, 2012). A variety of mechanisms are evolved in development of AR; such as mutant selection, formation of inactivating enzymes and continuous evolution to multidrug inactivating forms, changes in entry of and/or accelerated efflux of antibiotics due to evolutional changes in proteins of bacterial cell walls. Recently, (Ryan, 2017) reported that alterations in bacterial metabolizing enzymes can inactivate antibiotics faster leading to AR.

3. Factors responsible for development of antibiotic resistance

There are three broad categories of factors involved:

A) Environmental and occupational factors

B) Host related factors

C) Inappropriate antibiotic use

A. Role of Environment in propagation of AR

1. Water Bodies

The freshwater bodies are the main sites for evolution and the rise of new AR. In water bodies like waste water effluents, lakes, and rivers or streams, there are many drug resistant bacteria from different sources, e.g., industrial, urban, and agricultural waste. These environmental species are provided with intrinsic antibiotic resistance mechanisms. In addition, these resistant organisms are selected by over-expression of broad range of defensive mechanisms, such as efflux pumps proteins. These selected strains are mixed with environmental drug sensitive species. Thus, the mixing of these two types in water bodies leads to enormous genetic exchange within same species and within interspecies by processes such as transduction, transformation and conjugation. Transfer of genes is facilitated by plasmids, phages and transposons. Plasmid transfer from a donor to a recipient cell occurs at a low frequency in bulk water (Sengeløv G, 1998). Similarly, filter feeding organisms that collect bacteria belonging to different species and concentrate them at high density in a reduced space, facilitate gene exchange (Taylor NG, 2011). Biofilm matrix in water habitats also creates favourable conditions both for plasmid exchange and transformation process (Molin S, 2003). (Gillings MR, 2009) have provided evidences that the clinical Class-I integrons originated from environmental bacterial communities. Class-I integrons are found in sewage waste water and other polluted water bodies containing disinfectants, quaternary ammonium compounds and heavy metals. This increases the risk of selection and spread of integron structures. These genetic structures may be acquired by bacterial species that play role as shuttle between environment and hospital associated infections and constitutes gene vectors for further dissemination in nosocomial bacteria.

Antibiotic resistance acquired by opportunistic and pathogenic bacteria evolve by means of Darwinian forces, i.e., bacterial genetic mutations are induced as a result of environmental forces (Gullberg E, 2011). Mutations within the chromosome can be responsible for the decreased affinity of antibiotics to their targets. Furthermore, some resistance mechanisms (e.g., efflux pumps, chromosomal AmpC β-lactamases) confer a naturally reduced susceptibility to the antibiotics (See Box-1).

Gene transfer occurs both horizontally and vertically. Resistant genes can be transferred by bacteria to progeny during cell division. This is vertical transmission. The cells can also transfer resistant genes such as AmpC and ELBS-genes by exchange of genetic material through special gene sections called as plasmids (non chromosomal genetic material) between bacteria of same species or other species by a process of conjugation. This is called as horizontal spread. In fact, most of AmpC β-lactamases resistant genes (*AmpC*) and some of ESBL-genes are carried in plasmids. This is how normal intestinal flora carrying resistant genes can transmit on the multidrug resistant (MDR) genes for ESBL and/or AmpC to pathogenic bacteria, such as Salmonella.

(Aminov, 2011) has reviewed the role of horizontal gene transfer mechanisms and found that transduction has an important role in genetic exchanges among environmental bacteria, found in freshwater. Horizontal gene transfer results in transfer in-species and among different species of bacteria and allows spread from normal commensals and pathogenic bacteria. This type of gene exchange is promoted in hospitals, community-farms, and aquacultures where the usage of antibiotics selects for resistant bacteria. Similarly, water bodies such as rivers, streams, waste water effluents, and lakes facilitate the transport and transfer of the antibiotic resistance genes. Liberal use of disinfectants and low-cost pharmaceuticals, contribute significantly to the emergence of bacterial drug resistances (Depledge M. , 2011). Inadequate waste-management of the pharmaceuticals causes alarming pollution of the environmental habitats such as agricultural soils and rivers, which probably contributes to the selection of antibiotic resistant bacteria and speeds up the emergence of new resistances. Furthermore, rivers often receive bacteria from different sources, e.g., waste water treatment plants or water originating from urban effluent, industrial, or agricultural activities, thus constituting potential compartments where environmental, human, and/or animal related bacteria can coexist, at least temporally. This mixing can result in two main risks: (i) Environmental bacterial species carrying intrinsic antibiotic resistance genes mix and act as donors for human pathogens which, in turn, could introduce new acquired resistance mechanisms in the hospitals (Wright, 2010); (ii) Extensive usage of antibiotics in medicine, agriculture, and poultry, human or animal related bacteria acquire antibiotic resistance, directly by the presence of antibiotics and indirectly through co-selection induced by other pollutants (Martinez, 2009). Recent studies suggest that the spread of resistant bacteria in natural fresh water systems can reach drinking water supplies and thus enter the human food chain (Walsh TR, 2011). These factors indicate that water sanitation is crucial for a better control of the spread of antibiotic resistances.

2. Use of antibiotics in Poultry and Livestock

Overuse of antibiotics in animal farms endangers us all as it multiplies drug resistance in the environment. It is estimated that 80% of all antibiotics consumed in the United States are used in food animals. Antibiotics are used in animals as animal feed supplements to promote animal growth. They are also spread on fruit trees to prevent and treat infection. Enerofloxacin was used in animals in many countries, which resulted in development of Ciprofloxacin resistant Salmonella infections. It is estimated that antibiotic consumption in livestock is likely to double from 2010 to 2030 (Hellen Gelband, 2015). A recent survey in Punjab showed that two third of eighteen poultry farms used antibiotics for growth promotion; 1,556 Escherichia coli isolates from 530 birds from 18 farms were tested for susceptibility to 11 antimicrobials; 510 of these E coli isolates produced ESBL - enzymes that confer resistance to most beta-lactam antibiotics.

A similar report was obtained in samples from National Capital Region (NCR) by Centre for Science and Environment (CSE) in 2014. The Pollution Monitoring Laboratory of CSE tested 70 samples of chicken in Delhi and NCR (36 samples were picked from Delhi, 12 from Noida, 8 from Gurugram and

7 each from Faridabad and Ghaziabad). Three tissues —muscle, liver and kidney tested positive for the presence of six antibiotics widely used in poultry: Oxytetracycline, chlortetracycline, doxycycline, enrofloxacin and ciprofloxacin (class fluoroquinolones) and neomycin, an aminoglycoside. Antibiotics are frequently administered into chicken during its life cycle of 35-42 days: they are regularly mixed with feed to promote growth and routinely administered to all birds for several days to prevent infections.

Similarly, meat-producing farms were found to have twice the rates of antimicrobial resistance as compared to egg-producing farms, as well as higher rates of multidrug resistance. High levels of resistance was shown to several antibiotics ranging from 39 per cent for ciprofloxacin, used to treat respiratory infections, to 86 per cent for nalidixic acid, used to treat urinary tract infections. Almost 60 per cent of the E. coli samples exhibited "resistance conferring" genes (Ramakant Sahu, 2014).

Extended Spectrum β-Lactamases (ESBL) and/or AmpC producing bacteria occur in all livestock species as well as in many animals kept as pets (dogs, cats etc). In foods, these are detected particularly often in broiler meat, beef and pork as well as plant based foods. Most of the bacteria detected on foods originate from agricultural livestock farming and are transmitted to the food in the course of food production (milking and slaughtering). Studies have shown that many E. coli isolates from calves are cephalosporin-resistant E. coli. In examinations of healthy animals, the proportion of cephalosporin-resistant E. coli was highest among broilers.

B. Host related Factors (Table-1)

A number of factors related to animals or humans favour development of AR. In pus pockets and cavities, as in pulmonary tuberculosis, the bacteria multiply slowly and thus are less amenable to conventional doses of antibiotics. A given antibiotic may not reach at the site in adequate bactericidal concentration because biofilm barriers do not allow access. Other factors are summarized in Table-1.

C. Inappropriate Use

By far it is the most important acquired cause of AR in human beings which can be prevented by proper education and training.

1. **Overuse:** In many countries in the absence of standard treatment guidelines, inadequate knowledge and regulatory control, antibiotics are overprescribed (to an extent that 50% use is considered as inappropriate). 30% of all hospitalised patients receive one or more than one antibiotics (Ventola, 2015). Often fever of undetermined cause is treated with antibiotics. (Sumanth Gandra, 2017) examined, as part of the Global Antimicrobial Resistance, Prescribing, and Efficacy in Neonates and Children (GARPEC) project, prevalence of and indications of antimicrobial use, as well as antimicrobial agents used in hospitalized children by conducting four point prevalence surveys in six hospitals. They found overuse of third generation cephalosporins for lower respiratory tract infections. This inappropriate use has caused emergence of resistance

because of selection of resistance strains of common pathogens. The ease with which antibiotics can be accessed without a prescription further promotes inappropriate use and its consequences.

2. **Inappropriate prescribing and usage:** Inadequate doses, less frequent dosing intervals, shorter duration of use than recommended, multiple antibiotics, lack of instructions and failure to complete therapy promote AR. Sub inhibitory concentrations contribute to selection of resistant types of organism.
3. **Less availability of newer antibiotics:** Ever since the advent of penicillin in 1940, new antibacterials have been developed and used. However, almost all developed so far have shown loss of efficacy due to bacterial resistance against them. Academia and industry have failed to meet with the demand for newer antibiotics (*antibiotic famine*). About 6 newer antibacterials, mostly newer fluoroquinolones, and penems, came in market in 2014, two anti-tubercular drugs (Delamanid and Bedaquiline) are now available after about four decades of research. Currently, industry feels that newer antibacterial drug development is less profitable activity because of huge investment and regulatory constraints. The irony is, emergence of multidrug resistant bacteria has increased demand for newer antibacterials. WHO (WHO, 2017) has prioritised the list of those pathogens for which there is an urgent need of newer drugs (Table-2).

4. Mechanisms of Development of AR

A. Role of Integrons, Transposons and Insertion Sequences

These DNA sequences play pivotal role in genesis of AR. The characteristic features of these DNA sequences are shown in the Table-3.

B. Process of Gene Transfer

Transfer of genetic material occurs during bacterial cell division or passage of genes from one bacterium to another of the same species or other species (Table-4).

5. Resistance to Individual Antibiotics

A. β-lactam Antibiotics

The antibiotics have different chemical structures. A major group of antibiotics, β-lactams, belongs to a chemical class having a common 4-member ring called as β-lactam ring (Figure-1). β-Lactams constitute 60% of antibiotics used clinically. Therefore, it is necessary to understand the underlying mechanisms of development of bacterial resistance against them.

1. Role of β-lactamase Enzymes

a. Conventional β-lactamase Enzymes

Many bacteria have ability to synthesize antibiotic destroying enzymes (penicillinases, cephalosporinases and carbapenemases), that hydrolyse β-lactam antibiotics. These are collectively called as β-lactamases. The evolution and complexity of classification of these bacterial enzymes is well described by (Karen

Bush, 2010) and a simplified classification is shown in Table-5. Bacterial β-lactamases hydrolyze and inactivate the β-lactam antibiotics by cleaving the amide bond of β-lactam ring (O=C-N) in an acylation-deacylation based process. Inactivation of many beta lactam antibiotics by such hydrolysis is an important cause of innate and acquired AR. Cefazolin (Ist generation) can easily be hydrolysed by β-lactamases of S. aureus. The Cefoxitin (IInd generation) is less susceptible to hydrolysis and retains significant antibacterial activity against anaerobes. The IIIrd generation Cephalosporins such as cefotaxime, ceftazidime and cefoperazone are still active against gram-negative bacilli but can be hydrolysed by inducible chromosomal type-I β-lactamases. The IVth generation (Cefepime) drugs are less susceptible to type-I β-lactamases but can be hydrolysed by metallo-β-lactamases such as New Delhi metallo β-lactamase(NDM-1) and KPC class-A type-I β-lactamases.

Gram-positive organisms produce larger amount of enzymes than gram-negative rods. However, in the latter, the enzyme is located between outer and inner membranes and thus can easily inactivate the incoming antibiotic through porin channels. The β-lactamases of gram-positive organisms are inducible, encoded in plasmids and transmitted by bacteriophages. In gram-negative bacteria, the enzymes are coded either in chromosomes or in plasmids and are constitutive or inducible. Many bacteria have shown increasing level of drug resistance with passage of time. Often, there is across resistance to similar antibiotics of the same or different classes of antibiotics. This is called as multidrug resistance and is a serious health problem today. Most worrisome are AmpC β-lactamases (AmpC) and extended spectrum β-lactamases (ESBL) producing bacteria.

Amp-C β-lactamases are clinically important cephalosporinases produced by many Enterobacteriaceae strains which are resistance to cephalothin, cefazolin, cefoxitin, most penicillins and co-amoxiclav. The plasmid-mediated *AmpC* genes are derived from inducible chromosomal genes that have become mobilized and are major cause of concern to clinicians. Commonly reported genotypes are ACC, FOX, MOX, DHA, CIT and EBC. These enzymes confer a resistance pattern similar to the overproduction of chromosomal AmpC β-lactamases, which may involve all β-lactam antibiotics except for carbapenems and cefepime. In India, AmpC β-lactamases prevalence has been reported in Klebsiella spp (24.1%) and E coli (37.5%). In another Indian study, 3.3 per cent of isolates produced AmpC β lactamases (Manoharan A, 2012).

b. Extended Spectrum Β-Lactamases (ESBLs):

The ESKCAPE Organisms (**E**nterococcus faecium, **S**taphylococcus aureus, **K**lebsiella pneumonia, **C**lostridium difficile, **A**cinetobacterspp, **P**seudomonas aeruginosa, **E**nterobacter spp) and Enterobacteriaceae are clinically worrisome group of pathogens which show resistance due to production of ESBLs and are resistant to IIIrd generation cephalosporins. The Klebseilla produces a unique carbapenemase {New Delhi Metallo β-lactamase-1 (NDM-1)} and thus has become carbapenem resistant. These bacteria and salmonella spp are resistant to aminopenicillins (e.g. ampicillin), cephalosporins (third and fourth generation) and monobactams.

c. Metallo β-lactamases (MBLs)

First chromosomally encoded MBL was identified in Bacillus cereus in 2008 and since then a variety of MBLs have posed a global antibiotic resistance threat. The most important variant is New Delhi Metallo-β-lactamase (NDM-1). It is a highly potent carbapenems-hydrolyzing zinc dependent MBL. E. coli and Klebsiella were initial bacteria producing NDM-1, resistant to carbapenems but due to horizontal transfer of resistance gene (medical tourism, travel across continents), more bacterial strains are exhibiting NDM-1 production and carbapenem resistance. Phylogenetically, NDM-1 has similarities in Zn^{++} binding motifs with marine bacteria Erythrobacterlitoralis (ElBla2), Haliangium ochraceum and Hirschiabaltica (Daiyasu H, 2001). . It is suggested that NDM-1 might have appeared via horizontal gene transfer from environmental reservoirs, further confirming role of environmental factors in development of bacterial drug resistance. The Lancet Infectious Diseases reported 37 strains of superbugs producing NDM-1 from UK and 99 strains from India in (Kumarasamy KK, 2010). The source of origin was found from water bodies (drinking and river water). This report took every one by storm and alerted one and all across the globe, because of in-effectiveness of available antibiotics such as pencillins, IIIrd generation cephalosporins and carbapenems.

(Avneet Saini, 2012) reviewed the three dimensional structure of the enzyme to identify potential target site NDM-1 for development of effective inhibitors. The NDM-1 is important because bacteria of enterobacteriaceae (K. pneumonia, E. coli, E. cloacae, Proteus spp., Citrobacterfreundii, K. oxytoca, M. morganii and Providenciaspp) have evolved capacity to produce NDM-1 and there is really no effective antibiotic left to kill these organisms called as *superbugs*.

2. Role of Penicillin Binding Proteins (PBPs) in β -lactam resistance

Both gram-positive (Staphylococci) and gram-negative rods (E. coli) have varying amounts of PBPs. The cell wall synthesizing enzymes (transpeptidases and carboxypeptidases) are found in PBPs and thus synthesis of bacterial cell wall peptidoglycan involves PBPs. Penicillins and cephalosporins inhibit transpeptidation by targeting PBPs. The bacteria may be intrinsically resistant because PBPs are structurally different. Some organisms which are initially sensitive may become resistant due to reduced affinity by development of high molecular PBPs (homologous recombination between PBP genes of different species of bacteria), not amenable to β-lactams. This is way of resistance shown by S. aureus, Streptococci viridans and Methicillin Resistant S. Aureus (MRSA).

The outer membrane of gram-negative rods is impenetrable barrier except porin channel through which ampicillin, amoxicillin and cephalosporins enter. Pseudomonas aeruginosa lacks such permeable pores and thus inherently resistant to a number of penicillins and cephalosporins. Gram-negative organisms (P. aeruginosa, N. gonorrheae and E. coli) have rapid efflux cell membrane mechanisms to extrude incoming antibiotics

3. Role of Efflux Pump Mechanisms in development of AR

The efflux pumps are important way by which bacteria, parasites, and fungi remove harmful chemicals. There are five types of transporter proteins involved in extrusion of toxins and antibiotics from bacteria. These are ATP-binding cassette (ABC) transporter, the major facilitator super family (MFS), the small multi-drug resistance (SMR), the multi-drug and toxic-compound extrusion (MATE), and the resistance nodulation division (RND) families. The ABC transporter is coded in falciparum gene {Plasmodium falciparum Multidrug Resistant Gene-1 (*pfmdr*-1)} and confers resistance to most common antimalarial drugs chloroquine, quinine, mefloquine, halofantrine, lumefantrine and artemether. The transporter genes form the main efflux systems families (*Tet and the CmlA/FloR)* which are efflux pumps for tetracycline and chloramphenicol causing acquired resistance. Some RND efflux genes exhibit a basal level of expression, and therefore contribute to intrinsic resistance in Acenobacter spp (Coyne S, 2011).

Efflux pumps in Salmonella spp., conferring resistance to antibiotics, is able to extrude bile salts in intestines. This allows colonization and survival of salmonella in human or animal intestines (Lacroix FJ, 1996). Here, there is horizontal gene transfer to other bacteria living in the same habitat. (Nikaido H, 2012) have observed that the rise of resistance due to efflux pumps mechanisms in hospital settings is tightly linked to the sub-inhibitory concentration of the antibiotics during clinical therapies. Other selective factors such as heavy metals, naturally present in the soil, and solvents produced as consequences of metabolic activities, have been shown to be substrates of several efflux pumps conferring multi-drug resistance. There could be a causal relationship between pollution of the water environment by antibiotics, antiseptics (Triclosan) or pollutants, and the selection of bacteria expressing efflux pumps (Hernández A, 2011).

B. Resistance to Aminoglycosides

There are three mechanisms operating:

1. Failure of antibiotic to penetrate inner membrane of gram-negative organisms.
2. Inactivation by aminoglycoside modifying enzymes located in periplasmic space. Resistance to many aminoglycosides except amikacin is by this mechanism and is clinically important. The enzyme-genes are transmitted by conjugation (plasmid transfer). Often inactivating enzymes are bifunctional. Thus, gentamicin resistance confers resistance to tobramycin, amikacin, kanamycin and netilmicin. Streptomycin may still be effective in gentamicin resistant bacteria because it is inactivated by different enzyme.
3. Low affinity of antibiotics to ribosomal proteins which synthesize vital bacterial proteins.

C. Resistance to other antibiotics (Table-6)

The AR may develop due to changes in ribosomal structures responsible for synthesis of vital proteins or mutations in genes responsible for enzymatic inactivation of antibiotics. A summary of different mechanisms involved for currently use other antibiotics is given in Table-6.

6. Strategies to Contain Antibiotic Resistance:

A multipronged action is required to preserve the efficacy of available antibiotics. This is because the sources of resistance are of various types. AR-bacteria are found in humans, animals, food, and the environment (in air, water and soil). They can spread between people and animals, and from person to person. Apart from inappropriate use in health care settings, poor infection control, inadequate sanitary conditions and inappropriate food-handling encourage the spread of antimicrobial resistance. Thus, several measures are required to control above conditions. These can be categorized in two broad groups

A. Reducing Clinical Antibiotic Resistance Burden:

1. **Antibiotic Stewardship Program (ABSP):** Antibiotic Stewardship program is a coordinated intervention among infection physicians, nurses and microbiologists to promote appropriate use of antibiotics in hospitals. ABSP is found to be a powerful tool to limit unrestricted antibiotic use in hospitals. It has shown impact in reducing antibiotic use by 11%-38% (Bartlett JG, 2013).

2. **Rational antibiotic prescribing:** Educating prescribers about sound pharmacokinetic principles and providing health care workers about the necessary information on rational use of medicines are important tools for change in prescribing behaviour.

3. **Standard Treatment Protocols and Guidelines:**

   Use of hospital formularies, restriction on use and monitoring use of newer antibiotics are can reduce use of IVth generation cephalosporins, imipenem and newer fluoroquinolones. The protocols and antibiotic guidelines are prepared and used by a number of tertiary care centres in India, but widespread use is required at all levels of health care delivery. NDM-1 resistant organisms are difficult to treat and therefore, recently (2017), Indian Council of Medical Research (ICMR) has advised tertiary care hospitals to avoid liberal use of three antibiotics carbapenems, polymyxin and colistin, which are effective against these pathogens.

   Formulations and use of guidelines in critical care settings can reduce the antibiotic overuse. In India, *National Policy for containment of antimicrobial resistance in India-2011,* was released by the Director General of health Services, Govt of India, to identify nature and type of resistant organism induced infections and suggestions for pragmatic antibiotic use. *National Treatment Guidelines for Antimicrobial Use in Infectious Diseases* were prepared in 2016 by National Centre for Disease Control, Directorate General of Health Services, Ministry of Health & Family Welfare, Government of India, which provide guidelines to clinicians for appropriate use of antibacterials in common and resistant organisms and implementation of preventive strategies.

   The Indian Council of Medical Research (ICMR) established AR surveillance network in 2012 to collect nationally representative data on trends and patterns of AR to the commonly used antibiotics. A working group on Antimicrobial Stewardship Program (AMSP) was simultaneously constituted in late 2012 to provide overall direction to development of

AMSP in the country. One of the key recommendations of the group was to devise standard treatment guidelines, based on Indian data, which can guide antibiotic usage in the country. The data emanating out of the ICMR network were shared with all the teams. The document was compiled in the form of *Treatment Guidelines for Antimicrobial Use in Common Syndromes* (Kamini Walia V. C., 2017). This manual is very handy in selecting specific antibiotic for common infectious diseases seen in routine clinical practice. Recently, a retrospective study have shown the positive effect of Antibiotic policy (2014) on NICU mortality and antibiotic consumption (Jinka DR, 2017). There was decrease in use of IIIrd generation Cephalosporins and increased use of Ist line agents such as ampicillin and gentamicin, without change in mortality and outcomes in neonates.

4. **Improved diagnosis before treatment:**

The biggest challenge to clinicians is to differentiate viral from bacterial causes of diseases and convince patient that antibiotic therapy is not needed. Usually, empiric treatment of suspected infection is started with one or more than one antibiotics. Practitioners use successive antibiotics until fever abates and the cause remains unknown. Such diagnostic uncertainty promotes use of multiple antibacterial agents which results in emergence of drug resistant bacteria. A US study reported that only in 7.6% cases of community acquired pneumonia requiring hospitalization, was the microbiological diagnosis available for antibacterial therapy. There is a need of rapid diagnostic tools and techniques to provide microbiological results in less than 24 hours so that appropriate antibiotic can be started. Availability of newer diagnostic tools such as real time PCR, mass spectrophotometry and molecular techniques that identify unique nucleic acid sequences and biomarkers of bacteria can provide pathogen specific diagnosis at the time of initiating antibiotic therapy or modifying empiric therapy within 24 hours. Instruments that use multiple diagnostic platforms, such as PLEX-ID, can identify over 5000 pathogens within hours (Bartlett JG, 2013). A recent meta-analysis reported role of procalcitonin-guided antibiotic treatment in acute respiratory infections. High procalcitonin levels suggested bacterial cause of respiratory infections requiring antibiotics (Schuetz P, 2017).

5. **Prevention of bacterial infection:**

Use of universal precautions and adequate cleanliness are time-tested techniques to reduce infection rate. The ICU inpatients are exposed to drug resistant organisms transmitted by health workers and fomites. Careful hand hygiene before and after examination of such patients reduces inter-patient transmission. Hospital infection control guidelines and committees can play important role in prevention of spread of drug resistant organisms. Periodic disinfection of hospital environment and equipments and automated hand washing techniques are shown to reduce infections. Regular use of vaccines to health care providers is important way to prevent spread of disease. Newer techniques of self cleaning of rooms and robotic technology would further reduce nosocomial infection rates.

6. **Role of Regulatory bodies (Indian initiatives):**

In February 2016, Union Health Minister launched campaign *'Medicines with the Red Line"* to increase awareness and reduce misuse of antibiotics (Figure-2). The schedule H1 was included in Drugs and cosmetic Rules, 1945 so that antibiotics were not dispensed without a prescription. Schedule H1 imposes restrictions on sale of 46 antibiotics, which include 3rd and 4th generation cephalosporins, newer fluoroquinolones, carbapenems and anti-tubercular drugs, and other medicines. The chemist has to maintain register for three years with information of patient, prescriber and dispensed quantity of antibiotic. However, many antibiotics, such as piperacillin, tazobactam, tigecycline, gentamicin, linezolid, co-amoxyclav, ciprofloxacin and ofloxacin, have not been included. It is hoped that augmentations of provisions of Schedule H1 would further contain over-the-counter sale of antibiotics. Other initiatives taken are shown in Table-7.

7. **Role of WHO**

WHO is providing technical assistance to help countries develop their national action plans, and strengthen their health and surveillance systems so that they can prevent and manage antimicrobial resistance. It is collaborating with partners to strengthen the evidence base and develop new responses to AR global threat. WHO is working closely with the Food and Agriculture Organization of the United Nations (FAO) and the World Organisation for Animal Health (OIE) in a 'One Health' approach to promote best practices to avoid the emergence and spread of antibacterial resistance, including optimal use of antibiotics in both humans and animals.

A global action plan on antimicrobial resistance was adopted by Member States at the Sixty-eighth World Health Assembly and supported by the governing bodies of FAO and OIE in May and June 2015. The goal of the global action plan is to ensure, for as long as possible, continuity of successful treatment and prevention of infectious diseases with effective and safe medicines that are quality-assured, used in a responsible way, and accessible to all who need them. A manual on Global Antimicrobial Resistance Surveillance System (GLASS) is available in different languages at www.who.int. WHO also publishes list of critically important antimicrobials periodically and its 5th revision is currently available online (Advisory, 2016). The list is intended to assist in managing antimicrobial resistance, ensuring that all antimicrobials, especially critically important antimicrobials, are used prudently both in human and veterinary medicine.

8. **Role of people participation:**

a) **Increasing Public Awareness:**

Everyone has a role to play. Educational awareness to public about the use and misuse of antibiotics and explaining that "antibiotics save lives but too few are available" is an important aspect. The patients, healthcare workers, hospitals, clinics and nursing homes, healthcare quality organizations, professional organizations, Government and local health agencies, can contribute significantly in promoting pragmatic use of antibiotics. Patients and their families should be educated to-

- Use antibiotics as prescribed by a doctor
- Complete the full antibiotic course, even if they feel better
- Not to share antibiotics with others or using left over prescriptions
- Not to use antibiotics as growth promoters in farm animals
- World Antibiotic Awareness week is observed every year since 2015 and this year will be held between 13th-19th November, 2017. The theme is *"Seek advice from a qualified healthcare professional before taking antibiotics"*. WHO encourages member countries and partners to disseminate awareness by poster and infographics.

b) **Role of healthcare workers, quality organizations and pharmacists:**

They can assist by:

- Enhancing infection prevention and control
- Prescribing and dispensing antibiotics only when they are truly needed.
- Strictly observing a ban on over the counter sale of antibiotics
- Developing and implementing standards for stewardship programs
- Complying with rules and regulations

The role of various stakeholders is described in a recent US document on Antibiotic use (CDC, 2017).

B. Development of Newer Antibiotics

Whereas only 5 new antibiotics were approved between 2000-2010, the efforts at international and national levels have resulted in an spurt in the development thereafter Thus during 2014-15, five newer drugs were released for clinical use (Table-8).

C. Alternative Approaches

To overcome the different cellular barriers approaches for treating infection include the development of nanoparticles, anti-microbial peptides, anti-senseoligonucleotides, which control gene expression through targeting RNA, and also novel use of a topical antibacterial polymer polyhexamethylenebiguanide. The formation of biofilms presents problems for treating bacterial infection, and approaches to either inhibit or prevent biofilm formation using light treatment as well as chemical and biological means through bacteriophage are reviewed (Hughes G, 2017). The cholesterol degradation pathway supplies nutrients for intracellular M. Tuberculosis, and mycobacterial cholesterol metabolism is discussed as providing a route for targeting intracellular infection by M. Tuberculosis infection.

Marine bacterial products are explored by *ichip* technology to identify substances with antibacterial properties. Thus, Teixobactin was identified in 2015 and is being evaluated further. Another exciting field is to reduce pathogenicity of bacteria by starving, inhibiting ability to release endotoxins and modulating host response by probiotic use.

7. Conclusions

Antibiotic Resistance is an ever increasing public health problem which has evolved from environmental mixing of genes and is further aggravated by unrestricted use of antibiotics in livestock husbandry and poultry farming. Inappropriate use of antibiotics at all levels of health care delivery; poor sanitation and lack of awareness of seriousness of the AR are increasingly realized as modifiable factors. These issues are taken care at global, national and local levels. Strategies are designed to curb the menace of AR by regulating availability and access, improving prescribing habits and monitoring the antibiotic use. It is hoped that these measures would curtail the increasing emergence of multidrug resistant organisms. Simultaneous development of newer agents should satisfy the need of antibiotics in nosocomial infections.

Box-I: Mutation Selection

AR is most frequently due to selection of mutant bacteria which propagate in nature. Mutations occur in genes responsible for (a) Altered antibiotic binding proteins-PBPs, (b) altered formation of structural protein and (c) Altered enzymes which inactivates antibiotics. Mutations occur randomly and such mutant strains have survival advantage in environment. Exposure to pollutants with low antibacterial activity and heavy metals favours selection and propagation of mutant strains, many of which are resistant bacteria and thus humans are exposed to such resistant bacterial strains inadvertently. In Mycobacteria, single step mutation can cause Isoniazid resistance. Sometimes, there is mutational defect in DNA repair mechanism. This leads to a high degree of alteration in many genes in bacteria. These bacteria are hyper mutable phenotypes and may lead to evolution of Multi Drug Resistance (MDR) bacteria.

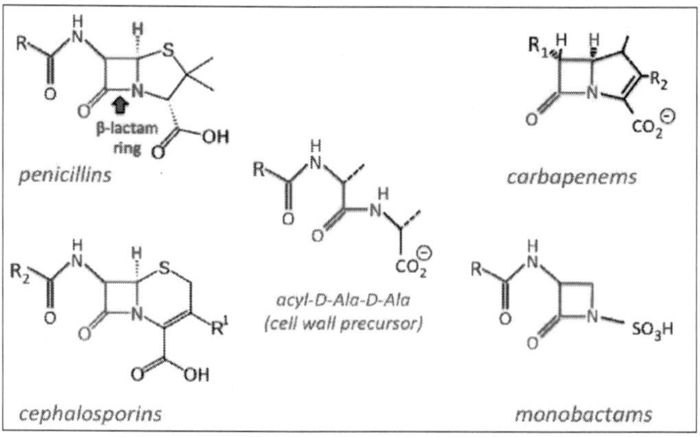

Fig. 1: Structure of β-lactam antibiotics, similarity between β-lactam structure with cell wall precursor and site of inactivation by β-lactamase enzyme (Arrow). The 4-member β-lactam ring is shown in red.

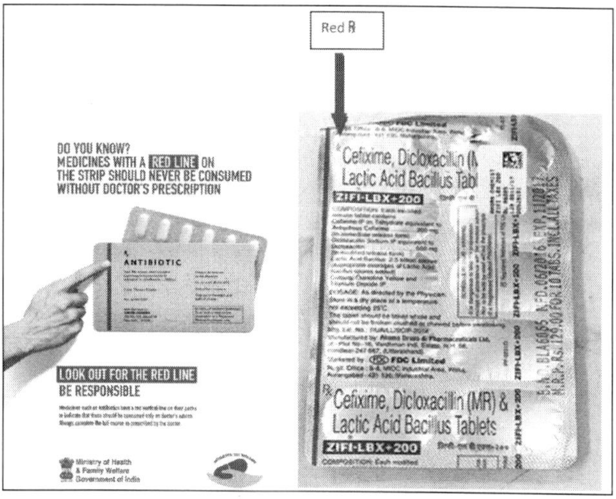

Fig. 2: Increasing Public Awareness

Table 1: Host factors in development of AR

Host/Bacterial Interaction		**Mechanism**
Size of Inoculum	Larger inoculums	More number of resistant mutants
Biofilms	Implants, Prosthetic heart valves, catheters	Bacteria produce polysaccharides in biofilms and have reduced growth rates so the sensitivity to antibiotics is reduced. Reduced access to antibiotics.
Age of infection	Acute versus chronic	Bacteria multiply slowly in chronic infections. The antibiotic more effective during log growth phase are rendered less effective.
Additional Interference	Pus (Abscess)	Low pH and lower pO_2 reduce bactericidal action of penicillins.
Level of Immunity	Immunocompromised Host	HIV, MDR-TB occur commonly

Table 2: Priority List of Pathogens for Drug Research (WHO, 2017)

1. Mycobacterium tuberculosis
2. Critical Priority Pathogens: Carbapen resistant organisms:
   a. Acenobacter, Pseudomonas, Enterobacteriaceae
3. High priority Pathogens
   a. Vancomycin resistant: Enterococci, S. aureus (MRSA)
   b. Fluoroquinolone resistant: Salmonella and Comylobacter
   c. IIIrd Generation Cephalosporin Resistant: Neisseria
4. Medium priority Pathogens:
   a. Penicillin resistant S pneumonia
   b. Ampicillin resistant H influenza
   c. Fluoroquinolone resistant Shigella

Table 3: Characteristics of different DNA sequences

Element	Characteristics	Function
Insertion Sequences (IS)	Short DNA segments which encode for a specific enzymatic function. Can copy themselves and insert into chromosomes or plasmids.	Assist in development of active integration site on plasmid or transposons.
Transposons	Mobile elements, like IS, that can shuttle between chromosome and plasmids.	Bidirectional transfer of resistance genes between chromosomes and plasmids.
Integrons	Like IS but are non-mobile and cannot copy themselves. Integrons can localize within transposons or plasmids.	Provide site (Promoter site) for integration of mobile gene cassettes carrying resistance determinants to form downstream sequences in bacteria
Class-I Integrons	Sites for gene aggregation on plasmids or transposons	Favour the spread of several genes (MDR) by transfer to other microbes.

Table 4: Different mechanisms of Gene transfer

	Gene transfer Process	Diagram
Transduction	Transfer of genetic information from a donor to a recipient bacterium of same or different species by way of a bacteriophage- a virus that propagates in bacteria and has carried DNA (including resistant genes) from previous bacterium in its outer coat.	Transduction is important in development of AR in S. aureus. 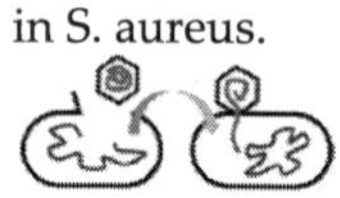
Conjugation	Transfer of DNA from a donor to a recipient bacterium by direct physical contact between the bacteria by forming sex pillus or bridge and is unidirectional. Donor bacteria have F factor or fertility factor or sex factor. The F factor is a circular piece of DNA that can replicate autonomously in the cell (independent replicon). Plasmids are extra-chromosomal pieces of DNA that can replicate autonomously. An episome is a plasmid that can integrate into the bacterial chromosome. Conjugation is a major way of transfer of multidrug resistant genes in gram-negative organisms.	Conjugation is exchange of resistance genes between intestinal commensals and pathogens (Enterococci) in GIT of humans and animals. 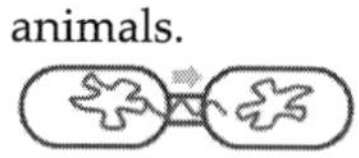
Transformation	Uptake of a naked DNA from a donor bacterium by a recipient bacterial cell. It is a common phenomenon in nature. Certain bacteria (e.g. Bacillus, Haemophilus, Neisseria, Pneumococcus) can take up double stranded DNA segments from the environment sources and this DNA is incorporated into the recipient's chromosome when there is degree of homology between donor and recipient DNAs.	Transformation is responsible for pneumococcal penicillin resistance. It is used in recombination technology nowadays. 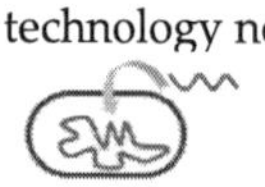

Table 5: Simplified Classification of β-lactamase enzymes

Nature	Class	Example	Resistance
Serine β lactamases	Class-A	ESBLs, Carbapenemase	Inhibited by Clavulanate and Tazobactam
Metallo-β lactamases (Zn binding thiol Gp)	Class-B	Carbapenemases	All β-lactams except Aztreonam
Serine β lactamases	Class-C	AmpC (Chromosomal)	Cefoxitin and IIIrd generation Cephalosporins resistance
Serine β lactamases	Class-D	Cloxacillin degrading enzymes, AmpC (Plasmid encoded)	All β lactams

Table 6: Mechanisms of development of resistance in other antibiotics

Antibiotic	Type of resistance	Bacterial site	Mechanism
Tetracyclines	Plasmid mediated and inducible	Cell wall	Reduced influx or enhanced efflux
		Production of ribosomal protection proteins	Displacement of tetracyclines from ribosomal binding sites
		Inactivation of tetracyclines	
Fluoroquinolones	Mutations in topoisomerase-II/IV genes	Reduced binding on DNA targets	Reduced introduction of negative supercoils in pathogens
	Plasmid mediated resistance	Mutation in genes	Reduced binding, increased inactivation of aminoglycosides and Increased efflux
Macrolides	Mutations in 23s ribosomal RNA(rRNA) and genes for ribosomal proteins	Reduced drug binding to ribosomal fractions and methylation of rRNA by acquired *ermgenes**	Resistance in pneumococci and E coli
	Changes in inactivating enzymes	Macrolide phosphor-transferase and esterase hydrolysis	Inactivation by pneumococci and staphylococci
	Mutation in genes for Efflux pumps	Transporters malfunction	Pneumococcal resistance
Spectinomycin	Mutation	16s ribosomes	Reduced binding
Vancomycin	Through transposons of plasmids	Altered cell wall targets of enterococci which bind vancomycin (van-A,B and C phenotypes)	E faecalis resistance

Antibiotic	Type of resistance	Bacterial site	Mechanism
		Conjugative plasmid mediated van-A transposon transmitted from E faecalis to MRSA	Staphyloccocal resistance
Antitubercular Drugs			
Rifampicin	Mutation in codon 526 and 531 of rpoB gene which synthesizes DNA dependent RNA polymerase enzyme (BP, 2014)	No suppression of chain formation	Important for tuberculosis and E. coli
Isoniazid	Spontaneous single point mutations of katG	Altered activity of catalase peroxidase gene (katG)	Cross resistance to ethionamide
		Enhanced efflux	Cross resistance with ethambutol
Pyrazinamide		Altered Pyrazinamidase activity due to single point gene mutations	Less activation (deamination) of pyrazinamide in Mycobacteria

**erythromycin ribosomal methylation gene*

Table 7: Initiatives taken in India

S. No.	Initiative	Year	Objectives
1	12th five year plan – Containment of AR	2012-2017	To generate awareness, to establish surveillance system and to strengthen infection control guidelines.
2	The National Policy for Containment of AR	2011	To monitor sale of antibiotics by introduction of schedule H1 in Drug and cosmetic Rules. To constitute Antibiotic Management Team to develop Hospital antimicrobial policy. To establish co-ordination among CSIR, MOHFW, ICAR and Department of Animal Husbandry.
3	National AR Research and Surveillance Network (AMRRSN)	2011	To set up Antimicrobial surveillance network for common pathogens. To develop national repository of bacterial strains.
4	Jaipur Declaration (a WHO initiative)	2011	To formulate multisectoral national alliances against antimicrobial resistance. To strengthen legislation and regulate use of antibiotics. To strengthen infection control practices. To encourage basic and operational research.

S. No.	Initiative	Year	Objectives
5	Chennai Declaration	2012	To take initiatives to formulate national policy. To improve infection control standards. To make necessary curricular changes at UG and PG level. Strict implementation of hospital infection control policy. To standardize microbiology laboratories in India. To involve NGOs to disseminate information.
6	The Drugs and Cosmetic Rule, 1945	Amended in 2013	To control unrestricted use of antibiotics in India. The packaging of these drugs will have mandatory Schedule H1 warning printed on a label in a box with red border and the Rx symbol in red.
7	National Treatment Guidelines for Antimicrobial Use in Infectious Diseases	2016	To restrict inappropriate use of antibiotics, optimize selection and reduce adverse events and cost.

Table 8: Newer antibiotics approved and in development

Name	Year	Chemical class
Doripenem	2007	Carbapenem
Telavancin	2008	Glycopeptide
Ceftaroline	2010	Vth Generation Cephalosporin
Tedizolid	2014	Oxazolidinone
Delbavancin, Oritavancin	2014	Glycopeptide
Ceftazolone+Tazobactam	2014	Cepahlosporin+Betalactamase Inhibitor (BLI)
Ceftazidime+Avibactam	2015	IIIrd generation Cephalosporin +BLI
Plasmomicin	Phase-III trials	Aminoglycoside
Delafloxacin	Approved June, 2017	Broad spectrum Quinolone
Vaborbactam+Meropenem	Aug,2017	meropenem, a penemand vaborbactam, a beta-lactamase inhibitor
Omadacycline	Phase-II trials	Tetracycline
Pseudouridimycin	Early phase studies	Bacterial RNA polymerase inhibitor
Teixobactin	Clinical Trials	Macrocyclic Depsipeptide

References

Advisory, G. W. (2016). *Integrated Surveillance of Antimicrobial Resistance (AGISAR).* Raleigh: WHO.

Aminov, R. I. (2011). Horizontal Gene Exchange in Environmental Microbiota. *Frontiers in Microbiology, 2,* 158.

Avneet Saini, R. B. (2012). Insights on the structural characteristics of NDM-1: The journey so far. *Advances in Biological Chemistry,* 323-34.

Baquero F, M. J. (2008). Antibiotics and antibiotic resistance in water environments. *Current Opinion in Biotechnology, 19*(3), 260-5.

Bartlett JG, G. D. (2013). Seven ways to preserve the miracle of antibiotics. *Clinical Infectious Diseases, 56*(10), 1445-50.

BP, G. (2014). Resistance to rifampicin: a review. *The Journal of Antibiotics, 67*(9), 625-30.

CDC. (2017). *Antibiotic Use in the United States: Progress and Opportunities.* Atlanta: US Department of Health and Human Services.

Coyne S, C. P. (2011). Efflux-mediated antibiotic resistance in Acinetobacter spp. *Antimicrobial Agents and Chemotherapy, 55*(3), 947-53.

Daiyasu H, O. K. (2001). Expansion of the zinc metallo-hydrolase family of the beta-lactamase fold. *FEBS Letters, 503*(1), 1-6.

Depledge, M. (2011). Pharmaceuticals: Reduce drug waste in the environment. *Nature, 478*(7367), 36.

Depledge, M. (2011). Pharmaceuticals: Reduce drug waste in the environment. *Nature, 478*(7367), 36.

Gillings MR, X. D. (2009). Gene cassettes encoding resistance to quaternary ammonium compounds: a role in the origin of clinical class 1 integrons? *ISME J, 3*(2), 209-15.

Gullberg E, C. S. (2011). Selection of resistant bacteria at very low antibiotic concentrations. *PLoS Pathog, 7*(7), 1-9.

Hellen Gelband, M. M.-P. (2015). *THE STATE OF THE WORLD'S ANTIBIOTICS 2015.* Washington, D.C.: CDDEP.

Hernández A, S. M. (2011). Quinolone resistance: much more than predicted. *Frontiers in Microbiology, 2,* 22.

Heynick, F. (2009). The original 'magic bullet' is 100 years old - extra. *British Journal of Psychiatry, 195*(5), 456.

Hughes G, W. M. (2017). Novel approaches to the treatment of bacterial biofilm infections. *British Journal of Pharmacology, 174*(14), 2237-46.

Jinka DR, G. S.-U. (2017). Impact of Antibiotic Policy on Antibiotic Consumption in a Neonatal Intensive Care Unit in India. *Indian Pediatrics, 54*(9), 739-41.

Kamini Walia, V. C. (2017). *Treatment Guidelines for Antimicrobial Use in Common Syndromes.* New Delhi: Indian Council of Medical Research Department of Health Research.

Kamini Walia, V. O. (2015). Antimicrobial stewardship programme (AMSP) practices in India. *Indian Journal of Medical Research, 142*, 130-8.

Karen Bush, G. A. (2010). Updated Functional Classification of β-Lactamases. *Antimicrobial Agents and Chemotherapy, 54*(3), 969-76.

Kumarasamy KK, T. M. (2010). Emergence of a new antibiotic resistance mechanism in India, Pakistan, and the UK: a molecular, biological, and epidemiological study. *The Lancet infectious diseases, 10*(9), 597-602.

Lacroix FJ, C. A. (1996). Salmonella typhimurium acrB-like gene: identification and role in resistance to biliary salts and detergents and in murine infection. *FEMS microbiology letters, 135*, 161-7.

Manoharan A, S. M. (2012). Phenotypic & molecular characterization of AmpC β-lactamases among Escherichia coli, Klebsiella spp. & Enterobacter spp. from five Indian Medical Centers. *Indian Journal of Medical Research, 135*, 359-64.

Martinez, J. (2009). Environmental pollution by antibiotics and by antibiotic resistance determinants. *Environmental Pollution, 157*(11), 2893-902.

Molin S, T.-N. T. (2003). Gene transfer occurs with enhanced efficiency in biofilms and induces enhanced stabilisation of the biofilm structure. *Curr Opin Biotechnol, 14*(3), 255-61.

Nikaido H, P. J. (2012). Broad-specificity efflux pumps and their role in multidrug resistance of Gram-negative bacteria. *FEMS microbiology reviews, 36*(2), 340-63.

Otten, H. (1986). Domagk and the development of the sulphonamides. *The Journal of antimicrobial chemotherapy, 17*(6), 689-96.

Petri, W. (2011). *Penicillins, Cephalosporins, and other β-lactam antibiotics.* (C. B. Brunton L, Ed.) New Delhi: McGraw Hill.

Ramakant Sahu, P. S. (2014). *Antibiotics in Chicken Meat.* New Delhi: Centre for Science and Environment.

Ryan, E. S. (2017). Drug metabolism and antibiotic resistance in micro-organisms. *British Journal of Pharmacology, 174*, 2159-60.

S. Koike, I. G.-S. (2007). *Applied and Environmental Microbiology, 73*(15), 4813-23.

Schuetz P, W. Y.-C. (2017). Effect of procalcitonin-guided antibiotic treatment on mortality in acute respiratory infections: a patient level meta-analysis. *The Lancet Infectious Diseases*, 30592-3.

Sengeløv G, S. S. (1998). Methods for detection of conjugative plasmid transfer in aquatic environments. *Curr Microbiol, 37*(4), 274-80.

Sumanth Gandra, S. K. (2017). Point Prevalence Surveys of Antimicrobial Use among Hospitalized Children in Six Hospitals in India in 2016. *Antibiotics, 6*(3), 19.

Taylor NG, V.-J. D.-A. (2011). Aquatic systems: maintaining, mixing and mobilising antimicrobial resistance? *Trends Ecol Evol, 26*(6), 278-84.

Ventola, C. L. (2015). The Antibiotic Resistance Crisis, Part 1: Causes and Threats. *Pharmacy & Therapeutics, 40*(4), 277-83.

Walsh TR, W. J. (2011). Dissemination of NDM-1 positive bacteria in the New Delhi environment and its implications for human health: an environmental point prevalence study. *The LANCET Infectious Diseases, 11*(5), 355-62.

WHO. (2017, June 1). IMPLEMENTATION OF THE GLOBAL ACTION PLAN. *WHO GAP AMR Newsletter*, pp. 1-4.

WHO. (2017). *Prioritization of Pathogens to Guide Discovery, Research and Development of New Antibiotics for Drug-Resistant Bacterial Infections, Including Tuberculosis.* Geneva: WHO.

Wright GD, P. H. (2012). Antibiotic resistance is ancient: implications for drug discovery. *Trends Microbiol, 20*(4), 157-9.

Wright, G. (2010). Antibiotic resistance in the environment: a link to the clinic? *Current Opinion in Microbiology, 13*(5), 589-94.

Chapter 13

Stem Cells its Emerging Biology, Clinical Applications and Challenges

Kanjaksha Ghosh, Avani Shah and Kanchan Mishra

Institute: Surat Raktadan Kendra & Research Centre, Gujarat, India.

Email:avanishaho8@gmail.com

Abstract

Every organ in our body generally lasts the whole of our lifetime measuring nearly 60-80 years at present. Rarely due to continued damage or due to some genetic factors or various contributing factors in the environment i.e. drugs, infections, diet and toxins .Sometimes one or other of these organs fail prematurely or cause different diseases endangering our life. We needed technology to advance to help us. Radioisotopes (radiobiology) and advances in cell culture provided us in the middle of 20th century the requisite technology to understand and count at least some form of stem cells. Now a days stem cells can be banked for long period of time using a process called cryopreservation. These cells are processed through a rate controlled freezing process and are preserved in liquid nitrogen with some cryoprotective chemical like Dimethyl sulphoxide.

Stem cell expansion in culture in vitro is one of the advancing technology and is improving every day we need to expand stem cells in vitro because of various reasons , however one of the challenges in-vitro expansion is the right kind of environmental set up for such expansion is still being searched. Stem cell based gene therapy has its own challenges and hazards. However the dividend for this kind of therapy is likely to be very great hence we will continue to circumvent these challenges and finally develop its multitude of applications towards human service.

Introduction

Every organ in our body generally lasts the whole of our lifetime measuring nearly 60-80 years at present. Rarely due to continued damage or due to some genetic factors or various contributing factors in the environment i.e. drugs, infections, diet and toxins .Sometimes one or other of these organs fail prematurely or cause different diseases endangering our life. However who repairs or regenerates these damaged organs in most of the time and whole of our lifetime? This question has troubled many scientists, doctors and biologists through the bygone era.

Hematologists were initially investigated the fact , that every day several billion red blood cells , white cells and platelets are destroyed in our body but we still keep their number constant in blood. So there has to be some kind of cells in our hematopoietic system which can produce all kind of blood cells throughout our whole life and if we lose those cells no blood cells can be produced and we get a fatal disease called Aplastic anemia. Hematologists at that time (turn of 19th century and beginning of 20th century) named these hypothetical cells haemopoietic stem cells (Maximov & Bloom). Similarly in many animals and even in man if half of the liver is removed by operation these livers grow back again in short time. Every few days whole of our body skin cells, gastrointestinal tract epithelial cells and genitourinary tract epithelial cells are totally replaced. Hence a consensual was beginning to emerge that such cells must be there in ever organ or tissue which are capable of regeneration and replacement of cells in that organ damaged due to various reasons. Moreover from the animal world striking regenerative capability of the animals ie a lizard growing back its tail after it was damaged, a spider similarly growing back its legs if damaged or removed. How for a long time in 20 th century nobody has an idea how these cells must look like and how to count their number amongst many cells seen in any organ including blood and bone marrow as a part of haemopoietic system. We needed technology to advance to help us. Radioisotopes (radiobiology) and advances in cell culture provided us in the middle of 20 th century the requisite technology to understand and count at least some form of stem cells. In the present chapter we will broadly discuss definition of stem cells, how are they measured? Which are the sources today for this kind of cells? What is possible to do with these cells and what are the challenges in using these cells for medical and other purposes and what the future of stem cell research may mean to us i.e. humankind.

Stem Cells definition, properties and classification (1-3)

Definition: Stem cells are characterized by its extensive capability of multiplication, capability of being differentiated under various chemical and environmental cues and finally it can also produce daughter stem cells with all the properties of mother stem cells. The mitosis of stem cells could be asymmetric where each stem cell divides into one daughter stem cells and another cell which is going to be differentiated or symmetric where one stem cell gives rise to two daughter cells both capable of differentiation and loss of this stem cell is sensed by the stem cell compartment leading to division of another stem cell into two daughter stem cells marinating the constant number in the stem cell compartment as shown below in figure 1. There is a hierarchy of stem cells and its differentiated offspring, this hierarchy of differentiation has been well worked out for haemopoietic stem cells and presented in figure 2.

This ability to produce daughter stem cells is very important and protects in normal health from stem cell exhaustion in the lifetime of the individual. Stem cells normally remain in quiescent state and in special microenvironment called 'Niche'. This niche is composed of different types of cells e.g. fibroblasts, adiposities, special cells immunocompetent cells of certain subtypes and, extracellular matrix of different composition. Quiescence of stem cells is maintained by interaction of the stem cells with stromal cells through various integrin and other adhesion molecules. Various growth factors, cytokines, hormones and perturbation of stem cell compartments by drugs and by diseases influence the nature of stroma and stem cell interaction influencing the level of quiescence or activity. When stroma stem cell interaction becomes lose then stem cells becomes active and is in a position to circulate and can translocate itself in another place initiating tissue regeneration.

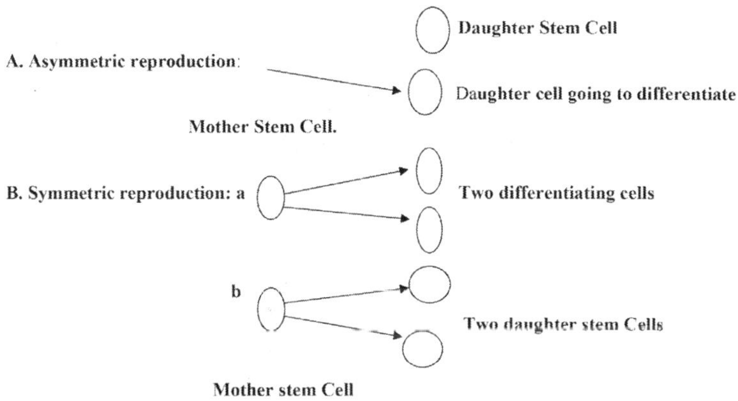

Fig. 1: Differentiation of stem cells

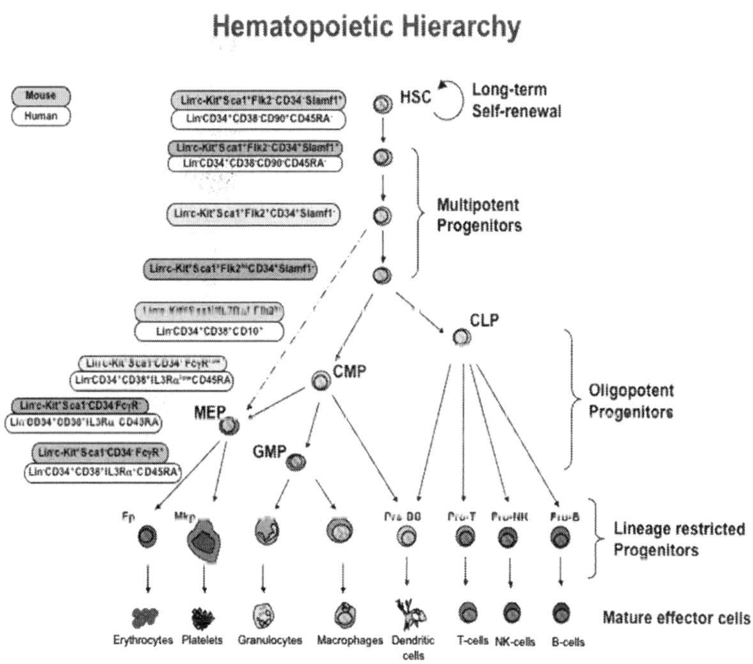

Fig. 2: Differentiation scheme of haemopoietic stem cells (4)

Properties of stem cells: Basic properties of stem cells have been well incorporated in its classification. Stem cells have receptors on its surface for various growth factors and adhesion molecules. These growth factor and adhesion molecules differ for different types of stem cells and its degree of differentiation. The pattern and nature of adhesion molecules expressed on the stem cell provides a kind of bar code address telling the body where these cells will eventually find its home (niche) where stromal cells express reciprocal receptors for the adhesion molecules. The density of expression of different growth factor receptors determines how this particular cell will execute its differentiation programmers in response to different growth factors. Stem cell can also secrete growth factors or growth inhibitors to attract or repel different types of cells which will help in tissue regeneration, repair and immunomodulation.

Various types of antigens expressed on the surface of stem cells can be classified as (i) Lineage dependent antigens (ii) stage (immaturity) dependent antigens (iii) activation dependent antigens. Nowadays Fluorescent dye tagged monoclonal antibodies to different cellular antigens (currently almost 300 antibodies against various such antigens denoted as CD1, CD2 etc are available) can be used by flowcytometry to define different types of stem cells. These antibodies can also be used for histological staining of solid tissues. There are certain subsets of cells which come between fully differentiated cells in any tissue and its cognate stem cells. These cells have lost most of the properties of stem cell but can divide and differentiate into cells of the lineage, these cells are called committed progenitor cells they cannot replenish its own compartment. The compartment is to be replenished by stem cell division of that organ or tissue. Table 1 presents some of the antigens expressed in different types of stem cells and these cells can be identified by using the antibodies to these antigen using a machine called flowcytometer. These antibodies can also help in purifying stem cells from a mixture of different cells by a process called immunoafiinity purification.

Table 1: Immunophenotypic profile of different classes of circulating stem cells

Marker	pCMC	BM-MSC	HSC	EP_C	BD-MSC	MOMCs
CD14	–	–	–	–		+
CD34	+	–	+/–	+	–	+
CD44	+	+	+/–	–	+	–
CD45	–	–	+	–	–	+
CD90	+	+	+	+	+	–
CD105	–	+	+	+	+	+
CD106	+	+	+	+	+	–
CD133	+	–	+	+		–
CXCR4	–	+	+	+		–
HLA-DR/SLA-DR +		–	–	–		+
Collagen I	+	+	–	+		+
α-SMA	+	+	–	–		–
vWF	–	–	–	+		–

Notes: +, expression; -, no expression (5).

Abbreviations: pCMC, porcine circulating multipotent cells; BM-MSC, bone marrow mesenchymal stem cells; HSC, hematopoietic stem cells; EPc, endothelial progenitor cells; BD-MSC, blood-derived mesenchymal stem cells; MOMCs, monocyte-derived multipotential cells; CXCR4, C-X-C chemokine receptor type 4; HLA-DR, human leukocyte antigen; SLA-DR, swine leukocyte antigen DR; α-SMA, alpha-smooth muscle actin; vWF, von Willebrand factor.

Recently it has been demonstrated that stem cells which can differentiate into limited cell repertoire of a particular germ layer (Ectoderm, Endoderm or Mesoderm) can under suitable in vitro condition be made to differentiate into cells of alternative or another germ layer. This phenomenon is called transdifferentiation. Transdifferentiation is a very important property and this quality of a stem cell opens the way to use one type of stem cells for repair / regenerative purpose of any tissue.

Classification of stem cells (3)

a) **Classification based on tissue of origin:** Depending on tissues or organs from which the stem cells are obtained they can be classified as Haemopoietic (bone marrow or peripheral blood), Neural, Liver, Renal, Mesenchymal , cord blood , adipose tissue, placental stem cells etc.. On surface marker study they usually carry one of the marker of Stem Cells like CD 34 or CD 133, and several antigen which denotes the lineage of the tissue and finally antigen denoting the levels of maturity e.g. DR antigens for haemopoietic stem cells. Maturity can also be detected by the level of expression as well as the site of expression of the antigen e.g a cell membrane antigen is initially synthesized inside a cell cytoplasm hence a cell showing cytoplasmic positivity for that antigen but no cell membrane or poor cell membrane positivity denotes the cell to be in the earlier stage of differentiation than one strongly expressing the cell membrane positivity for the same antigen.

b) **Classification based on potency** (ability of the cells to differentiate into a spectrum of diverse kinds of differentiated cells) **Totipotent** e.g a cell which can produce every cell or every organ of the body classical example is fertilized ovum or cells obtained from first 3 4 cell division of this fertilized ovum. These cells are often called embryonic stem cells. **Pluripotent** e.g. when these stem cells are capable of making most but not all the cells or tissues of the body.

   Now a day's science has advanced to such a degree that in the laboratory any fully differentiated cell like epithelial , mesenchymal can be made Pluripotent stem cell by activating /expressing three or four genes exemplified by c myc , Oct 4, Sox2, Klf4, Nanog , Lin28. These artificially constructed pluripotent cells has a lot of application probabilities in medicine and and related sciences. This kind of cells is called **Induced Pluripotent Cells (IPSc)**. Stem cells could also be **multipotent or committed** to only one or few lineage of cells.

c) **Classification based on culture or harvest conditions or characteristics:** Originally haemopoietic stem cells were demonstrated in the form of colonies in the spleen of irradiated mouse and it was called **CFU-S (colony forming unit in spleen).** Later on such colonies could be grown in soft agar , methyl cellulose containing culture platelets much like we grow bacterial colony where they were named on the cell of origin or characteristic appearance in culture e.g. **CFU-G**(Colony Forming unit Granulocyte), **BFU E** (Burst Forming Unit Erythrocyte) , **CFU-GEMM** (Colony Forming Unit Granulocyte, Erythrocyte , Megakaryocyte , Monocyte) etc.

d) **Classification depending on the donor of stem cells usage:**

If the patient's own stem cells are used it is called **autologous.** If stem cells from another animal of the same species as the recipient is used it is called **allogeneic.** When stem cells from one species is injected in another species it is called **Xenogenic,**

Stem Cell Expansion and Banking (3, 6)

Now a days stem cells can be banked for long period of time using a process called cryopreservation. These cells are processed through a rate controlled freezing process and are preserved in liquid nitrogen with some cryoprotective chemical like Dimethyl sulphoxide.

This way these cells can be preserved for more than 10 years and can be used in times of need. Once umbilical cord blood or blood trapped in placenta after the baby is born was found to be a good source of haemopoietic stem cells and umbilical cord itself was also found to contain mesenchymal stem cells in good amounts. These stem cells are banked either by the use of the same baby in future if need be but more often these stem cells are used in many unrelated patients across the world to treat serious hematological or immunological disorders. Today almost 100,000 such transplantations are done across the world. Like cord blood stem cells bone marrow or peripheral blood stem cells from the patient or from another donor can be cryopreserved for future use.

Stem cell expansion in culture in vitro is one of the advancing technology and is improving every day we need to expand stem cells in vitro because of various reasons , however one of the challenges in-vitro expansion is the right kind of environmental set up for such expansion is still being searched. However several expansion programs in the world using bioreactor and only synthetic culture material has produced expanded cells which has been used for haemopoietic stem cell transplantations with successful marrow reconstitution.

Possible clinical application of stem cells (3)

Stem cells have tremendous potential clinical application. However significant challenges need to be overcome before these cells can be used for many clinical situations.

Presently haemopoietic stem cell transplantations for serious hematological, immunological and certain genetic disorder is an accepted procedure. However stem cell therapy for many degenerative and malignant conditions is in serious research phase.

Some of the areas of this therapy are given below. Another potentially developing area is marriage of molecular biology with stem cell therapy. In this condition autologous stem cells from patients with genetic disorders can be gene corrected and then transplanted. At animal level such corrections have been possible for thalassemia, sickle cell anemia etc. However human trial is still having various hurdles to cross. Pharmaceutical industry has a challenge in developing new drugs and testing its toxicity in animals. Animal ethicists have been pressing for alternate ways for testing chemical compounds. Stem cells provide an option to develop organ on chip for drug effect and toxicity testing. Marriage of engineering technology with stem cell biology has produced a completely new branch of biological sciences where efforts are made to develop tissues and organs using stem cells on artificial scaffolds using 3D printing technology to spray stem cells in different location of the scaffold in requisite quality. In a similar way haemopoietic stem cells are being harnessed to produce universal red cells for transfusion. Each of this development when fully realized have the potential to totally change the medical care for various diseases which are incurable today.

Stem Cell therapy and various types of cell therapies having clinical application

1. Ischemic and Non Ischemic Cardiomyopathy leading to heart failure resistant to maximum medical therapy (7-10):

Ischemic heart disease is a leading cause of heart failure in the world today. In addition dilated Cardiomyopathy or cardiac muscle diseases of various etiologies eventually lead to heart failure resistant to treatment with current combination of drugs. Several clinical combinations of drugs like ACE Inhibitors, Diuretics and beta blockers and vasodilators have been used for the purpose. But there is a subset of patients who resist maximum combinations of these drugs. Inotrops were not of much use in chronic heart failure and many of the present day heart failures are diastolic failures where increased ventricular wall stiffness as a result of fibrosis and deposition of other extracellular matrix is the major contributor for which no satisfactory therapy as yet is available.

Several clinical trials which involved injecting either bone marrow mononuclear cells (which contains around <1% CD 34 + haemopoietic stem cells), growth factor stimulated peripheral blood stem cells at varying dosages i.e. from 10^5cells/Kg to 10^6 cells/kg has shown significant benefit (5-10%) in improvement of ejection fraction, systolic volume, end diastolic volume and 6 minutes walking distance at varying period after intravenous / intra coronary injection of these cells.

This effect tends to persist beyond one year and no serious side effects were seen for this autologous stem cell therapy. It is believed that these stem cell do not persists in the myocardium as shown by myocardial biopsy But probably these cells helps through production of various growth factors or produce immunomodultory effect leading to structural changes and dissolution of fibrosis in the myocardium. The effects of mononuclear stem cell therapy can have an additive effect on maximally tolerated anti failure regimes. The therapy was also found to be useful in refractory angina pectoris.

2. Mononuclear Cell / Stem cell therapy for limb ischaemia (11):

Vascular insufficiency in the limbs particularly in the lower limbs leading to claudication pain and eventually gangrene happens in a subset of patients with diabetes or atherosclerotic vascular disorder and there number is increasing every day as people are living long and prevalence of diabetes and atherosclerosis is increasing in the population.

When limb ischemia is due to a thrombus or obstructed embolus then surgical procedure through thrombo embolectomy is the procedure of choice. But progressive limb ischemia due to various reasons responds well to CD34+ haemopoietic stem cell therapy from autologous bone marrow samples. The procedure is safe and can be quickly performed. The mononuclear cell preparation on or CD34+ stem cell preparation can be injected intra muscularly or in the close proximity across the length of the culprit vessels (several injection) 10^4-10^5 cells at each sites and at a time in over 15-20 sites.

There are many studies on peripheral vascular insufficient and success of stem cells or bone marrow derived mono nuclear cell infusion in the condition. The success has been demonstrated by angiography thermography and functional recovery. The treatment can be repeated as required.

Cell Therapy for Diabetes Mellitus (12-14):

Insulin Dependent (IDDM) and Non Insulin dependent diabetes mellitus where controlling the diabetes was difficult has been treated by various groups either by using autologous bone marrow derived mononuclear cells or CD34+ stem cells with improvement of glycaemic control. These patients have also been treated with umbilical cord based stem cell therapy with positive results i.e. reduction in insulin requirement, increased C peptide secretion and lower HbA1c levels with better control of disease in short and medium term (upto two years) has been documented in innumerable studies. No. serious side effects were noticed. Both immunomodultory effect paracrine effect and transdifferentiation of haemopoietic stem cell into insulin secreting β cells of the islets have been theorized to be the mechanism of action of stem cells in the disease.

Probably a combination of factors work. These stem cells most commonly is given by simple intravenous injection or else it can be given through celiac artery for homing into the pancreas. General application of all types of stem cells and bone marrow derived mononuclear cells produced positive effect in both types of diabetes mellitus with significantly increased C-peptide levels in plasma suggesting requirement of insulin reduction and secretion of additional insulin by cell therapy. Of all the cells Intravenous infusion of CD34+ cells harvested from bone marrow gave the best result as shown in an extensive meta analysis where 58.9% treated patient become insulin independent at least for a mean period of 16 months. It was also shown that the effect of stem cell therapy in diabetes patient is better when offered during the early stage of the disease.

3. Treatment of painful osteoarthritis knee with haemopoietic stem cell from marrow or platelet rich plasma.(15,16):

Osteoarthritis of knee joints is common clinical condition and is seen in many people above the age of 55-60 years. It is common and occurs early in those patients who injures their Knee joint at some point in life i.e. sports person those who have to life weight regularly, daily passengers and others who have to stand for a long time and ankle joint which has suffered other types of inflammatory arthritis before.

Essential pathology of osteoarthritis in this complex weight bearing joint is (i) Tear /injury of various ligaments (ii) Tearing and degeneration of articular cartilage (iii) diminished production of high molecular weight viscous lubricating synovial fluid. (iv) Eburnation (due to repeated friction) and osteophyte formation in the bone (v) non inflammatory effusion in the joint.

The present therapy of OA of knee joint is far from satisfactory and generally it involves (i) pain relief by NSAIDS (ii) physiotherapy to strengthen the muscles around the joint (iii) supports with various kind of orthotic materials and bandages (iv) well designed shoes for shock absorbing weight and certain unproven but frequently used medications like:

i) Chondroitin sulphate / heparan sulphate tablets orally (ii) injection of high molecular weight heparrinoid in the Knee joint

Finally when everything else fails and pain is not bearable knee replacement surgeries of various types are undertaken.

There are studies to show that autologous platelet concentrates properly prepared (**which we can do**) in our own laboratory can significantly alleviate pain and improve joint function. If we prepare these platelets from patients own blood, there are no chance of transfusion transmitted infection. Minor side effects like slight increase in local pain, swelling, dizziness have been noticed during injection of this material but these side effects are short lasting.

In the event the platelet concentrate does not work. Mesenchymal stem cell and other mononuclear cells obtained from the bone marrow were shown to have significant moderately long lasting (2 years+) effect of this therapy. Considering the large number of such available patients' orthopedic surgeries may be approached from such therapy.

5. Use of Fetal liver cells in acute and chronic liver injury (17-19):

Quite a few studies from m India has shown good effect of fetal liver cell therapy in acute and chronic liver in jury both in human and in animal models and this avenue is worth exploring because many of the end stage liver disease patients have no other option but allogenic liver transplantation. Apart from horrendous cost this surgery is a major undertaking and nor available in Surat where as cell therapy can be made easily available. Even autologous bone marrow derived stem cells are useful for the condition.

6. Use of Limbal stem cells for corneal injury or diseases (20):

Chemical injury of the cornea is one of the important causes of blindness and require cornea grafting which is not available to everybody , but now a day's use of allogeneic corneal limbal cells is in craesingly used for epithelisation of damaged cornea. In our country this procedure is used in several hospitals with great success.

Cancers as disease of stem cells (21)

One of the interesting concepts which have evolved from study of Stem cell biology is cancer as a stem cell disease. We all know that it is very difficult to eradicate cancer. It has the habit of relapsing and travelling to distant places leading to metastasis. Why do the cancers relapse even after killing most of the cells by surgery? Chemotherapy and radiotherapy or various combinations thereof. It is believed now that most of the relapse in cancer is related to proliferation of cancer stem cells and most of the therapy today hardly touches cancer stem cell. Hence in future there will be technique to identify the size of this compartment in every cancer. These cells need to be isolated and treatment should be targeted to these cells.

Challenges

What are the challenges we have to overcome before we can harness the unimaginable power of stem cell therapy and other applications? We have to know which disease, which kind of stem cells, what time window, how much of it and which route of administration?

Most of these informations related to stem cell therapy is not known and this hampers rational use of these cells. We don't know what exactly attracts stem cells to the site where they are needed to do their job ie homing cues and time windows during which these cues work. We don't know whether this time window can be increased. For example now a days we know very well that a heart attack patient needs to have his treatment started within 2 hours of attack , so called golden hour. Similar Golden hour may be operative for stem cell therapy too. This golden hour may be different in different types of disorders. We are capable of expanding in vivo the stem cells in a limited manner we don't have very good idea whether in vitro expansion faithfully mimick invivo expansion or multiplication of cells. It is quite likely we are far off the mark.If these stem cells are surviving inside the patients we also need to have data to show that these cells donot undergo malignant transformation. Particularly if these cells have gone through several cycles of expansion in- vitro. Stem cell based gene therapy has its own challenges and hazards. However the dividend for this kind of therapy is likely to be very great hence we will continue to circumvent these challenges and finally develop its multitude of applications towards human service.

References

Ghosh K. Haemopoietic stem cells: Surprises never end. Science Letters. 2003 26(7A-8):188-195. (National Academy of Science: Allahabad, India).

K Ghosh, M Madkaikar. Haematopoietic Stem Cells-present perspective and future directions. Proc Nat Acad Sci Ind 2004; 124 Part B (III-IV) : 195- 210.

Essentials of Stem Cell Biology (Third Edition)2014 *Edited by:*Robert Lanza and Anthony Atala. Elsevier ISBN: 978-0-12-409503-8.

Bryder D, Rossi DJ, Weissman IL. Biological Perspectives: Hematopoietic Stem Cells; the Paradigmatic Tissue-Specific Stem Cell. The American J Pathol 2006; 169: (2), 338-46.

Liddo DI, Aguiari P, Barbon S, et.al. Nanopatterned acellular valve conduits drive the commitment of blood-derived multipotent cells. International J Nanomed 2016; 11.

Madkaikar M, Ghosh K, Gupta M, Swaminathan S, Mohanty D.Ex vivo expansion of umbilical cord blood stem cells using different combinations of cytokines and stromal cells.Acta Haematol. 2007; 118:153-9.

Bhargava B, Narang R, Ray R etal. The ABCD (Autologous Bane Marrow Cells in Dialated cardiomypathy) Trial: A long term fellow upstanding. J. Amer. Coll. Cardiol 2010, 55: 1642-44.

Henng TD, Schaer GL, Traverse JH etal. Autologous CB34+ cell therapy for refractory angina: 2 yr. outcome form ACT 34 – CMI study. Cell Transplant 2016, 25: 17001-17011.

Quyymi AA, Vazquez Z, Kereiakes D etal. PreSERVEAMI: A ranomised double blind placebo controlled clinical trial of intracoronay administration autologous CD34+ cells in patients with left ventricular drugs function post STEMI. Circ – Res 2016.

Vrtovec B, Poglajen G, Sever M etal. CD34+ stem cell therapy in non ischaemic dilated cardiomyopathy patients. Clinical pharmacology and Therapeutics 2013, P.P. 1-7. Nature Publication.

Raval Z. Losordo DW. Cell therapy of peripheral arterial disease: From experimental founds to clinical trials cric. Res 2013; 112: 1288-1302.

EL. Badawy A, EL Badri N. Clinicl efficacy of stem cell therapy in diabetes mellitus: A meta analysis. Plos. One 2016.

Bhansali A, Asokumar P. Walia R etal. Efficacy and safety of autologus bone moarrow derived stem cell transplantation with type 2 diabetes: a randomised placebo controlled study. Cell transplant -2014; 23: 1075-85.

Lilly MA , Davis MF et al Current stem cell based therapies in diabetes. Am J Stem Cells 2016; 5: 87-98. IF: 4.30.

Patel S, Dhillon MS et al. Treatment of platelet rich plasma in more effective than placebo for knee ostearthitis Am. J. Sports Med. 2013

Cui GH, Wang YY etal. Efficacy of measenchynal stem cells in treating patients with osteoarthrits of the knee: A meta analysis. Exp Ther Med 2016; 12: 3390-3400.

Khan AA, Shaik MV, Parveen N, Rajendraprasad A, Aleem MA, Habeeb MA, Srinivas G, Raj TA, Tiwari SK, Kumaresan K, Venkateswarlu J, Pande G, Habibullah CM.Human fetal liver-derived stem cell transplantation as supportive modality in the management of end-stage decompensated liver cirrhosis.Cell Transplant. 2010;19:409-18.

Khan AA, Parveen N, Mahaboob VS, Rajendraprasad A, Ravindraprakash HR, Venkateswarlu J, Rao SG, Narusu ML, Khaja MN, Pramila R, Habeeb A, Habibullah CM.Safety and efficacy of autologous bone marrow stem cell transplantation through hepatic artery for the treatment of chronic liver failure: a preliminary study.Transplant Proc. 2008 ;40:1140-4.

Khan AA, Habeeb A, Parveen N, Naseem B, Babu RP, Capoor AK, Habibullah CM. Peritoneal transplantation of human fetal hepatocytes for the treatment of acute fatty liverof pregnancy: a case report.Trop Gastroenterol. 2004 ;25:141-3.

Iyer G, Srinivasan B, Agarwal S, Tarigopula A. Outcome of allo simple limbal epithelial transplantation (alloSLET) in the early stage of ocular chemical injury.Br J Ophthalmol. 2017; 101:828-833.

Mayol JF, Loeuillet C, Herodin F, Wian D. Characterisation of normal and cancer stem Cells : one experimental paradigm for two kinds of cells. BioEssays 2009; 31:993-1001.

Chapter 14

Molecular Approaches along with Conventional Hemagglutination for Multitransfused Patients

Avani Shah[1], Preeti Sharma[2], Keyur Patel[1], Kanjaksha Ghosh[1] and Kanchan Mishra[1]

[1]Surat Raktadan Kendra & Research Centre, Surat, Gujarat, India.

[2]Department of Biotechnology, Veer Narmad South Gujarat University, Surat-395007, Gujarat, India.

Email: awanishaho8@gmail.com

Abstract

The evolution of blood transfusion services was one of the most important of medical advances derived from World War I. A well-organized Blood Transfusion Service (BTS) is a vital component of any health care delivery system. For quality, safety and efficacy of blood and blood products, well-equipped blood centers with adequate infrastructure and trained manpower are essential requirements. Blood Transfusion Service (BTS) is an essential part of modern health care system without which medical care is impossible. However, provision of safe and quality blood for a country like India involves a highly complex operation involving various stakeholders and the magnitude and complexity of issues raises several challenges. Molecular testing can be extended to platelet antigens, a useful tool for patients with platelet refractoriness or cases of neonatal allo-immune thrombocytopenia and post transfusion purpura. This methodology can also be done with HLA A and B typing. As from long period of time molecular techniques have been introduced to detect transfusion transmitted infections and that is why it is easy to adapt PCR based techniques in day to day activity of blood banks.

1. History of Blood Transfusion

The evolution of blood transfusion services was one of the most important of medical advances derived from World War I [1]. A well-organized Blood Transfusion Service (BTS) is a vital component of any health care delivery system. For quality, safety and efficacy of blood and blood products, well-equipped blood centers with adequate infrastructure and trained manpower are essential requirements [2].

The practice of blood transfusion, that is the transference of blood from the circulation of one individual to that of another for practical therapeutic purposes, is of relatively recent origin. Although it only became a practical possibility during and shortly after the Second World War, the concept of 'transfusion' has a longer history.

The transfusion time line highlights many of the discoveries, inventions, observations, and practices, which, since ancient times, have led to remarkable progress and resulted in the effective treatments that are now taken for granted. The 20th Century has witnessed the most progress in the enumerable transfusion practices, activities and safety.

Table: 1 Series of event in the history of blood transfusion [3]

Year	Events
1628	English physician William Harvey discovers the circulation of blood.
1665	Physician Richard Lower keeps dogs alive by transfusion of blood from other dogs.
1667	Jean-Baptiste Denis in France and Richard Lower in England separately report successful transfusions from lambs to humans.
1795	In Philadelphia, American physician Philip SyngPhysick, performs the first human blood transfusion,
1818	James Blundell, a British obstetrician, performs the first successful transfusion of human blood to a patient for the treatment of postpartum hemorrhage.
1840	Samuel Armstrong Lane, aided by consultant Dr. Blundell, performs the first successful whole blood transfusion to treat hemophilia.
1867	English surgeon Joseph Lister uses antiseptics to control infection during transfusions.
1900	Karl Landsteiner, an Austrian physician, discovers the first three human blood groups, A, B, and C. Blood type C was later changed to O. His colleagues Alfred Decastello and Adriano Sturli add AB, the fourth type
1907	Hektoen suggests that the safety of transfusion might be improved by cross matching blood between donors and patients to exclude incompatible mixtures. Reuben Ottenberg performs the first blood transfusion using blood typing
1908	Moreschi describes the antiglobulin reaction. The antiglobulin is a direct way of visualizing an antigen-antibody reaction that has taken place but is not directly visible
1912	Roger Lee, a visiting physician at the Massachusetts General Hospital, along with Paul Dudley White, develops the Lee-White clotting time.
1914	Long-term anticoagulants, among them sodium citrate, are developed, allowing longer preservation of blood.
1927-1947	The MNSs and P systems are discovered. MNSs and P are two more blood group antigen systems — Just as ABO is one system and Rh is another.
1932	The first blood bank is established in a Leningrad hospital.
1939-40	The Rh blood group system is discovered by Karl Landsteiner, Alex Wiener, Philip Levine, and R.E. Stetson and is soon recognized as the cause of the majority of transfusion reactions.
1943	P. Beeson publishes the classic description of transfusion-transmitted hepatitis.
1945	Coombs, Mourant, and Race describe the use of antihuman globulin (later known as the "Coombs Test") to identify "incomplete" antibodies.

Year	Events
1950	In one of the single most influential technical developments in blood banking, Carl Walter and W.P. Murphy, Jr., introduce the plastic bag for blood collection.
1971	Hepatitis B surface antigen (HBsAg) testing of donated blood begins.
1979	A new anticoagulant preservative, CPDA-1, extends the shelf life of whole blood and red blood cells to 35 days.
1981	First Acquired Immune Deficiency Syndrome (AIDS) case reported.
1984	Human Immunodeficiency Virus (HIV) identified as cause of AIDS
1985	The first blood-screening test to detect HIV is licensed and quickly implemented by blood banks to protect the blood supply.
1987	Two tests that screen for indirect evidence of hepatitis are developed and implemented, hepatitis B core antibody (anti-HBc) and the alanine aminotransferase test (ALT).
1989	Human-T-Lymphotropic-Virus-I-antibody (anti-HTLV-I) testing of donated blood begins.
1990	Introduction of first specific test for hepatitis C, the major cause of "non-A, non-B" hepatitis.
1992	Testing of donor blood for HIV-1 and HIV-2 antibodies (anti-HIV-1 and anti-HIV-2) is implemented.
1996	HIV p24 antigen testing of donated blood begins. Although the test does not completely close the HIV window, it shortens the window period.
1999	Blood community begins implementation of Nucleic Acid Amplification Testing (NAT) under the FDA's Investigational New Drug (IND) application process. NAT employs a testing technology that directly detects the genetic materials of viruses like HCV and HIV.
2002	West Nile virus identified as transfusion transmissible.
2002	Nucleic acid amplification test (NAT) for HIV and HCV was licensed by the Food and Drug Administration.

2. Blood Transfusion Services in India

Blood Transfusion Service (BTS) is an essential part of modern health care system without which medical care is impossible [4]. The provision of safe and adequate blood and blood products at national level is the responsibility of the government / national health authority of each country [5]. Blood safety is essential to ensure that a patient who comes for treatment is not made sicker by another illness [6]. These products must be safe, clinically effective and of appropriate and consistent quality [7].

However, provision of safe and quality blood for a country like India involves a highly complex operation involving various stakeholders and the magnitude and complexity of issues raises several challenges [8]. This requires a holistic and comprehensive approach in planning, designing and operationalizing the BTS services. It is important to ensure coordination between the blood transfusion services, health services and hospitals, educational institutes, religious, social and industrial organizations, mass media and other stakeholders including general public. The system should also ensure adequate input into the legislative, regulatory, technical, social and cultural aspects of making this life saving product accessible and safe.

The Blood Safety Program in India has developed as a component of the National AIDS Control Programme that has led to several advancements in terms of better policies, increased infrastructure, facilities, quality and access to blood transfusion services. In contrast to many western countries, Blood services have been a highly decentralized and fragmented structures and operations in India [5].

3. Different Blood Group Systems

Karl Landsteiner has been credited for the discovery of ABO blood group system in 1900 [9]. His extensive research on serology based on simple but strong scientific reasoning led to identification of major blood groups such as O, A, and B types, compatibility testing, and subsequent transfusion practices.

The International Society of Blood Transfusion (ISBT) has instituted a numerical system of nomenclature to help standardize red cell blood group terminology. This convention mandates that each system and collection has been given a number and letter designation, and each antigen within the system is numbered sequentially in order of discovery. The 36 human blood group system genes have been identified and sequenced and all the polymorphisms are now known [10].

Most blood group polymorphisms result from single nucleotide polymorphisms. (SNPs) encoding amino acid substitutions in either a glycosyl transferase or extracellular domain of a red cell membrane protein. A blood group system consists of one or more antigens controlled at a single gene locus, or by two or more very closely linked homologous genes with little or no observable recombination between them. Currently recognized antigens within blood group systems are shown in the table 2 and fall into one of four classifications:

- systems
- collections (200 series)
- low incidence antigens (700 series)
- high incidence antigens (901 series)

Table 2: Different blood group systems [10]

S. No.	System name	System symbol	Gene name(s)*	Chromosomal location	CD numbers
001	ABO	ABO	ABO	9q34.2	
002	MNS	MNS	GYPA, GYPB, (GYPE)	4q31.21	CD235a CD235b
003	P1PK	P1PK	A4GALT	22q13.2	CD77
004	Rh	RH	RHD, RHCE	1p36.11	CD240
005	Lutheran	LU	BCAM	19q13.2	CD239

S. No.	System name	System symbol	Gene name(s)*	Chromosomal location	CD numbers
006	Kell	KEL	KEL	7q33	CD238
007	Lewis	LE	FUT3	19p13.3	
008	Duffy	FY	ACKR1	1q21-q22	CD234
009	Kidd	JK	SLC14A1	18q11-q12	
010	Diego	DI	SLC4A1	17q21.31	CD233
011	Yt	YT	ACHE	7q22	
012	Xg	XG	XG,MIC2	Xp22.32	CD99†
013	Scianna	SC	ERMAP	1p34.2	
014	Dombrock	DO	ART4	12p13-p12	CD297
015	Colton	CO	AQP1	7p14	
016	Landsteiner-Wiener	LW	ICAM4	19p13.2	CD242
017	Chido/Rodgers	CH/RG	C4A,C4B	6p21.3	
018	H	H	FUT1	19q13.33	CD173
019	Kx	XK	XK	Xp21.1	
020	Gerbich	GE	GYPC	2q14-q21	CD236
021	Cromer	CROM	CD55	1q32	CD55
022	Knops	KN	CR1	1q32.2	CD35
023	Indian	IN	CD44	11p13	CD44
024	Ok	OK	BSG	19p13.3	CD147
025	Raph	RAPH	CD151	11p15.5	CD151
026	John MiltonHagen	JMH	SEMA7A	15q22.3-q23	CD108
027	I	I	GCNT2	6p24.2	
028	Globoside	GLOB	B3GALNT1	3q25	
029	Gill	GIL	AQP3	9p13	
030	Rh-associated glycoprotein	RHAG	RHAG	6p12.3	CD241
031	FORS	FORS	GBGT1	9q34.13-q34.3	
032	JR	JR	ABCG2	4q22.1	CD338
033	LAN	LAN	ABCB6	2q36	
034	Vel	VEL	SMIM1	1p36.32	
035	CD59	CD59	CD59	11q13	CD59
036	Augustine	AUG	SLC29A1	6p21.1	

Blood group antigens [11]

Blood groups are antigens and, by definition, a molecule cannot be an antigen unless it is recognized by an antibody (or T cell receptor); therefore, all blood group specificities are defined by antibodies. Most adults have antibodies to the A or B antigens, or to both; that is, they have 'naturally occurring' antibodies to those ABO antigens they lack. Blood group antigens may be:

- Proteins;
- Glycoproteins, with the antibody recognizing primarily the polypeptide backbone;
- Glycoproteins, with the antibody recognizing the carbohydrate moiety;
- Glycolipid, with the antibody recognizing the carbohydrate portion. Blood group polymorphisms may be as fundamental as representing the presence or absence of the whole macromolecule (e.g. RhD), or as minor as a single amino acid change (e.g. Fy^a and Fy^b) or a single monosaccharide difference (e.g. A and B).

Blood group proteins and glycoproteins are integral structures of the red cell membrane. Diagrammatic representations of some blood group proteins and glycoproteins in the membrane are shown in Fig 1. Because of these differences in structure, conformation, and molecular nature, not all blood group substances are equally immunogenic in vivo as shown in table 3.

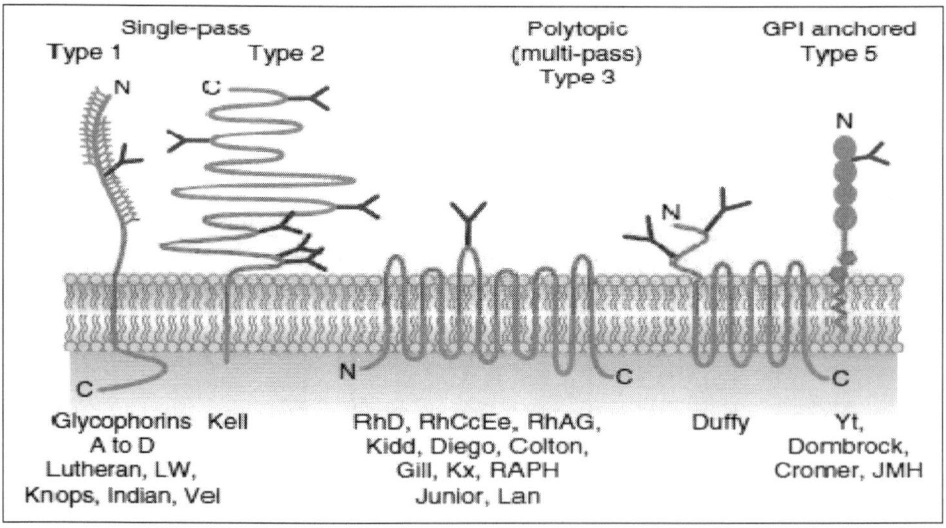

Fig. 1: Diagram of different types of blood group active proteins and glycoproteins based on their integration into the red cell surface membrane. Listed are examples of blood group antigens for each type. (Type 4 proteins are cytoplasmic and not present in red cells.)

Table 3: Immunogenicity of different blood group antigens

Blood group antigen	Blood group system	Immunogenicity (%)
D (Rh)	Rh	50
K	Kell	5
c (hr′)	Rh	2.05
E (rh″)	Rh	1.69
k	Kell	1.50
e (hr″)	Rh	0.56
Fy^a	Duffy	0.23
C (rh′)	Rh	0.11
Jk^a	Kidd	0.07
S	MNSs	0.04
Jk^b	Kidd	0.03
s	MNSs	0.03

Blood group antibodies [11]

Blood group antibodies are usually IgM or IgG, although some may be IgA. 'Naturally occurring' antibodies are usually predominantly IgM, whereas 'immune' antibodies are predominantly IgG. As a general rule, IgM antibodies will directly agglutinate antigen-positive red cells in a saline medium, whereas most IgG antibodies require potentiators or anti-human globulin to effect agglutination.

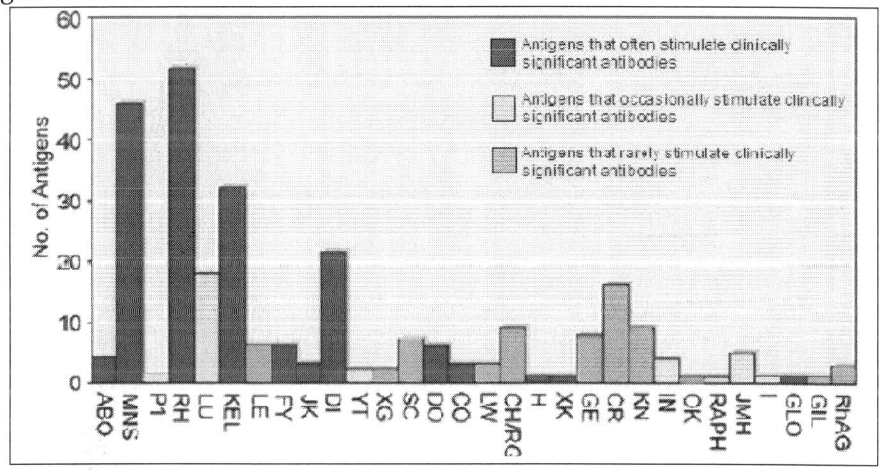

Fig. 2: Clinical importance of different blood group specific antibodies [12]

Most human antibodies with which we are familiar are polyclonal in origin, being of broader specificity than monoclonal antibodies, which can have single epitope specificity. These antibodies can be of importance in certain clinical situations such as the ones described briefly as follows:

1. Hemolytic transfusion reaction (HTR), when an antibody destroys antigen-positive transfused red cells. The most severe HTR are generally caused by antibodies to antigens of the ABO system, which are IgM in nature and initiate the complement cascade through to the membrane attack complex (MAC) causing lysis of cells intravascularly. Other antibodies, IgG in nature, generally either do not initiate complement activation or initiate only up to the C3 stage, and red cells are cleared extravascularly.
2. Hemolytic disease of the fetus and newborn (HDFN), when an IgG maternally derived antibody, which is directed against a paternally derived antigen present on the fetal/neonatal red cells, crosses the placenta and destroys the cells.
3. Hemolytic anemia (HA), when an autoantibody directed against 'self' antigens is produced and causes increased red cell destruction. These antibodies may be non-specific or may possess a defined specificity, often against a high incidence antigen. The antibodies may be warm reactive or react optimally in the cold.

Clinically important blood group systems [11]

- **ABO system**

  Among the 36 systems, ABO remains the most important in transfusion and transplantation since any person above the age of 6 months possess clinically significant anti-A and/or anti-B antibodies in their serum. Blood group A contains antibody against blood group B in serum and vice-versa, while blood group O contains no A/B antigen but both their antibodies in serum.

- **H-antigen**

  H-antigen is the precursor to the ABO blood group antigens. It is present in all RBCs irrespective of the ABO system. Persons with the rare Bombay phenotype are homozygous for the H gene (HH), do not express H-antigen on their RBCs. As H-antigen acts as precursor, its absence means the absence of antigen A and B. However, the individuals produce iso-antibodies to H-antigen as well as to antigens A and B.

- **Rhesus system**

  Rhesus-system is the second most important blood group system after ABO. Currently, the Rh-system consists of 50 defined blood group antigens out of which only five are important. RBC surface of an individual may or may not have a Rh factor or immunogenic D-antigen. Accordingly, the status is indicated as either Rh-positive (D-antigen present) or Rh-negative (D-antigen absent). In contrast to the ABO system, anti-Rh antibodies are, normally, not present in the blood of individuals with D-negative RBCs, unless the circulatory system of these individuals has been exposed to D-positive RBCs. These immune antibodies are immunoglobulin G (IgG) in nature and hence, can cross the placenta. Prophylaxis is given against Rh immunization using anti-D Ig for pregnant Rh-negative mothers who have given birth to Rh-positive child.

- **Kell system**

  These erythrocyte antigens are the third most potent immunogenic antigen after ABO and Rh system, and are defined by an immune antibody, anti-K. It was first noticed in the serum of Mrs. Kellacher. She reacted to the erythrocytes of her newborn infant resulting in hemolytic reactions. Since then 25 Kell antigens have been discovered. Anti-K antibody causes severe hemolytic disease of the fetus and newborn (HDFN) and hemolytic transfusion reactions (HTR).

- **Duffy system**

  Duffy-antigen was first isolated in a patient called Duffy who had hemophilia. It is also known as Fy glycoprotein and is present in the surface of RBCs. It is a nonspecific receptor for several chemokines and acts as a receptor for human malaria parasite, *Plamodiumvivax*. Antigens Fya and Fyb on the Duffy glycoprotein can result in four possible phenotypes, namely Fy (a+b−), Fy (a+b+), Fy (a−b+), and Fy (a−b−). The antibodies are IgG subtypes and can cause HTR.

- **Kidd system**

  Kidd antigen (known as Jk antigen) is a glycoprotein, present on the membrane of RBCs and acts as a urea transporter in RBCs and renal endothelial cells. Kidd antibodies are rare but can cause severe transfusion reactions. These antigens are defined by reactions to an antibody designated as anti-Jk^a, discovered in the serum of Mrs. Kidd who delivered a baby with HDFN. Jk^a was the first antigen to be discovered by Kidd blood group system, subsequently, two other antigens Jk^b and Jk3 were found.

- **MNS antigen system**

  MNS antigen system, first described by Landsteiner and Levine in 1927 is based on two genes: Glycophorin A and Glycophorin B. The blood group is under control of an autosomal locus on chromosome 4 and also under control of a pair of co-dominant alleles LM and LN. Anti-M and anti-N antibodies are usually IgM types and rarely, associated with transfusion reactions.

- **Lutheran system**

  Lutheran system comprised of four pairs of allelic antigens representing single amino acid substitution in the Lutheran glycoprotein at chromosome 19. Antibodies against this blood group are rare and generally not considered clinically significant.

4. Traditional Serological Investigation for Blood Group Antigens and Antibodies

Many different types of tests are available, and it is important to be familiar with the different purposes of each. In vitro testing for the detection of antigens or antibodies may be accomplished by commonly used techniques, including hemagglutination (a special type of agglutination), precipitation, agglutination inhibition, and hemolysis [13].

Routine blood grouping still relies primarily on hemagglutination reactions between antigens and antibodies that are read and interpreted either manually or by automated means. The principles behind hemagglutination reactions, the discovery of the biochemistry of blood group antigens, and the increasing knowledge of the properties of immunoglobulins associated with blood group antibodies led to the development of laboratory tests other than direct agglutination. Antiglobulin methods and enzyme technology were introduced as routine methods for the detection of antigen–antibody reactions and played a part in the discovery and expansion of knowledge of blood group systems in general. Since these advances, non-routine methods have become available for specialist investigations and as research tools, such as flowcytometry and analysis of antigens at the molecular level [11].

Factors affecting antigen-antibody reaction

1. Effect of pH

The ideal pH of a test system for antigen-antibody reactions ranges between 6.5 and 7.5, which is similar to the pH of normal plasma or serum. Exceptions include some anti-M and some Pr(Sp1) group antibodies that show stronger reactivity below pH 6.5 [14]. Acidification of the test serum may aid in distinguishing anti-M and anti-Pr(Sp1) antibodies from other antibodies.

2. Temperature

Different isotypes of antibodies may exhibit optimal reactivity at different temperatures. IgM antibodies usually react optimally at ambient temperatures or below 22°C at the immediate spin (IS) phase of testing, whereas IgG antibodies usually require 37°C incubation and react optimally at the antihuman globulin (AHG) phase of testing. Because clinically significant antibodies may be in both these temperature ranges, it is important to do testing with a range of temperatures.

3. Centrifugation

High-speed centrifugation is one of the most efficient methods used in blood banking. Under the right centrifugation conditions, sensitized RBCs overcome their natural repulsive effect (zeta potential) for each other and agglutinate more efficiently. Having RBCs in closer physical proximity allows for an increase in antigen-antibody lattice formation, which results in enhanced agglutination.

4. Antigen-Antibody Ratio

Antigen and antibody have optimal concentrations; in ideal reactive conditions, an equivalent amount of antigen and antibody binds. Any deviation from this decreases the efficiency of the reaction and a loss of the zone of equivalence between antigen and antibody ratio that is necessary for agglutination reactions to occur. An excess of unbound immunoglobulin leads to a prozone effect, and a surplus of antigen leads to a postzone effect.

5. Immunoglobulin Type

The IgM molecule has the potential to bind 10 separate antigen sites; however, an IgG molecule has only 2 binding sites per molecule, which implies that an IgG molecule would have to bind 2 RBCs with only 1 binding site on each cell [14]. IgM molecules rarely bind 10 sites, owing to the size and spacing of antigens in relation to the size and configuration of the IgM molecule.

6. Time and ionic strength

In order to speed up the interaction of antigen and antibody, the ionic strength of the test milieu can be lowered. This means that solutions of saline containing less Na+ and Cl– ions than normal isotonic salt solutions interfere less in the reaction between an antigen and antibody of complementary electrostatic charge. This is because the ions cluster around and neutralize the opposite charges on the antigen and antibody molecules. By reducing the number of free ions in solution, this 'neutralizing' effect is diminished, thus enhancing the speed at which the antigen–antibody complexes are formed. Such solutions are known in immunohematology's Low Ionic Strength Saline or LISS. However, the reduction in ionic strength must be controlled to prevent the non-specific uptake of immunoglobulins in 'sub-LISS' conditions.

Different hemagglutination tests used in blood banks [11, 15, 16]

In blood banks pre-transfusion tests include ABO and Rh (D) typing of the recipient's red blood cells and an antibody screen the latter is a method to detect clinically significant non-ABO antibodies in the recipient's plasma. Most clinically significant antibodies are IgG and develop following exposure to foreign red blood cell antigens during transfusion or pregnancy. Before a non-emergent transfusion, compatibility testing is performed in addition to blood grouping and antibody screening. The compatibility test may be a serological cross match or may involve the use of a validated computer program to ensure that an appropriate component has been selected for the intended.

Even though some of these classical methods are not highly sensitive, nonetheless, they still hold importance in ABO grouping tests. There is a wide range of blood typing techniques [16], which differ from each other interms of sensitivity, reagents and equipment required, the time of operation and throughput analysis. Herein, we describe some general approaches of blood grouping along with their inbuilt advantages and drawbacks.

1. Direct Hemagglutination tests

As the name suggests, this occurs as a direct result of an antigen–antibody interaction. Generally, the antibody is of the IgM immunoglobulin class and reactions take place optimally at low temperatures. Examples of IgG antibodies that can effect direct agglutination are known, such as anti-A and anti-B, and some IgG class anti-M.

In the routine laboratory, most direct agglutination techniques are used in ABO forward and reverse grouping tests or in the determination of other red cell antigens with human, polyclonal, or monoclonal directly-agglutinating antibodies.

These tests can be performed on slides, in tubes, by solid/liquid phase microplate technology, or by using a column agglutination technique, without the necessity of enhancing the reaction in order to visualize the hemagglutination. However, slide techniques are not recommended for initial or definitive antigen determinations, particularly when dealing with neonatal samples, as certain blood group antigens may not be fully developed at birth. The use of a relatively insensitive technique can therefore lead to mistyping in some cases.

a) **Slide technique**

The slide test is relatively the least sensitive method among others for blood group determination, but due to its prompt results, it is very much valuable in emergency cases. A drop of blood samples is mixed with respective antisera like anti-A, anti-B and anti-D separately on clean glass slide. The agglutination or pattern can be visually observed from which the ABO and rhesus D (RhD) type of blood can be determined.

b) **Tube technique**

In comparison to the slide test, the tube test is more sensitive and reliable; therefore, it can be used conveniently for blood transfusion. In this method, both forward (cell), as well as reverse (serum) grouping is carried out. The forward grouping suggests the presence or absence of A and B antigens in RBCs, whereas reverse grouping indicates the presence or absences of anti-A and anti-B in serum. In forward grouping, blood cells are placed in two test tubes along with saline as a diluents media, and then one drop of each anti-A and anti-B is added separately in these samples. These tubes are subjected to centrifugation for few minutes, and then, the resultant matrix is gently shaken for observing agglutination.

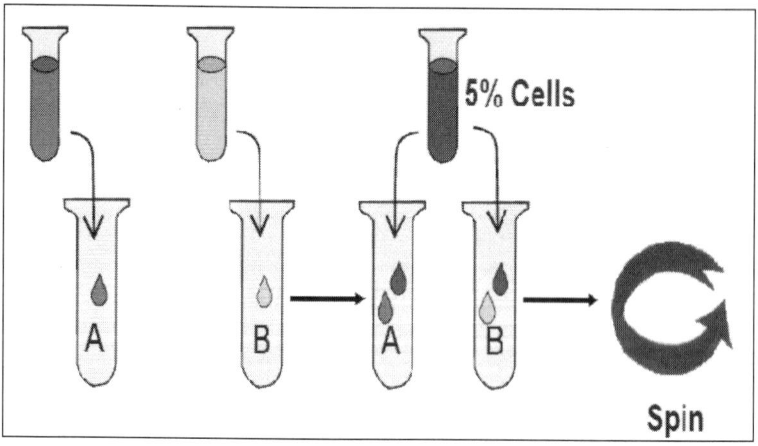

Fig. 3: ABO forward grouping

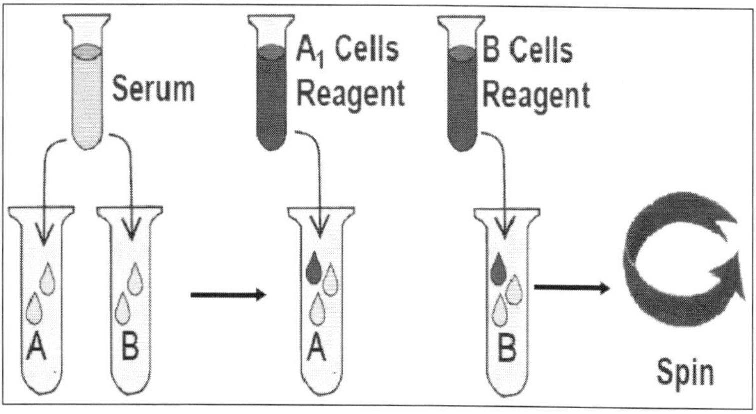

Fig. 4: ABO reverse grouping

c) Microplate Technology

Among classical methods, microplate technology is a further step towards more sensitive and fast blood typing analysis with the feasibility of automation. In this technique, both antibodies in blood plasma and antigens on RBCs can be determined. Typical microplates consist of a large number of small tubes that contain a few μL of reagents, which are treated against the blood samples. Following centrifugation and incubation, the subsequent agglutination can be examined by an automatic readout device.

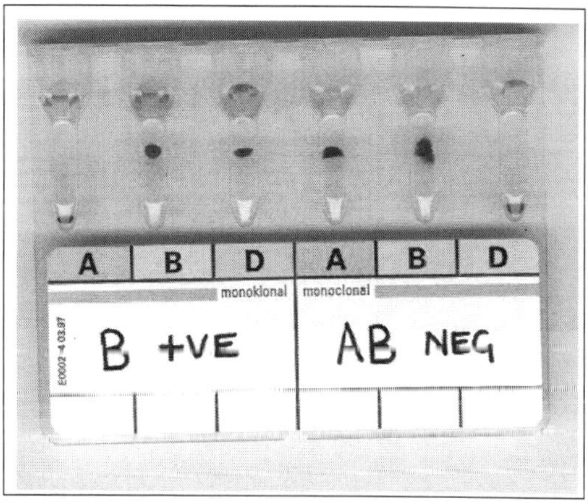

Fig. 5: Gel cards showing blood grouping

d) Column/Gel Centrifugation

Column agglutination technology or gel centrifugation is a relatively modern approach that has gained substantial interest in ABO blood grouping, as it intends to establish a standard procedure for quantifying cell agglutination. In gel matrix blood serum or cells are mixed with anti-A, anti-B and anti-D reagents [Figure 3] in microtubes under controlled incubation and centrifugation. The gel particles trap the agglutinates, whereas non-agglutinated blood cells are allowed to pass through the column. The analysis time can be reduced by using glass beads in place of gel material, since in this way, faster centrifugation speeds can be achieved, which leads to rapid results. This technology is sensitive, straightforward and relatively easy to operate for less trained personnel.

2. Indirect Hemagglutination test

Antibodies that cannot directly agglutinate cells are detected by means of enhanced test systems, notably the use of enzyme treatment of red cells or by the Antiglobulin test.

a) **Enzyme techniques**

Enzyme-treated cells are used in antibody screening and importantly, in antibody identification procedures. They are particularly useful for determining specificities within mixtures of antibodies, where one or more are directed against enzyme-sensitive antigens.

b) **Antiglobulin test**

The Antiglobulin test also known as Coomb's test refers to two clinical blood tests used in immunohematology which are done to find certain antibodies that cause autoimmune hemolysis of red blood cells. The two types of Coombs tests are:

- Direct Coombs test
- Indirect Coombs test
- **Direct Antiglobulin Test [DAT] or Direct Coomb's test [DCT]**

The direct Coombs test is used to detect if antibodies or complement system factors have bound to RBC surface antigens in vivo. A blood sample is taken and the RBCs are washed and then incubated with antihuman globulin. If this produces agglutination of RBCs, the direct Coombs test is positive, a visual indication that antibodies are bound to the surface of red blood cells. This is the test that is done on the newborn's blood sample, usually in the setting of a newborn with jaundice. The test is looking for "foreign" antibodies that are already adhered to the infant's RBC's, a potential cause of hemolysis.

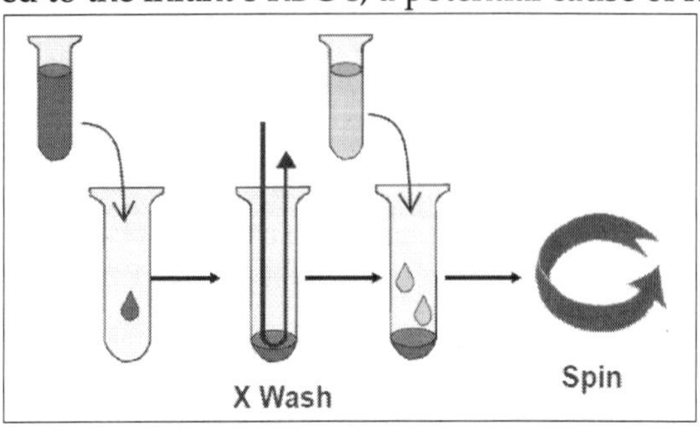

Fig 6: Direct Coomb's Test [DCT]

- **Indirect Antiglobulin Test [IAT] of Indirect Coomb's test [ICT]**

  The indirect Coombs test is used to detect in-vitro antibody-antigen reactions. It is used to detect very low concentrations of antibodies present in a patient's plasma/serum prior to a blood transfusion. In antenatal care, this test is used to screen pregnant women for antibodies that may cause hemolytic disease of the newborn. The IAT can also be used for compatibility testing, antibody identification, RBC phenotyping, and titration studies.

Step 1

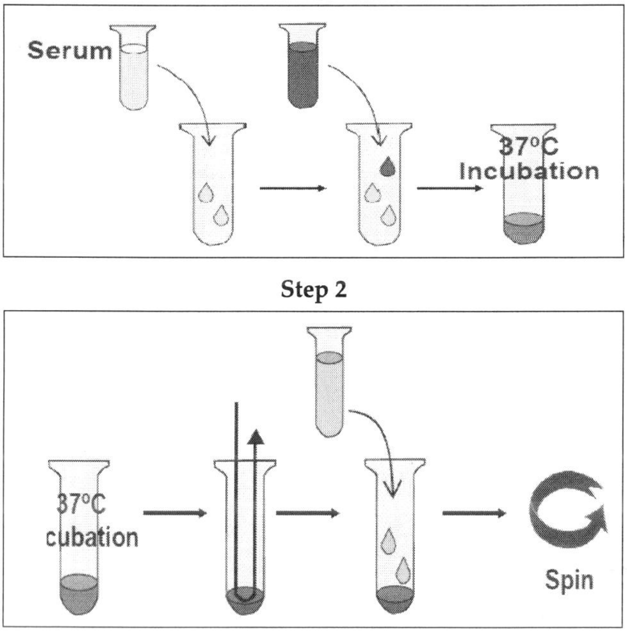

Fig. 7: Indirect Coomb's test (ICT)

- **Test additives used to enhance the antigen-antibody reaction rate**

  Protein Media

  There are several colloidal solutions currently utilized in blood bank testing, and they are all used to enhance agglutination reactions. Colloids include albumin, polyethylene glycol (PEG), polybrene, polyvinyl pyrolidone (PVP), and protamine. These substances work by increasing the dielectric constant (a measure of electrical conductivity), which then reduces the zeta potential of the RBC.

  Proteolytic Enzymes

  Certain enzymes have been found to modify various blood group antigens and are useful in testing, Enzymes used in the detection and identification of blood group antibodies include **ficin** (isolated from fig plants), papain (from papaya), **trypsin** (from pig stomach), and **bromelin** (from pineapple). It is thought that treating RBCs with enzymes results in the release of sialic acid from the membrane with a subsequent decrease in the negative charges and zeta potential of the RBCs. It has also been suggested that enzyme treatment removes hydrophilic glycoproteins from the membrane of RBCs, causing the membrane to become more hydrophobic, which would allow RBCs to come closer together.

3. Elution tests

A subsidiary test that may be performed in the elucidation of weak antigens, separation of mixtures of antibodies, detection of causative antibody in Hemolytic Disease of the Fetus and Newborn (HDFN), and investigation of a transfusion reaction or the specificity of an auto antibody in Auto Immune Hemolytic Anemia (AIHA), is an elution technique. Where an antigen is suspected to be present, but cannot be demonstrated by routine methods, the cells are incubated with appropriate antibody and the antibody subsequently eluted from the cells and identified. For example, this technique is required for detection of some very low subgroups of A, especially Ael, and for the very weak D antigen, DEL.

4. Automation in test procedures

For all serological testing requirements, there are several systems well established that employ microplate technology and / or column agglutination such as ID-System. The choice of automation depends upon the technology routinely use, the through put required, the number, and mix of laboratory staff.

5. Flow cytometry

Flow cytometry can be applied in special circumstances: when investigating the cause of double cell populations or for identifying weakly expressing antigens. It can also be used to assess the amount of feto-maternal hemorrhage (FMH) in RhD-negative mothers who required anti-D prophylaxis and for circulating the concentration of anti-D in immunized RhD-negative antenatal women.

Limitation of traditional serological methods

The classical method of testing for blood group antigens and antibodies is hemagglutination. This technique is simple and when done correctly, has a specificity and sensitivity that is appropriate for the clinical care of the vast majority of patients. Indeed, direct and indirect hemagglutination tests have served the transfusion community well for, respectively, over 100 and over 50 years. However, in some aspects, hemagglutination has limitations. For example, it gives only an indirect measure of the potential complications in an at-risk pregnancy, it cannot precisely indicate RHD zygosity in D-positive people, it cannot be relied upon to type some recently transfused patients, and it requires the availability of specific reliable antisera.

5. Molecular Testing for Blood Group Genotyping

The discovery of the ABO blood group system by Karl Landsteiner in 1900 was naturally one of the most important marks in medicine in the 20th century [9, 17]. More than 700 inherited blood group antigens have been described on the surface of human red cells [10]. Until the 1990s, blood screening, typing and diagnostics depended entirely on serological techniques. For over a century, hemagglutination has been the gold standard for red blood cell (RBC) antigen detection used in all blood services. The classical method of testing for blood group antigens and antibodies is hemagglutination, which has certain limitations [18, 19].

Molecular genotyping methods were introduced to the transfusion medicine community over a decade ago. Implementation of DNA-based methods in the blood bank environment benefits from the ability to validate a specific SNP/ antigen association by testing a large number of samples with concurrent red blood cell (RBC) serologic and DNA testing [20]. The molecular bases for all the polymorphisms have been determined; with the exceptions of P1 / P2, Xg, and MER2 [21].

Many blood group antigens are the result of single nucleotide gene polymorphisms or SNPs (pronounced 'snips') inherited in a straight forward Mendelian manner [20]. However, other variations exist, such as gene deletions, single nucleotide deletion, insertion of sequences, and polymorphisms impacting the expression of proteins [21, 22, 23]. The application of this knowledge has currently an impact on transfusion medicine [18–24], as well as, in prenatal diagnosis of hemolytic anemia of the newborn [25].

Table 4: Molecular events that gives different blood group antigen and phenotypes

Event	Mechanism	Blood group phenotype
Promoter mutation	Nucleotide change in GATA box	Fy(b-)
Alternative spicing	Nucleotide change in splice site	S-s-, Gy(a-)
Premature stop codon	Deletion of nucleotides	Fy(a-b-), Rh null, Ge2, Ge3, Ge4, K0
	Insertion of nucleotides	D-, Co(a-b-)
Amino acid change	Missense mutation	D-, Rh null, K0
Hybrid genes	Crossover	GP.Vw, GP.Hil
	Gene conversion	GP.Mur, GP.Hop, D --
Interacting protein	Absence of RHAG	Rh null
	Absence of Kx	Weak expression of Kell antigen
Modifying gene	IN(LU)	LU(a-b-)

It is now possible to predict blood group phenotypes from tests on genomic DNA, with a high degree of accuracy. In the beginning, the laboratory developed assays PCR-RFLP (polymerase chain reaction-restriction fragment length polymorphism) and PCR-SSP (polymerase chain -sequence specific polymorphism) were labor intensive, with discrepancies that required extensive serologic and molecular genetics investigation [26-29].The molecular methods available for red cell genotyping can be divided into the following categories: low to medium-throughput: PCR, PCR-RFLP, PCR-SSP or PCR-ASP (PCR- allele specific polymorphism), Real-time PCR, DNA sequencing and pirosequencing and high throughput with Microarrays-based systems (e.g. BloodChip, BeadChip and Genome Lab SNP stream) [26].This article aims to indicate some of the technologies currently available and often used for genotyping of red blood cells.

Need of molecular testing in transfusion medicine

Development of alternative methods to determine blood groups is not just of academic interest. There are situations in which the genotype is a superior, or the only, approach. For example, serologic RBC agglutination tests have limitations when patients are multiply transfused or have RBCs coated with immunoglobulin. In addition, agglutination tests depend on the availability of specific and potent reagents, but these are not available for many blood group antigens, such as Dombrock (Doa, Dob), Colton (Coa, Cob), etc., or for low-frequency antigens in the majority of blood group systems. Furthermore, discrepancies in serologic reactivity between different manufacturers' reagents can occur, complicating determination of the antigen status of RBCs. Genotyping can resolve these. Finally, D-zygosity testing and fetal typing from amniocytes or from cell-free fetal DNA present in maternal plasma can only is done by molecular testing [20].

One to two percent of all patients who receive transfusions develop antibodies to RBC antigens. In patients receiving chronic transfusion (e.g., for sickle cell disease [SCD]), the frequency of alloimmunization is higher, affecting ≈20 percent to 30 percent of recipients, [30, 31] though most patients who develop alloantibodies do so before the 15th transfusion [32]. For patients with hematologic malignancies, the incidence of RBC alloimmunization is estimated at nine percent to 15 percent [32, 33] despite the immuno suppressive effects of the chemotherapy most patients receive. Thus, alloimmunization to RBC antigens in hematology patients is relatively common.

Once alloimmunization occurs, the likelihood of additional antibody responses is also relatively high. In surgical, pregnant, and non–hematologic malignancy patients, once RBC antibodies have been induced, 20 percent to 25 percent of patients form additional antibodies after subsequent transfusions and thus become multiply alloimmunized. In a retrospective study from the Netherlands that covered a 24-year period, 25 of 115 immunized patients (21.7%) formed 30 additional antibodies after receiving a median of seven additional RBC transfusions. The median interval between primary and additional antibody detection was four months. Interestingly, diagnosis or treatment intensity did not significantly influence development of additional antibodies [34].

Application of molecular testing in transfusion medicine

Molecular genotyping is being increasingly used in immunohematology reference laboratories in western countries and has now become more efficient and cost-effective. Some of the important applications of molecular blood group genotyping in transfusion setting and in prenatal diagnosis are shown in table 5.

a. Prediction of blood group genotype

Prediction of a blood group antigen by testing DNA is easy and reliable if the antigen is encoded by a common or "normal" functional allele. However, the many uncommon alleles make this approach imperfect. There are far more alleles than phenotypes [35].

b. Identify a fetus at risk for anemia of the neonate

Hemagglutination, including antibody titers, gives only an indirect indication of hemolytic disease of the fetus and newborn (HDFN) risk and severity. Antigen prediction by DNA assays can be of value in the prenatal setting to identify the fetus who is NOT at risk of HDFN (i.e., predicted to be antigen-negative) so that the mother need not be aggressively monitored. Another value is to predict the D type of a fetus to aid in the evaluation of whether Rh-immune globulin need, or need not, be administered [35].

Table 5: Clinical application of molecular analysis

Antigen typing a patient
• To identify a fetus at risk for HDN
• When antibody is weak or not available, e.g., anti-Do^a, -Do^b, -Js^a, -V/VS
• Who has recently received a transfusion
• Whose RBCs are coated with immunoglobulin (+DAT)
• To distinguish an alloantibody from an autoantibody
• To detect weakly expressed antigens (e.g., Fy^b with the Fy^X phenotype); where the patient is unlikely to make antibodies to transfused antigen-positive RBCs
• Identify molecular basis of unusual serologic results, especially Rh variants
• To determine zygosity, particularly *RHD*
Antigen typing for donors
• To screen for antigen-negative donors
• When antibody is weak or not available, e.g., anti-Do^a, -Do^b; -Js^a, -Js^b; -V/VS
• Mass screening to increase antigen-negative inventory and to find donors whose RBCs lack a high-prevalence antigen
• To resolve blood group A, B, D, C, and e discrepancies
• To detect genes that encode weak antigens
• To type donors for reagent RBCs (antibody screening and identification panels)
Other applications
• One-step, automated, objective antibody detection and identification
• Use of transfected cells as immunogens for production of monoclonal antibodies
• Conversion of IgG monoclonal antibodies to IgM direct agglutinins

c. Prediction of blood group antigens in multi-transfused patients

To know the RBC phenotype of a patient is an invaluable part of the antibody identification process. When a patient receives transfusions, the presence of donor RBCs in the patient's peripheral blood makes RBC phenotyping by hemagglutination complex, time consuming, and possibly inaccurate [35]. To overcome this problem, PCR-based assays using DNA isolated from WBCs, buccal smear, or urine sediment can be used to predict the antigen type of patients. In the way the PCR-based assays are performed for this purpose, any donor WBCs in a transfused patient's circulation do not interfere with the interpretation [35-38].

d. Typing of an antigen-negative blood donors

Screening for rare donors by analysis of DNA is valuable for typing for "minor "antigens and Rh variants. Those antigens that are predicted to be negative should be confirmed by hemagglutination. In this manner, precious antibodies are conserved for the confirmation of DNA typing interpretations. The value of access to larger numbers of antigen-negative RBC components is multifaceted. If antigen-negative inventories were sufficient, several uses of antigen-matched blood could be contemplated to improve patient care. Obviously, as with hemagglutination, the rare antigen-negative donor will likely only be found by screening thousands of donors.

e. Typing for low-prevalence antigens

The "low-prevalence" antigens are not on antibody screening RBCs, the corresponding antibodies are not available to screen for suitable donors, and the crosshatches not always reliable for their detection. PCR-based assays provide a tool to mass screen donors, thereby increasing the antigen-negative inventory and improving patient care.

f. Typing for high-prevalence antigens

As anti-Lub, -Dib, -Yta, -Sc1, and -Coa are inconsistently available, testing DNA is adesirable alternative. The ready availability of anti-k, -Kpb, -Jsb, and -Fy3 often makes hemagglutination the method of choice for these antigens. On the other hand, as probes for various nucleotide changes can be added to a microchip at little incremental cost, all of the above antigens could be assayed simultaneously. Detection of Vel–, Lan–, At(a–), or Jr(a–)donors is restricted to hemagglutination because the molecular bases of these antigens are not yet known. Detection of null phenotypes such as Rh-null, K0, Gy(a–), Ge–, or McLeod is complex due to multiple molecular bases associated with each of these phenotypes [39].

g. Prediction of ABO and RHD alleles

DNA analysis is not suited for routine ABO and D determination of donor blood as it is more time-consuming, more expensive, prone to misinterpretation, and thus, not an improvement over hemagglutination. The reasons include the following: the naturally occurring anti-A and/or anti-B in the plasma of most people who lack the corresponding antigens provides a built-in check when performing ABO typing by hemagglutination; potent, well-standardized monoclonal antibodies are available for ABO and D typing; hemagglutination is relatively simple and rapid; and systems are in place to test and record, relatively efficiently, the ABO and D type of a donor. In both ABO and Rh systems, there are few antigens and many alleles. PCR-based assays may be useful to define some Rh variants and to precisely match D and e antigen status of a donor to a recipient, especially in the case of patients with sickle cell disease (SCD) [35, 36].

Molecular techniques used for genotyping of blood group antigens

As the molecular basis of a blood group antigen has been determined, the precise area of DNA can be analyzed to predict the presence or absence of a blood group antigen on the surface of an RBC. Fortunately, as the majority of genetically defined blood group antigens are the consequence of a single nucleotide change, simple PCR-based assays can be used to detect a change in a gene encoding a blood group antigen. Innumerable DNA-based assays have been described for this purpose. Figure 1 illustrates readout formats for all PCR-based assays.

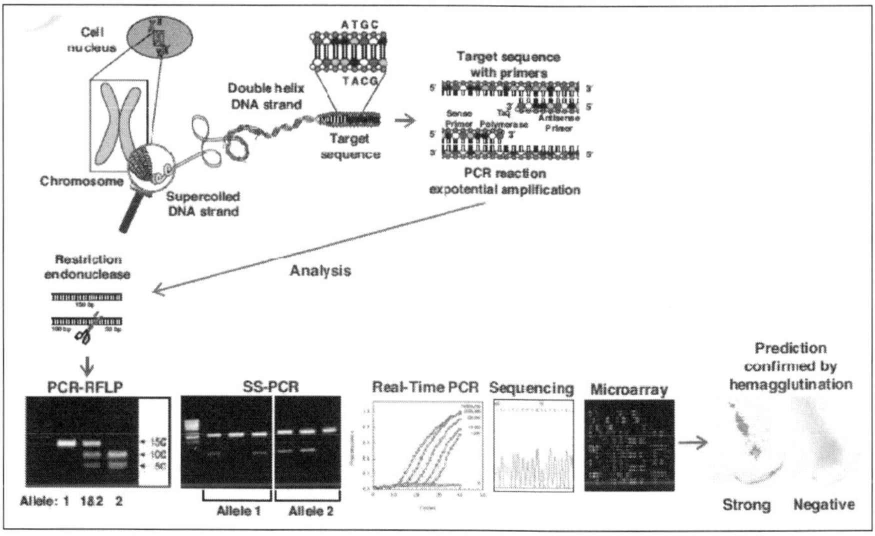

Fig. 8: From DNA to PCR based assay readouts. Schematic representation of DNA isolated from nucleated cell with a particular sequence targeted and amplified in PCR amplification. The readout formats of some of the various techniques available to analyze the results are shown.

Table 6: Different molecular techniques used for blood group genotyping

	Low throughput	Medium throughput	High throughput
Technique	PCR-SSP, PCR -RFLP, Nested PCR, Multiplex PCR etc.	PCR-Sequencing, Quantitative PCR etc.	Microarrays, Mini sequencing etc.
Applications	Genotyping common antigens of Rh, Duffy, Kell, Kidd etc., weaker variants etc.	Identification of weaker variants of ABO & Rh, non-invasive fetal RhD typing, Rh zygosity testing, SNP genotyping etc.	Genotyping of multiple blood group and platelet antigens
Advantages	Simple and easy, Cost effective	More sensitive, no post PCR processing required	Large scale donor typing for many antigens in a single test, automated

The molecular methods available for red cell genotyping can be divided into the following categories: low to medium-throughput: PCR, PCR-RFLP, PCR-SSP or PCR-ASP, Real time PCR, DNA sequencing and pirosequencing and high-throughput with Microarrays-based systems (e.g. BloodChip, BeadChip and Genome Lab SNP stream) [27].The various molecular methods used for red cell typing has been reviewed by Monteiro *et al.*, [40] and summarized in Table 6.

1. Low throughput assay based on classical PCR

PCR is used to amplify a specific sequence of DNA. The reaction consists in tree steps: denaturation, annealing and extension. These steps are repeated for 25-35 times and give the exponential increase in the number of copies. The PCR products can be analyzed using different methods, which can include electrophoresis to separate the fragments, based on size, through an agarose gel. Various PCR assays commonly used include AS-PCR, PCR-SSP; PCR-RFLP; and multiplex PCR.

a) PCR-RFLP

The alleles are differentiated after PCR by digestion of the products with a restriction enzyme. These enzymes are highly specific and cleave a unique sequence of nucleotides. Alleles are discriminated by the fragment pattern visualized by gel electrophoresis after digestion and the fragment pattern compared with known controls tested in parallel. Normally the controls used are homozygous samples for each allele and a heterozygote one [29, 30, 41]. Design of these tests was based on the introduction or loss of restriction sites by SNP of interest.

b) AS-PCR or PCR-SSP

This assay requires two reactions to be set up for each DNA sample. Each reaction tube has one primer that is gene-specific (common to both alleles), and one primer that is specific for one of the two possible alleles present. When the non- complementary sequence is present, annealing does not occur and there is no amplification. The amplicon of the two reactions are visualized by agarose gel electrophoresis. Internal control is required as lack of PCR product indicates absence on an allele. ABO variants, RHD /RHCE variants and other blood group genes such as K1 / K2, FYA/ FYB and JKA/JKB [42, 43] can be tested using this method.

c) Multiplex PCR

Multiplex PCR enables simultaneous amplification of many target alleles or regions of DNA in one reaction by using multiple primer pairs. This allows a reduction in the number of different assays performed, which saves time, reagents and cost. Based on the technical platform and design of the process, multiplex PCR can be set-up as a low or medium-throughput assay. This assay has been used for identifying common partial RHD variants. Common antigens of various minor blood group systems can also be detected simultaneously [44, 45].

2. Medium-throughput Assay

a) RT-PCR

Real-Time PCR method is based on detection of fluorescence signals in the PCR cycler. It measures the amplified DNA quantitatively in real time i.e. as the reaction progresses. Real-time PCR applications can be set-up as low or medium-throughput methods. This method has been implicated in determination of RhD zygosity and in noninvasive prenatal RHD typing. Melting curve analysis which involves the assessment of the dissociation-characteristics of double-stranded DNA(Tm) during heating in the presence of fluorophore has been applied to study various blood group polymorphisms [42, 43].

b) Sanger DNA sequencing

Sanger sequencing is being widely used in blood group genotyping. This method of DNA sequencing is based on the selective incorporation of chain terminating dideoxynucleotides (ddNTPs) by DNA polymerase during in vitro DNA replication. It gives the sequence of nucleotides in the target sequence [46].

c) Pyrosequencing

Pyrosequencing is a DNA sequencing method based on detecting pyrophosphate release rather than on strand termination. It has been successfully used for red cell genotyping, but presently limited to only few blood group systems [47].

3. High-throughput Arrays

There have been several large-scale studies to evaluate the performance of molecular high-throughput platforms for RBC typing. The BeadChip (Bioarray Solutions, Warren, NJ) and Genome Lab SNP stream (Beckman Coulter, Fullerton, CA) platforms have been used to genotype for multiple blood group antigens [49, 50, 51]. The BloodGen consortium was established to do mass-scale typing in the European Union on the BloodChip platform (Progenika) [52, 53].

a) BeadChip array, BloodChip and Genome Lab SNP Stream

These all are microarray based methods that integrate thousands of reactions in a single test and can be used to test multiple blood group antigens at different loci simultaneously [46-50]. In BeadChip a bead of 3 mm diameter accommodates approximately 106 oligonucleotide probes of 20 nucleotides in length for DNA analysis applications. In BloddChip selected SNPs, deletions, insertions corresponding to blood group alleles are incorporated in to the chip, whereas the Genome Lab SNP Stream method is based on a multiplex PCR followed by a single-base extension reaction using a gene-specific, tag-specific primer. A fluorescent label is incorporated and hybridization occurs in 384-well plates.

b) Fluidic microarray systems (Luminex XMAP)

The system detects PCR-amplified targets by direct hybridization to microspheres coupled to allele-specific oligonucleotides and can analyze up to 100 different analytes in a single reaction using a flow cytometer. Karpasitou et al. [54] adapted the technology to type for JKA / JKB, FYA / FYB,S / s, K1 / K2, KPA / KPB / JSA / JSB, COA / COB, and LUA / LUB.

c) TaqMan Open Array

The method is based in real-time PCR using TaqMan probes. The PCR includes a specific fluorescent dye labeled probe for each allele of the target SNP. The probes contain different fluorescent reporter dyes to differentiate each allele. The array consists of collection of 3072 reaction through-holes in the plate and provides genotyping and gene expression analysis of hundreds to thousands of samples and assays per day [55].

d) **MALDI-TOF MS (matrix-assisted laser desorption/ionization time-of-flight mass spectrometry)**

This technique has the capacity to discriminate DNA fragments that differ in a single nucleotide. It is a high-throughput, qualitative, and quantitative method that can analyze 36–40 multiple SNPS in a single reaction that takes approximately eight hours. This method has been used for genotyping of some of the Kell blood group system genes and for platelet antigens [52].

e) **Mini-sequencing or SNaPshot assay**

Cyclic mini-sequencing reactions with fluorescently labeled dideoxynucleotides are performed in solution using multiplex PCR product as template and detection primers that are designed to anneal immediately adjacent and upstream of the SNP site. Following the hybridization and extension steps, the fluorescent signals from the array are measured and the genotypes are deduced by cluster analysis. Mini-sequencing is used for typing of common ABH alleles while SNapShot method is used for antigens like Fya/ Fyb, Doa/ Dob, Joa, Hy,LWa/ LWb, Coa/ Cob, Sc1 / Sc2, Dia/ Dib, Jka/ Jkb, Lua/ Lub, MNSs, and K/ k [56].

Limitations of molecular techniques

To apply molecular approaches to clinical situations, several areas of knowledge are needed. For example, a knowledge of molecular techniques, of gene structure and processing, of the molecular bases of blood groups, of hemagglutination techniques, of the expression of blood group antigens, of factors that may affect interpretation of genotype (eg, chimeras), and of regulatory compliance (cGLP, IRB, FDA). In addition, it is important to be able to correlate DNA and serological results to the clinical problems being addressed.

From a practical perspective, not all blood group polymorphisms can be analyzed: like, in situations when a large number of alleles encode one phenotype (eg, ABO, Rh, and null phenotypes in many blood group systems); alleles with a large deletion (eg, GE: – 2,3 and GE:–2–3–4); or a hybrid alleles (eg, in the Rh and MNS systems); or when the molecular basis is not yet known (eg, Vel, Lan, Jra). Detection of null phenotypes, eg, Rh-null, 10;24 K0,25 McLeod,26 Kidd,27 and the p phenotype28 is complex by DNA analysis because of multiple molecular bases, but is easy by hemagglutination. For example, to detect D- test RBCs with anti-Rh17 (or -C & -c), to detect Fy(a-b-) test RBCs with anti-Fy3, and to detect Jk(a-b-) test RBCs with anti-Jk3 or test for the resistance of such RBCs to lysis by 2 Murea.[57].

When appropriate and feasible, an assay to detect a nucleotide change that silences a gene should be part of the DNA-based testing; e.g, GATA box and FY*265 (for Fyx) analyses with FYA/FYB typing, [58] presence of RHD pseudo gene with RHD typing, [59] and exon 5/ intron 5 analysis with GYPB*S typing [60]. While a nucleotide change (t>c) in the GATA-1 binding motif is the basis of the Fy (a-b-) phenotype in blacks, the Fy (a-b-) phenotype in Caucasians is very rare and associated with silencing of FY*A or FY*B by at least 4 different molecular bases [58]. Given the large number of alleles that silence various blood groups, the question is how much testing is practical or feasible. The limited DNA testing used for clinical utility will not allow accurate interpretation of all alleles; thus, in this scenario, the "genotype" may not be the phenotype and confirmation of predicted antigen-negativity by hemagglutination or a crosshatch is recommended.

The major limitations of molecular testing include: time, availability, expense, and correlation between genotype and phenotype. Most laboratories are not equipped to perform this testing at the present time, and specimens must be shipped to reference laboratories. The test can be completed in a matter of hours, but typically the turnaround time is one day. Serology by contrast can be performed in every laboratory, relatively inexpensive and testing can commence immediately. Even so, these limitations should not be a deterrent for ordering the test that may aid the blood bank for future management of a patient.

6. Future Perspective of Molecular Genotyping in Transfusion Medicine

Considerable work remains before genotyping is routinely implemented. But a future in which all donors have their blood genotyped is not an unreasonable expectation. Further, this could lead to a better match for a typed recipient, the so-called individualized transfusion treatment, thus reducing many transfusion complications. Even though we cannot match for every antigen, the blood supply is limited, and time constraints sometimes lead to urgent transfusion, molecular testing has the potential to improve patient care. Such testing is pending approval by the Federal Drug Administration (FDA) as donor units cannot be officially labeled with the genotype information. Transfusion services can choose to accept genotype information; however, FDA-approved serologic testing must be performed for phenotypic confirmation prior to labeling and dispensing blood as antigen negative for a patient. Furthermore, if there was a simple, inexpensive way to positively identify a donor at subsequent donations should DNA typing of a donor be performed only once?

Hemagglutination is the gold standard technique to type RBCs for the presence or absence of blood group antigens. PCR-based assays, used as an adjunct to hemagglutination, [Table 7] will be a powerful tool that could radically change approaches used to support patients in their transfusion needs. However there are certain events happens at genetic level where both these techniques differ [Table 8].

Other forms of molecular testing can also play a significant role in fetal and maternal care. For the fetus, genotyping can be of use in patients at risk for hemolytic disease of the fetus or newborn as this allows for Rh zygosity testing in the fetus and parents. Specifically, for women of childbearing age, weak and partial D may be of significant concern. A mother with a weak D will not form antibodies to the D antigen as opposed to a mother with partial D. Thus knowing the difference will influence whether to offer Rh negative blood and Rh immune globulin. While serology cannot distinguish between the two, techniques using

PCR for genotyping the RHD gene can. These techniques are currently only available in reference laboratories.

Table 7: Comparison of hemagglutination and PCR based assays for blood group antigens

	Hemagglutination	PCR based techniques
Value	Gold standard, Simple and quick, detects mixed populations of RBCs	Can be automated, high throughput
Reagents	Require Specialized monoclonal and polyclonal antisera, many antibodies are not commercially available, limited in volume, weakly reactive	Not require special reagent, readily purchasable
Limitations	Subjective test, use of reliable antisera, labor-intensive, small number of donors can be typed, difficult to type recently transfused patients, difficult in distinguish between allo and auto antibodies	Predicted antigen should be confirmed by hemagglutination, takes hours, results may not agree with hemagglutination in some cases, difficult to predict null phenotypes, expensive than hemagglutination

Table 8: Molecular events where genotype and phenotype will differ

Event	Mechanism	Blood group phenotype
Transcription	Nt change in GATA box	Fy(b-)
Alternative splicing	Nt change in splice site: Partial/complete skipping of exon	S-s-; Gy(a-)
	Deletion of nts	Dr(a-)
Premature stop codon	Deletion of nt(s) → frameshift	Fy(a-b-); D-; Rh_{null}; Ge: -2, -3,-4; Gy(a-); K_0; McLeod
	Insertion of nt(s) → frameshift	D-; Co(a-b-)
	Nt change	Fy(a-b-); r′; Gy(a-); K_0; McLeod
Amino acid change	Missense mutation	D-; Rh_{null}; K_0; McLeod
Reduced amount of protein	Missense mutation	Fy^x; Co(a-b-)
Hybrid genes	Crossover	GP.Vw; GP.Hil; GP.TSEN
	Gene conversion	GP.Mur; GP.Hop; D--; R_0^{Har}
Interacting protein	Absence of RhAG	Rh_{null}
	Absence of Kx	Weak expression of Kell antigen
	Absence of aas 59 to 76 of GPA	Wr(b-)
	Absence of protein 4.1	Weak expression of Ge antigens
Modifying gene	*In(LU)*	Lu(a-b-)
	IN(Jk)	Jk(a-b-)

Molecular testing can be extended to platelet antigens, a useful tool for patients with platelet refractoriness or cases of neonatal allo-immune thrombocytopenia and post transfusion purpura. This methodology can also be done with HLA A and B typing; a patient with platelet refractoriness can be offered HLA-matched platelets. More work needs to be done before a more thorough HLA analysis (classes I and II) can be offered for the transplant setting. Any blood banks can incorporate molecular techniques to do various PCR-based assays in transfusion medicine. As from long period of time molecular techniques have been introduced to detect transfusion transmitted infections and that is why it is easy to adapt PCR-based techniques in day to day activity of blood banks.

References

Hess JR, Thomas MJ. Blood use in war and disaster: lessons from the past century. Transfusion 2003; 43(11), 1622-1633.

Sarkar, R. S., Philip, J., Kumar, S., & Yadav, P. (2012). Evolution of the role of army transfusion services in the management of trauma patients and battle casualties with massive hemorrhage. Med J Armed Forces India, 68(4), 366-370.

Highlights of Transfusion Medicine History. Transfusion Medicine. American Association of Blood Banks (AABB).

Pal R, Kar S, Zaman FA, Pal S. The quest for an Indian blood law as of blood transfusion services regulatory framework. Asian J Transfus Sci 2011; 5(2): 171-174.

Ramani KV, Mavalankar D, Govil D. Management of Blood Transfusion Services in India: An Illustrative Study of Maharashtra and Gujarat States: Indian Institute of Ahmedabad, 2007.

Hemogenomics. Blood safety 2013. From http://www.hemogenomics.com/index.php/blood-safety.

WHO. (2012a). More voluntary blood donations essential [Press release]. Retrieved from http://www.who.int/mediacentre/news/releases/2012/blood_donation_20120614/ en/.

GOI. Transfusion Medicine 2003, Technical Manual. New Delhi: Director General of Health Services, Government of India.

Landsteiner K: Zur Kenntnis der antifermentativvenlytischen and agglutinierenden Wirkungen des Blutserums und der Lymphe. Sent Bact 1900; 27:357–362.

Red Cell Immunogenetics and Blood Group Terminology. Working Party area of the International society of blood transfusion (ISBT).

Daniels G, Bromilow I. Essential guide to blood groups. 3rd ed. Willy Blackwell publication.

Anstee DJ. Red cell genotyping and the future of pre transfusion testing. Blood 2009; 114:248-256.

Harmening DM. Modern Blood Banking and Transfusion Medicine. 6th ed.F. A. Davis Company.

Issitt, PD, and Anstee, DJ: Applied Blood Group Serology,4th ed. Montgomery Scientific, Durham, NC, 1998, pp 34–35.

Mujahid A, Dickert FL. Blood Group Typing: From Classical Strategies to the Application of Synthetic Antibodies Generated by Molecular Imprinting. Sensors; 2016: 16 (51).

Malomgrc,W.; Neumeister, B. Recent and future trends in blood group typing. Anal. Bioanal. Chem. 2009,393, 1443–1451.

Camp FR, Ellis FR: Selected Contributions to the Literature of Blood Groups and Immunology. Fort Knox, KY, US Army Medical Research Laboratory, 1966.

Reid ME: Transfusion in the age of molecular diagnostics. Hematology Am Soc Hematol Educ Program 2009; 171–177.

Avent ND: Large-Scale blood group genotyping – clinical implications. Br J Haematol 2008; 144:3–13.

Connie M. Westhoff. Molecular testing for transfusion medicine. Transfusion Med 2006; 13:471–475.

Daniels GL: The molecular genetics of blood group polymorphism. Hum Genet 2009; 126:729–742.

Cartron JP, Baily P, Le Van Kim C, et al.: Insights into the structure and function of membrane polypeptides carrying blood group antigens. Vox Sang 1998; 74(Suppl. 2):29–64.

Storry JR, Olsson ML: Genetic basis of blood group diversity. Br J Haematol 2004; 126:759–771.

Elizabeth Q: Blood-matching goes genetics. Science 2008; 319:1478–1479.

Mullis KB, Fallona FA: Specific synthesis of DNA in vitro via apolymerase catalysed chain reaction. Methods Enzymol 1987; 155:335–350.

Moulds JM: Future of molecular testing for red blood cell antigens. Clin Lab Med 2010; 30:419–429.

Hue-Roye K, Vege S: Principles of PCR-based assays. Immunohematology 2008; 24:170–175.

Storry JR: Molecular basis of erythrocyte blood group antigens and applications in transfusion medicine. Vox Sang 2002; 83(Suppl. 1):081–084.

Wagner FF, Frohmajer A, Ladewig B, et al.: Weak D alleles express distinct phenotypes. Blood 2000; 95:2699–2708.

Olujohungbe A, Hambleton I, Stephens L, et al. Red cell antibodies in patients with homozygous sickle cell disease: a comparison of patients in Jamaica and the United Kingdom. Br J Haematol. 2001; 113:661-665.

Rosse WF, Gallagher D, Kinney TR, et al. Transfusion and alloimmunization in sickle cell disease: The Cooperative Study of Sickle Cell Disease. Blood. 1990; 76:1431-1437.

Blumberg N, Ross K, Avila E, et al. Should chronic transfusions be matched for antigens other than ABO and Rho (D)? Vox Sang. 1984;47:205-208.

Sanz C, Nomdedeu M, Belkaid M, et al. Red blood cell alloimmunization in transfused patients with myelodysplastic syndrome or chronic myelomonocytic leukemia. Transfusion. 2013; 53:710-715.

Schonewille H, de Vries RR, Brand A. Alloimmune response after additional red blood cell antigen challenge in immunized hematooncology patients. Transfusion. 2009; 49:453-457.

Reid ME, Rios M, Powell VI, Charles-Pierre D, Malavade V. DNA from blood samples can be used to genotype patients who have recently received a transfusion. Transfusion 2000;40:48–53.

Wenk RE, Chiafari FA. DNA typing of recipient blood after massive transfusion. Transfusion 1997;37:1108–1110.

Legler TJ, Eber SW, Lakomek M, et al. Application of RHD and RHCE genotyping for correct blood group determination in chronically transfused patients. Transfusion 1999;39:852–855.

Rozman P, Dovc T, Gassner C. Differentiation of autologous ABO, RHD, RHCE, KEL, JK, and FY blood group genotypes by analysis of peripheral blood samples of patients who have recently received multiple transfusions. Transfusion 2000;40:936–942.

Reid, ME.; Lomas-Francis, C. Blood Group Antigen Facts Book. Academic Press; San Diego: 2004.

Monteiro F, Tavares G, Ferreira M, Amorim A,Bastos P, Rocha C, et al. Technologies involved in molecular blood group genotyping. Vox Sang. 2011;6:1–6.

Wu YY, Csako G: Rapid and/or high-throughput genotyping for human red blood cell, platelet and leukocyte antigens, and forensic applications. Clin Chim Acta 2006; 363:165–176.

Prager M: Molecular genetic blood group typing by the use of PCR-SSP technique. Transfusion 2007; 47:54–59.

Arau´ jo F, Pereira C, Aleixo A, et al.: Rapid genotyping of the major alleles at the Duffy (FY) blood group locus using real time fluorescence polymerase chain reaction. Immunohematology 2001; 17:42–44.

Arau´ jo F, Pereira C, Monteiro F, et al.: Blood group antigen profile predicted by molecular biology - use of real time polymerase chain reaction to genotype important KEL, JK, RHD, and RHCE alleles. Immunohematology 2002; 18:59–64.

Smith LM, Fung S, Hunkapiller MW, et al.: The synthesis of oligonucleotides containing an aliphatic amino group at the 5◎ terminus: synthesis of fluorescent DNA primers for use in DNA sequence analysis. Nucleic Acids Res 1985; 13:2399–2412.

Ferri G, Bini C, Ceccardi S, et al.: ABO genotyping by mini sequencing analysis. Transfusion 2004; 44:943–944.

Van Dronen J, Beckers EAM, Sintnocolaas K, et al.: Rapid genotyping of blood group systems using the pyrosequencing technique. Vox Sang 2002; 83:104–105.

Hashmi G, Shariff T, Seul M, et al.: A flexible array format for large-scale, rapid blood group DNA typing. Transfusion 2005; 45:667–679.

Beiboer SH, Wieringa-Jelsma T, Maaskant-Van Wijk PA, et al.: Rapid genotyping of blood group antigens by multiplexpolymerase chain reaction and DNA microarray hybridization. Transfusion 2005; 45:667–679.

Denomme GA, Van Oene M: High-throughput multiplex single nucleotide polymorphism analysis for red cell and platelet antigen genotypes. Transfusion 2005; 45:660–666.

Montpetit A, Phillips MS, Mongrain I, et al.: High-throughput molecular profiling of blood donors for minor red blood cell and platelet antigens. Transfusion 2006; 46:841–848.

Avent ND, Martinez A, Flegel WA, et al.: The BloodGen project: toward mass-scale comprehensive genotyping of blood donors in the European Union and beyond. Transfusion 2007; 47:40S–46S.

Avent ND, Martinez A, Flegel WA, et al.: The Bloodgen Project of the European Union, 2003–2009. Transfus Med Hemother 2009; 36:162–167.

Karpasitou K, Drago F, Crespiatico L, et al.: Blood group genotyping for Jka/Jkb, Fya/Fyb, S/s, Kpa/Kpb, Jsa/Jsb, Coa/Cob, and Lua/Lub with microarray beads. Transfusion 2008; 48:505–512.

Arau´ jo F, Cardoso M, Alves M, et al.: Determinac¸a˜o pre´-natal do geno´ tipo RHD por me´todos na˜o invasivos. Progr Diag Trat Prenat 2003; 15:126–132.

Palacajornsuk P, Halter C, Isakova V, et al.: Detection of blood group genes using multiplex SNaPshot method. Transfusion 2009; 49:740–749.

Heaton DC, McLoughlin K. Jk(a-b-) red blood cells resist urea lysis. Transfusion 1982;22:70–71.

Castilho L. The value of DNA analysis for antigens in the Duffy blood group system. Transfusion 2007; 47:28S–31S.

Westhoff CM. Rh complexities: serology and DNA genotyping. Transfusion 2007; 47:17S–22S.

Storry JR, Reid ME, Fetics S, Huang C-H. Mutations in *GYPB* exon 5 drive the S-s-U+^{var} phenotype in persons of African descent: Implications for transfusion. Transfusion 2003; 43:1738– 1747.

Chapter 15

Research & Developments in Medicinal Plants Sector: An Analysis from 36 States / Union Territories of India

Rahil Mathakia[3], Ashaba Rana[2] and Viralkumar B. Mandaliya[1*]

Assistant Professor (Research), [1]Gujarat National Law University, Gandhinagar, Gujarat, India.

Project Assistant,[3]Gujarat National Law University, Gandhinagar, Gujarat, India.

Lab. Tech., [2]Care Institute of Medical Service, Ahmedabad, Gujarat, India.

*Email: viral_mandaliya@yahoo.com

Abstract

Medicinal plants are known since centuries for its valuable capacity for ailments of livestock and human diseases. In India, various government organization has developed the database after a deep research and appropriate documentation to save the precious wealth for future generation. This chapter analyze the research and development in this sector from 36 States/Union Territories (UTs) of India. The Indian Citation Index (ICI) database is used to analyze the medicinal plants sector. Tamil Nadu, Uttar Pradesh, and Maharashtra were the top most State/UTs for highest contribution in this sector. The contribution of three authors, Deshpande Nirmala, Paulsamy S and Savithramma N were identified as top most in medicinal plants sector. This study will analyze various other parameters in this sector.

Keywords: bioinformatics database, human disease, ICI database, Indian Citation Index, livestock.

Introduction

Globally, the countryside people are basically depend on trees, shrubs, herbs, grasses and ferns and their product to fulfill their basic survival needed. Nowadays combination of traditional and scientific knowledge of plant and plant product is utilized as a medicine/drug for the prevention of number of diseases and ailments. Across all the developing countries, around 80 % of population is depends on medicinal plant[1]. It is documented that medicines used in Complementary and Alternative Medicine Therapies (CAMT) are medicinal plant origin[2]. Western

1 Ekor M (2013). The growing use of herbal medicines: issues relating to adverse reactions and challenges in monitoring safety. Front Pharmacol., 4: 177. doi: 10.3389/fphar.2013.00177.

2 Pan SY, Gao S. H., Zhou S. F. et al. (2012). New perspectives on complementary and alternative medicine: an overview and alternative therapy. Alter. Thera. Health Med., 18(4): 20–36.

Ghats, Himalaya, Andaman and Nicobar are rich in diversity of medicinal properties containing plants and around 45,000 medicinal plant species is found in India[3]. Among them only 3000 plant species are in use as therapeutics. Medicinal plant are play key important role in potential drug discovery because of medicinal plant contain various advantages like rich in availability, lesser side effects and highly economic in value[4].

In India, *Ocimum sanctum* (Tulsi), *Aloe barbadensis* (Ghritkumari), *Rauvolfia serpentine* (Sarpagandha), *Curcuma longa* (Haridra), *Commiphora wightii* (Guggulu), *Bacopa monnieri* (Brahmi), *Emblica officinallis* (Amla), *Withania somnifera* (Ashwagandha) and *Azadirachta indica* (Neem) are highly available and potentially used for various kind of medicine development[5].

Medicinal Plant are valuable source of therapeutics. A numerous number of research on animal and clinical studies indicate that biochemical in medicinal plant play key role in health benefit of human, such as[6] (i) Treat as antioxidant, antibacterial, antiviral and anti-inflammatory. (ii) Prevent various forms of cancer. (iii) Suppress cardiovascular diseases, respiratory diseases, liver disease, arthritis, and diabetes. (iv) Use in body maintenance, fat reduction, and boost immunity. (v) Increase quality of oral health, skin, and hair.

The Computational Databases on Medicinal Plants

A source of information, online or offline, computational tools that contain various information is called as database. Medicinal plant database provides various information related to medicinal plants like nomenclature in various languages and region, ecological interaction, biological characteristic, etc. Medicinal plant databases also provide numerous kind of benefits like screening and selection process for drug discovery. Table 1 summarizes the well-known databases on medicinal plants from India.

Table 1: The well-known databases on medicinal plants from India

S. No.	Name of Database	Web-Link	Information of Database
1	Encyclopedia on Indian Medicinal Plants	http://envis.frlht.org/indian-medicinal-plants-database.php	This database stores 7,637 botanical names (6,198 medicinal plants species) with 119183 vernacular names from 12 languages across India.
2	Indian Medicinal Plants Database	http://www.medicinalplants.in/	It incorporates 7263 botanical names of Indian medicinal plants and these botanical names have been correlated to more than 1,50,000 vernacular names in ten different languages of India.

3 Urana R (2017). A Study on Medicinal Flora of Yamunanagar. Inter. J. Sci. Res., 6(1): 112-114.

4 Nakum NM, Mandaliya VB, Pandya RV, and Thaker VS (2011). A simple and efficient protocol for high quality of DNA from *Vitis quandrangularis* L, Electro J of Plant Breeding, 2(1): 87-95.

5 Girnari SK, Bhatt KD, Mandaliya VB, Chariya LD, and Thaker VS (2011). RAPD markers studies in some medicinally important plant, J of Sci Agri Res, 72(1): 5-14.

6 Shakya AK (2016). Medicinal plants: Future source of new drugs. Inter. J. Herbal Med., 4(4): 59-64.

S. No.	Name of Database	Web-Link	Information of Database
3	Database on Medicinal Plants	http://nmpb-mpdb.nic.in	16 medicinal plants having high trade value in Indian market has been selected in the first phase.
4	Dravyaguna Database	http://www.bric-medplant.org/	This site is exclusively designed for people to know about Plant Wealth of Ayurveda (Dravyaguna Vignana) and applications for managing health and industrial applications.
5	Database on Ethno-medicinal Plants	https://www.dibru.ac.in/lifesciences/MedicinalPlant/index.php	This database was created and maintained by the Department of Life Sciences, Dibrugarh University, Assam, India. It contains information on medicinal plants of upper Brahmaputra valley, Assam.
6	Database of Medicinal and Aromatic Plants	http://bioinfo.bisr.res.in/project/domap/index.php	The Database of Medicinal and Aromatic Plants (DOMAP) in Rajasthan.
7	Medicinal Plants Unit - ICMR	http://www.icmr.nic.in/mpusite/	It contains the monograph on medicinal plants of India.
8	Neem Database	https://sites.google.com/site/neemdatabase1/home	It contains the information especially on neem plant.

Research & Developments in Medicinal Plants Sector from India

The present study is aimed to analysis on research and development in "medicinal plants sector" from India. India has developed Indian Citation Index (ICI) database[7] to conduct such analysis[8]. ICI database is covering about 1000 top Indian scholarly journals that covering all the disciplines. ICI enable a researcher to determine the status[9] of research and development from every States/Union territories of India[10]. The current data status of ICI as per their release note on 30th Nov 2017 is the current Index paper title count stands at 613 thousand, their paper wise reference count is at 11.62 million, and it were indexed from 1,031 total journals from India[11].

7 Parameshwar S, Goutami, and Patil DB (2016), Publication trends in library and information science: A bibliometric analysis of library herald. Library Herald, 54 (3), 316-330, DOI: 10.5958/0976-2469.2016.00023.3

8 Chand P (2011), Indian Citation Index (ICI): A dream of Indian research community comes true. Library Herald, 49(1), 34-47.

9 Ram S, Kataria S, and Ahmad S (2014), an assessment of the visibility of Indian Journals in Social Science Citation Index – Journal Citation Report. Journal of Information Management, 1(1), 1-16

10 Parameshwar S (2017). Publication Trends in Library and Information Science: A Bibliometric Analysis of Pearl: Journal of Library and Information Science. Pearl: A Journal of Library and Information Science, 11(2): 134-142.

11 Indian Citation Index, http://www.indiancitationindex.com

Material and Method

The complimentary access for one month was provided by IndianCitationIndex.com to access the database. Indian Citation Index database (www.indiancitationindex.com) was searched on 3rd November 2017 for the analysis on the sector "medicinal plants" from the year 2004-17 in special context to country India. The internet facility was provided by Information and Communication Technology (ICT) Division, Gujarat National Law University, Gandhinagar.

Results

Analysis of Total Record Counts on the Sector "Medicinal Plants" from year 2004-17

ICI database was searched on 6th December 2017 to analyze the total record counts on the sector "medicinal plants" from year 2004-17. The total record count observed was 3264 articles which includes the contribution from various countries in Indian journals. Then specific search was made in context to country India, and the total record counts observed was 2826 articles (Table 2). The highest number of record count observed in the year period of 2010-12 (Figure 1).

Table 2: Total record counts from year 2004-17 observed in the sector "medicinal plants" from Indian Citation Index

Year	Record counts	Year	Record counts
2004	74	2011	363
2005	88	2012	364
2006	92	2013	290
2007	110	2014	298
2008	140	2015	228
2009	210	2016	197
2010	324	2017	48

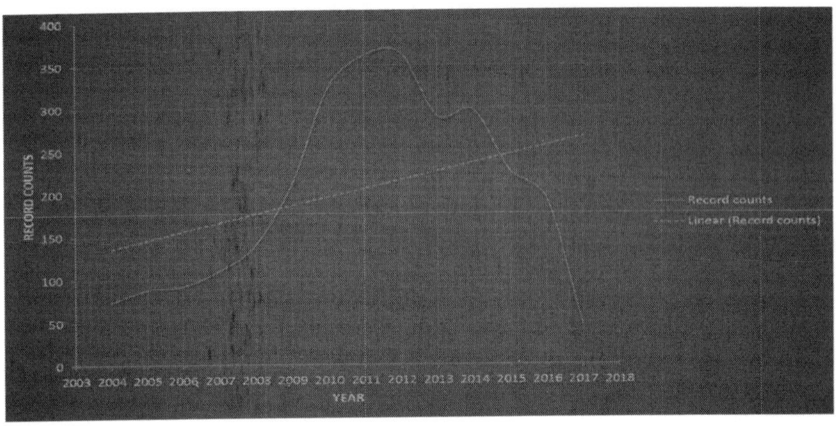

Fig. 1: Total record counts on the sector "medicinal plants" from Indian Citation Index (2004-17).

Analysis of Top Ten States/Union Territories of India in the Sector of "Medicinal Plants"

The important contribution of articles from the Indian territorial perspective were analyzed. The contribution was gathered from 36 state/union territories (UTs) across the nation (Table 3). Among total of 36 State/UTs, Tamil Nadu, Uttar Pradesh, and Maharashtra were the top most State/UTs (Figure 2) for contribution on "medicinal plants" and it was counted as about 50% of among all States/UTs (Table 4).

Table 3" The contribution from 36 state/union territories (UTs) across the nation on the sector of "medicinal plants"

S. No.	States	Counts	S. No.	States	Counts
1	Andaman and Nicobar Islands	6	19	Lakshadweep	0
2	Andhra Pradesh	131	20	Madhya Pradesh	147
3	Arunachal Pradesh	15	21	Maharashtra	301
4	Assam	69	22	Manipur	7
5	Bihar	26	23	Meghalaya	23
6	Chandigarh	13	24	Mizoram	6
7	Chhattisgarh	57	25	Nagaland	3
8	Dadar and Nagar Haveli	0	26	Orissa	63
9	Daman and Diu	0	27	Puducherry	22
10	Delhi	107	28	Punjab	5
11	Goa	5	29	Rajasthan	153
12	Gujarat	102	30	Sikkim	7
13	Haryana	77	31	Tamil Nadu	629
14	Himachal Pradesh	91	32	Telangana	96
15	Jammu and Kashmir	64	33	Tripura	7
16	Jharkhand	26	34	Uttar Pradesh	303
17	Karnataka	262	35	Uttarakhand	158
18	Kerala	145	36	West Bengal	109

Table 4: Top ten States/UTs in number of publication number on the sector "medicinal plants" (2004-17) identified from Indian Citation Index.

S. No.	States	Counts
1	Tamil Nadu	629
2	Uttar Pradesh	303
3	Maharashtra	301
4	Karnataka	262
5	Uttarakhand	158
6	Rajasthan	153
7	Madhya Pradesh	147
8	Kerala	145
9	Andhra Pradesh	131
10	West Bengal	109

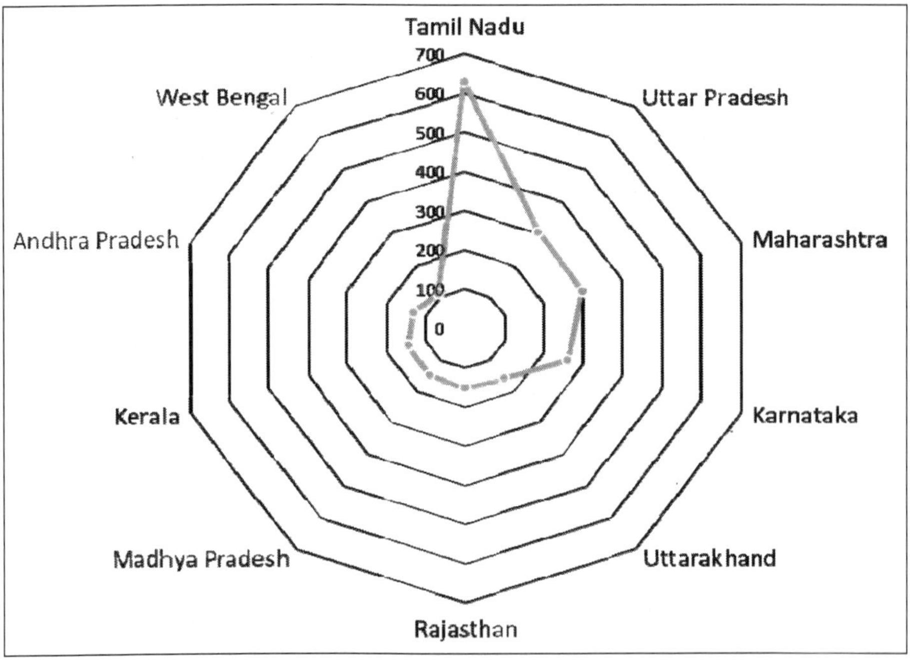

Fig. 2: Coverage of States/UTs in number of publication on the sector "medicinal plants" (2004-17) observed from Indian Citation Index.

Analysis of Top Ten Authors in the Sector of "Medicinal Plants"

Top authors who contributed on the sector "medicinal plants" were identified in this study (Table 5). Top author is who contribute the numbers of article in one topic in his/her career. The contribution of top three authors, Deshpande Nirmala, Paulsamy S and Savithramma N, have covered about 40% from top ten authors in "medicinal plants" (Figure 3).

Table 5: Top ten authors observed on the topic "medicinal plants" from Indian Citation Index (2004-17)

S. No.	Authors	Record Counts	Percent (%) Proposition
1	Deshpande Nirmala R	24	19.20%
2	Paulsamy S	16	12.80%
3	Savithramma N	14	11.20%
4	Verma R K	13	10.40%
5	Pullaiah T	12	9.60%
6	Kasera Pawan K	10	8%
7	Johri P K	10	8%
8	Singh S	9	7.20%
9	Sharma Ajit K	9	7.20%
10	Shendkar Chandrakant D	8	6.40%

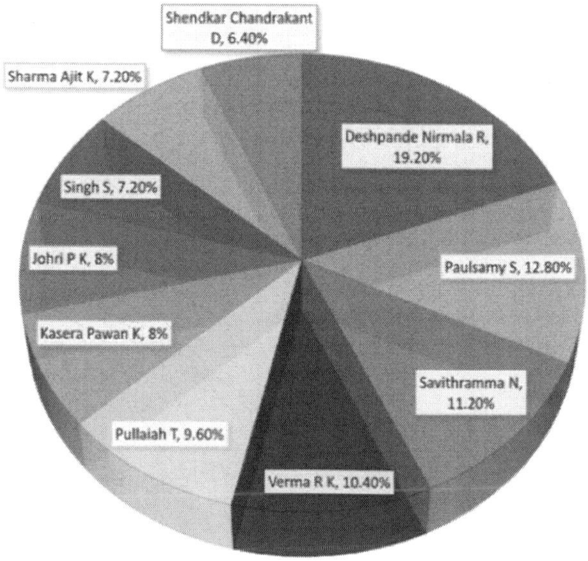

Fig. 3: Top ten authors on the sector "medicinal plants" identified from Indian Citation Index (2004-17).

Analysis of Top Ten Institutions in the Sector of "Medicinal Plants"

Top institutions in the sector "medicinal plants" were searched from ICI database. The highest number of record counts observed from University of Rajasthan (Figure 4). The total record counts from the state of Rajasthan is 153 from various institutions (Table 4), while University of Rajasthan alone has total counts of 43 in medicinal plants sector (Table 6).

Table 6: Top ten institutions searched for their work in the field of "medicinal plants" from Indian Citation Index (2004-17)

S. No.	Institutions	Record Counts
1	University of Rajasthan (UR)	43
2	Dr. Yashwant Singh Parmar University of Horticulture and Forestry (YSPUHF)	35
3	Sri Venkateswara University (SVU)	32
4	V I T University (VITU)	31
5	Sir Parashurambhau College (SPC)	30
6	CSIR - Central Institute of Medicinal and Aromatic Plants (CSIRCIMAP)	29
7	Kongu Arts and Science College (KASC)	29
8	ICAR - National Bureau of Plant Genetic Resources (ICARNBPGR)	28
9	Kuvempu University (KU)	27
10	Tamil Nadu Agricultural University (TNAU)	27

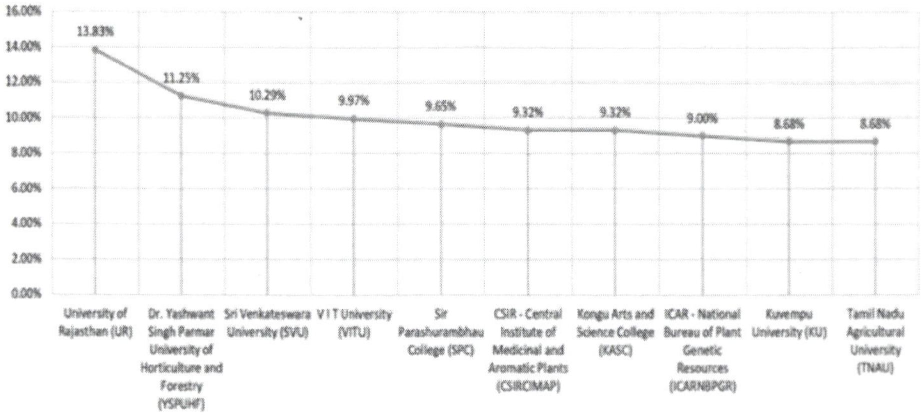

Fig. 4: Top ten institutions in the field of "medicinal plants" (2004-17) derived from ICI database.

Analysis of Top Ten Article in the Sector of "Medicinal Plants"

The citation of any article is generally referred as the article read and quoted in literature by an author. The number of citation of any articles represents the highest number of readability and weightage in that particular sector. In this study, top cited articles on the sector "medicinal plants" were identified and listed in Table 7. Here, an article published in Indian Journal of Physiology and Pharmacology in a year 2005 titled "Therapeutic uses of *Ocimum sanctum* linn (Tulsi) with a note on eugenol and its pharmacological actions: A short review." was cited 84 times by various authors.

Table 7: Top cited articles on the sector "medicinal plants" (2004-17) observed from Indian Citation Index

S. No.	Title	Total Citations	Total Citations per Year	Year	Publication Name
1	Therapeutic uses of *Ocimum sanctum* linn (Tulsi) with a note on eugenol and its pharmacological actions: A short review	84	6.46	2005	Indian Journal of Physiology and Pharmacology
2	Effect of pre-sowing treatment on seed germination and seedling vigour in *Angelica glauca*, a threatened medicinal herb	28	2.00	2004	Current Science
3	Phytochemical studies of *Strychnos potatorum* L.f. - A medicinal plant	27	2.45	2007	E-Journal of Chemistry
4	*Swertia chirayita* - An overview	26	2.00	2005	Current Science
5	Biological activities of crude extracts and chemical constituents of bael, *Aegle marmelos* (L.) Corr.	23	2.56	2009	Indian Journal of Experimental Biology

S. No.	Title	Total Citations	Total Citations per Year	Year	Publication Name
6	Hepatoprotective activity of *Pterocarpus santalinus* L.f., an endangered medicinal plant	19	1.58	2006	Indian Journal of Pharmacology
7	Impact of cadmium and lead on *Catharanthus roseus* - A phytoremediation study	19	1.73	2007	Journal of Environmental Biology
8	In vitro regeneration and mass multiplication of *Psoralea corylifolia*—An endangered medicinal plant	18	1.38	2005	Indian Journal of Biotechnology
9	The science behind sacredness of tulsi (*Ocimum sanctum* Linn.)	17	1.89	2009	Indian Journal of Physiology and Pharmacology
10	Antimicrobial activity of silver nanoparticles synthesized by using medicinal plants	17	2.43	2011	International Journal of Chemtech Research

Analysis of Top Ten Journal in the Sector of "Medicinal Plants"

The selection of journal for publication by author is majorly depends on the kind of articles it publishes and the institute/society from where the journal is published. Based on this study, top journals were identified for publication of the articles related to "medicinal plants" (Table 8). Here, three journals namely, International Journal of Pharmacy and Pharmaceutical Sciences, Journal of Pharmacy Research, and International Journal of Pharmaceutical Sciences: Review and Research, which has covered one half of total publication related to "medicinal plants" (Figure 5).

Table 8. Top publication on the sector "medicinal plants" (2004-17) identified from Indian Citation Index

S. No.	Publication Name	Record Counts	Percent (%) Proposition
1	International Journal of Pharmacy and Pharmaceutical Sciences	136	16.08%
2	Journal of Pharmacy Research	134	15.84%
3	International Journal of Pharmaceutical Sciences: Review and Research	94	11.11%
4	Asian Journal of Pharmaceutical and Clinical Research	84	9.93%
5	Advances in Plant Sciences	78	9.22%
6	Journal of Chemical and Pharmaceutical Research	71	8.39%
7	Indian Forester (The)	68	8.04%
8	Research Journal of Pharmaceutical, Biological, and Chemical Sciences	63	7.45%
9	Journal of Medicinal and Aromatic Plant Sciences	61	7.21%
10	Plant Archives	57	6.74%

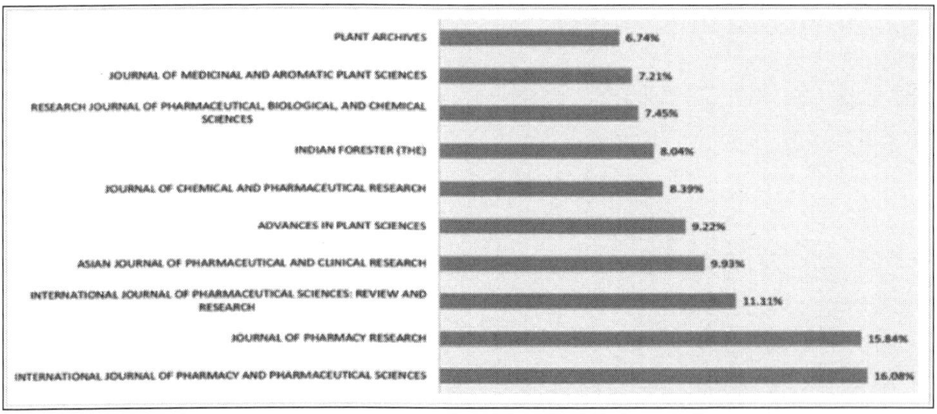

Fig. 5: Journal-wise publication on the sector "medicinal plants" prepared from Indian Citation Index (2004-17).

Analysis of Top Type of Document in the Sector of "Medicinal Plants"

From Indian Citation Index, the following are the document type generated on the selected topic: Research Article, Review Article, Short Communication and others (Table 9). Among all document type, the majority of articles were grouped a form of research articles (n=2471; 88%) (Figure 6).

Table 9: Top document types with record counts in the sector "medicinal plants" derived from Indian Citation Index (2004-17)

S. No.	Documents Type	Record Counts
1	Research Article	2471
2	Review Article	192
3	Short Communication	110
4	Others	45

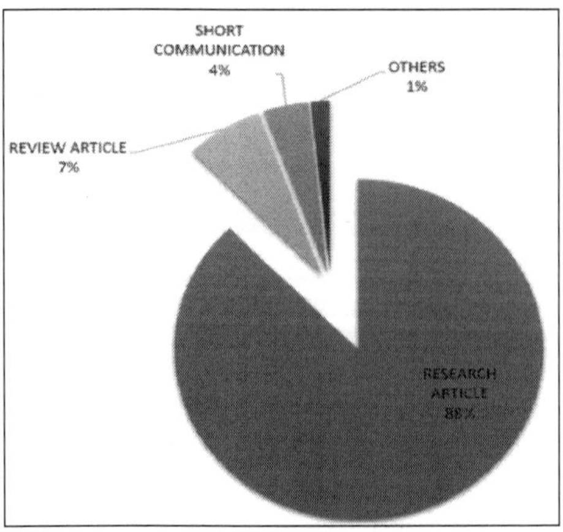

Fig. 6: Percent (%) proposition of types of documents on the sector "medicinal plants" derived from Indian Citation Index (2004-17).

Analysis of Top Ten Subject in the Sector of "Medicinal Plants"

The contribution of authors related to "medicinal plants" was classified into various subject category (Table 10). Here, Pharmacology & Pharmaceutical Science was top most subject category with highest number of record counts as 1133 number and about one third coverage (Figure 7).

Table 10: Subject wise categorization of the work related to "medicinal plants" inherited from Indian Citation Index (2004-17)

S. No.	Subjects	Record Counts	Percent (%) Proposition
1	Pharmacology and Pharmaceutical Science	1133	29.51%
2	Biological Science	582	15.16%
3	Botany	575	14.97%
4	Health Science	375	9.77%
5	Agriculture	286	7.45%
6	Biotechnology	215	5.60%
7	Environmental Science	194	5.05%
8	Chemistry	191	4.97%
9	Forestry	190	4.95%
10	General Science and Technology	99	2.58%

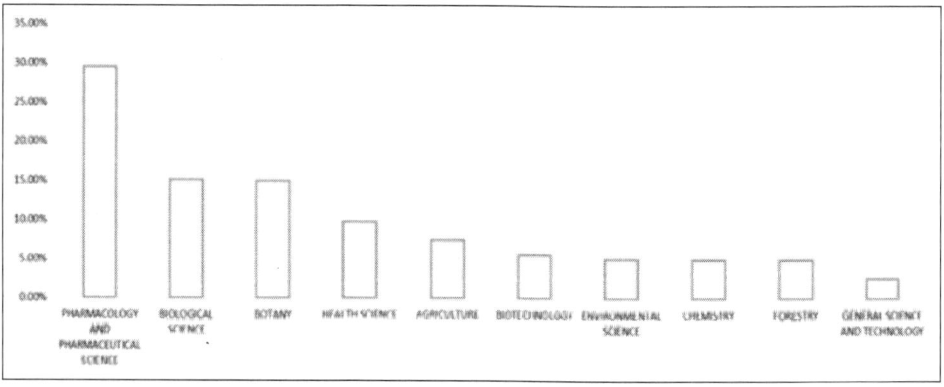

Fig. 7: Categorization of the work related to "medicinal plants" from year 2004-17 in subject category derived from Indian Citation Index.

Analysis of International collaboration in the Sector of "Medicinal Plants"

It is observed that the Indian authors are having their international collaboration to accomplish the work. Here, top five countries have been identified from ICI database which shown the international collaboration in the sector of medicinal plants (Table 11). From the USA highest number of collaboration were occurred which was total 14 in the sector of medicinal plants. (Figure 8).

Table 11: Collaboration of Indian authors with other countries in the sector of "Medicinal Plants" (2004-17)

S. No.	Countries	Record Counts
1	United States of America	14
2	Saudi Arabia	6
3	Malaysia	6
4	Ethiopia	5
5	Germany	4

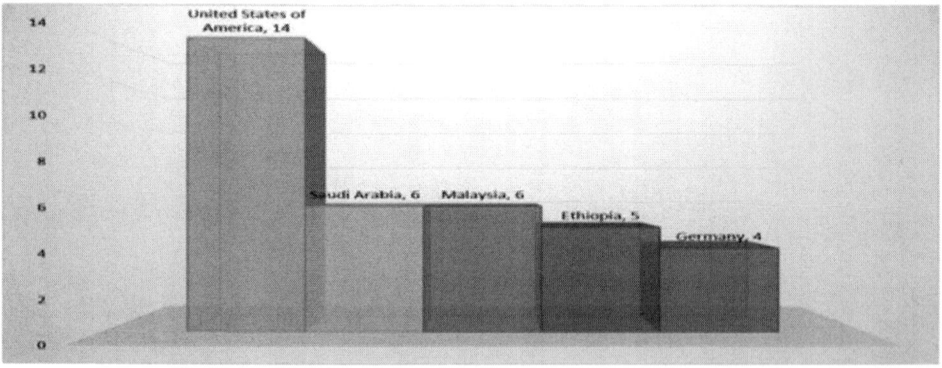

Fig. 8: Top countries for their collaboration in the sector of "Medicinal Plants" (2004-17)

Analysis of Top Ten Authors from Gujarat State in the Sector of "Medicinal Plants"

An additional search was made with the curiosity to know about the top most authors from Gujarat. Total number of 102 record counts was recorded from Gujarat. Figure 9 shows the top ten authors from Gujarat on the sector "medicinal plants". Here, Upadhyay S was identified as first top most author from Gujarat (Table 12).

Table 12: Top ten authors from Gujarat on the sector "medicinal plants" observed from Indian Citation Index (2004-17).

S. No.	Authors	Percent (%) Proposition
1	Upadhyay S	14.29%
2	Bansal Ruchi	11.43%
3	Jadeja B	11.43%
4	Upadhyay U	11.43%
5	Gajbhiye N	8.57%
6	Jat R	8.57%
7	Kumar Vimal	8.57%
8	Lambole Vijay	8.57%
9	Mishra S	8.57%
10	Odedra N	8.57%

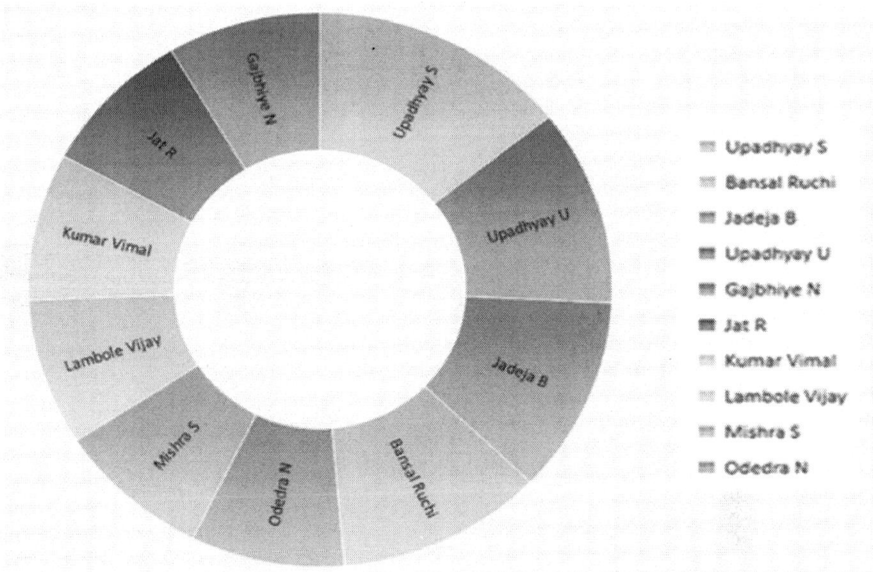

Fig. 9: Top ten authors from Gujarat on the sector "medicinal plants" identified from Indian Citation Index (2004-17).

Conclusions

The combination of medicinal plant extracts could be a huge source information to develop highly potential drug to curb various livestock and human diseases. Thus, there is an utmost scope to study the utilization of the plant and their product for the treatment of livestock and human diseases. The contributions from the state of Tamil Nadu was highest in all states/UTs. While University of Rajasthan has been observed as top most institution among all the institution in India working in the sector of medicinal plants. This study will help the readers, medicinal practitioner and authors to get the current status of research and development in the sector of "medicinal plants" across the nation.

Authors' contributions

R Mathakia has complied the dataset from IndianCitationIndex.com, A Rana has complied the various database on medicinal plants, and VB Mandaliya has prepared the manuscript.

Chapter 16

Antibiotic Resistance: Causes and Challenges

Dr. Anjali Soni*, Amee Patel, Vishma Shah and Juie Rana

Department of Biotechnology, Veer Narmad South Gujarat University, Surat, Gujarat, India

Email: anjalisoni@vnsgu.ac.in

Abstract

Antibiotic refers to any natural compound or synthetic chemical which has the ability to kill or inhibit the growth of microorganisms. Antibiotic resistance is a global problem which needs to be addressed among all countries. The first drug resistant strain was discovered in 1930 and later multidrug resistant among enteric bacteria was detected in late 1950s to early 1960s. It is therefore of paramount importance to understand the underlying resistant mechanisms of these organisms to design effective strategies and approaches to eliminate the spread of antibiotic resistant organisms. Thus, obtaining the data of increasing threat of antibiotic resistance, a slogan is coined by WHO in 2011- "No action today, no cure tomorrow", to implement new strategies to the use of designed drugs and to accelerate the discovery of new drugs. Another potential solution is to identify and develop new drug, which is very costly as well as complicating process.

Keywords: Antibiotic resistance, multidrug resistance, drug efflux, target modification, adaptive mutagenesis

Introduction

Antibiotic resistance is a major issue prevailing worldwide, which needs to be resolved now. The term antibiotic resistance refers to the ability of microorganisms to resist the effects of antibiotics, thus decreasing its efficiency. The first antibiotic discovery of Penicillin in 1943 by Alexander Flemming gave rise to the modern era of antibiotics. Antibiotics have revolutionized in the field of medicine and healthcare to a great extent but today it is going through an era in which it needs to address, the rapid emergence of resistance strains. Several factors contribute the resistance ability of an organism, which needs to be studied properly. Without effective antibiotics, diverse medical procedures such as surgery, care of premature infants, cancer chemotherapy, invasive diagnostic and treatment procedures, and transplantation medicine will be hampered with corresponding increase in morbidity and mortality from secondary microbial infections. WHO has highlighted antibiotic resistance as a "serious, global threat" in April 2014. Then the governing body of all member states of WHO launched National Action Plan

(NAP). Objectives of NAP are to combat antibiotic resistance by encouraging less reliance on antibiotics, and in the process preserve equitable access to medicines needed to treat serious infections. Among 151 countries (of WHO member), 85% of countries are or have developed NAPs, 19% have multisectorial antibiotic resistance action plan which reflects NAP objectives and 5% have multisectorial plan with monitoring processes in place[1]. The goal of this review is not just to give information regarding antibiotic resistance, but also reflect the aspects relates to antibiotic discovery, factors promoting resistance, mechanism of resistance and some views on the future aspects to combat this emerging resistance. To understand all the aspects of antibiotic resistance, it is of prime importance to study its mode of action by studying biochemical interaction between antibiotic and its target molecule. The first drug resistant strain was discovered in 1930 and later multidrug resistant among enteric bacteria was detected in late 1950s to early 1960s.It is therefore of paramount importance to understand the underlying resistant mechanisms of these organisms to design effective strategies and approaches to eliminate the spread of antibiotic resistant organisms.

Different Classes of Antibiotics and their Mode of Action

1. Aminoglycosides:
   - Family of over 20 antibiotics
   - Inhibition of protein synthesis (binds 30S ribosomal subunit, inhibits translocation of peptidyl tRNA and misreading of mRNA)
   - Examples: Streptomycin, neomycin, kanamycin, paromomycin
2. Tetracyclines:
   - Inhibition of protein synthesis and interferes with aminoacyl-tRNA binding
   - All contain for adjacent cyclic hydrocarbon rings
   - Examples: Tetracycline, doxycycline, limecycline, oxytetracyclin
3. Beta-lactams:
   - Most widely used antibiotics in the NHS
   - All contain a beta-lactam ring
   - Examples: Penicillin such as amoxicillin and flucloxacillin; Cephalosporin such as cephalexin
   - Inhibition of cell wall synthesis
   - Binds and inactivates PBPs
4. Sulfonamides:
   - First commercial antibiotics were sulfonamides -All contain the sulfonamide group
   - Examples: Prontosil, sulfanilamide, sulfadiazine, sulfisoxazole
   - Inhibition of folic acid synthesis

- Instead of killing bacteria, it just prevents their growth and multiplication.
- Causes allergic reactions in some patients

5. Fluoroquinolones:
   - Inhibition of DNA replication and transcription by inhibiting the activity of enzymes DNA gyrase and topoisomerase IV
   - All contains fused aromatic rings with a carboxylic acid group attached
   - Examples: Ciprofloxacin, levofloxacin, trovafloxacin
6. Polypeptides:
   - Disruption of cell membrane structure and permeability
   - Glycopeptides: Common "Drugs of last Resort", it consists of carbohydrate linked o a peptide formed of amino acids. Examples include: Vancomycin, teicoplanin
   - Lipopeptides: All contain a lipid bonded to a peptide. Examples: Daptomycin, Surfactin.
7. Chloramphenicol:
   - Commonly used in low income countries
   - Distinct individual compound
   - Inhibition of protein synthesis through binding of 50S subunit and inhibits peptidyl transferase
8. Streptogramin:
   - Two groups of antibiotics that act synergistically
   - Combination of two structurally differing compounds, from groups denoted A and B
   - Examples: Pristinamycin IIA, Pristinamycin IA
   - Inhibition of protein elongation
9. Macrolides:
   - Second most prescribed antibiotic in the NHS
   - All contain a 14, 15 or 16- membered macrolide ring
   - Examples: Erythromycin, Clarithromycin, azithromycin
   - Inhibition of protein synthesis and inhibits translocation of peptidyl tRNA
10. Lincosamides:
    - Inhibition of protein elongation
11. Oxazolidinones:
    - Potent antibiotics commonly used as 'Drugs of Last Resort'
    - All contain 2- oxazolidone somewhere in their structure
    - Examples: Linezolid, Posizolid, Tedizolid, Cycloserine

12. Ansamycins:
    - Can also demonstrate antiviral activity
    - All contain an aromatic ring bridged by an aliphatic chain
    - Examples: Geldanamycin, rifamycin, naphthomycin Thus, most possible targets for antibiotics are:
    - Inhibition of cell wall synthesis (inhibition of peptidoglycan structure and cross linking)
    - Disruption of cell membrane
    - Inhibition of protein synthesis
    - Inhibition of nucleic acid

Factors Responsible for Widespread of Antibiotic Resistance

1. Density of antibiotic usage that enhances the resistance selection:

   Patients do not follow dosage regimens as specified by doctor as well as discontinue treatment before pathogen is completely eliminated [2].
2. Contaminated water system which increases the frequency of environmental selection of antibiotic resistant organisms: Humans as well as animal waste from house, hospitals or offices contaminates streams, groundwater and other water resources, with resistant organisms.
3. Poor sanitation facilities
4. Over prescription of antibiotics:

   Lack of regulations in most countries enhances antibiotic resistance as drugs can be purchased without any medical prescriptions. Many pharmacies lack appropriate license and hence sell drug as a means of business.
5. Antibiotics overuse in agriculture and Animal industry:

   These antimicrobial drugs are often used as growth promoters/ pesticide in agriculture as well as for healthcare of livestock [3]. Therefore, consumption of these agricultural crops and livestock directly or indirectly transfers resistant microorganisms to humans. Multidrug resistant bacteria have been detected in the meat of these livestock animals in many countries like Africa and Kenya. Soil treated with fertilizers represents a "hotspot" of bacteria carrying antibiotic resistance genes (regardless of the fact that soil itself has natural reservoir of such resistant microorganisms).

Mechanism of Resistance

Major threatening organisms with multiple drug resistance genes in hospitals and community are reviewed within ESKAPE *(Enterococcus faecium, Staphylococcus aureus, Klebsiella pneumonia, Acinetobacter baumannii, Pseudomonas aeruginosa and Enterobacter spp.)* [4] These microbial pathogens are the leading cause of nosocomial infections throughout the world. All these organisms acquire resistance by different mechanism:

On Genetic Basis

Resistance is acquired among organisms either by mutation (spontaneous mutations/Adaptive mutagenesis) or by the means of mobile genetic elements such as plasmids or transposons (transferred by mechanism of Horizontal gene transfer). Some of these transposons contain integrons which consists of a site for integration of different antibiotic resistant genes). Example is the Tet (M), tetracycline resistance genes, commonly found on the transposon, Tn916. It is also found that, Multidrug-resistance (MDR) in bacteria is often the result of the acquisition of mobile genetic elements that contain multiple resistance genes.

Spontaneous mutations: It occurs by nucleotide point mutation during DNA replication process. Example is of *Escherichia coli* resistant to quinolone due to changes in seven positions in gyrA gene and three position changes in parC gene [5]. Resistance is also associated with the uptake and efflux systems caused by mutations in regulatory genes or their promoter regions. These mutations in efflux system also confer sometimes multidrug resistance to the organism. Example: mutations in the mar gene of *Escherichia coli,* affects the expression of about 60 different genes, including down-regulation of OmpF and up-regulation of AcrAB). This AcrAB is involved in the efflux of b-lactams, fluoroquinolones, chloramphenicol, and tetracycline. Overproduction of several antibiotic inhibiting enzymes is also a result of mutation.

Adaptive Mutagenesis: Adaptive mutations arise only in the presence of non-lethal selective pressure that favours them. This is the main feature that distinguishes them from spontaneous mutations. This type of mutation is often the main source of development of antibiotic resistant mutants under natural conditions.

Hypermutators: For integrity of any species, it is essential that genetic information of that particular organism is maintained stability. This stability is acquired by different molecular mechanisms during DNA replication process. However, many bacterial strains are found in natural environment and laboratories with an elevated mutation rate, which are referred as hypermutable strains. Mechanism is still unclear regarding the selective pressure that triggers such mutations in natural conditions. However, it appears that such kind of hypermutation in organisms is regulated by a special SOS-inducible mutator DNA polymerase (pol) IV. Examples of Hypermutable strains include - *Staphylococcus aureus, Streptococcus pneumonia, Haemophilus influenza, E.coli* and *Salmonella enterica* [5].

Different genetic elements involved in spread of resistance gene are:

1. Self -transmissible plasmid: Circular, autonomously replicating element. It carries genes needed for conjugal DNA transfer.
2. Conjugative transposon: Integrated elements that can excise to form a non- replicating circular transfer intermediate.
3. Mobilized plasmid: Circular, autonomously replicating element.
4. Transposon: Within same cell, it can move from one DNA segment to another.

5. Gene Cassette: circular, nonreplicating DNA segments containing only open reading frames. It integrates into integrons.
6. Integron: Integrated DNA segment that contains an integrase, a promoter, and an integration site for gene cassettes. Class one integrons are a common feature of soil and aquatic bacteria.

On biochemical basis

By reducing membrane permeability: Gram negative bacteria consist of outer membrane having lipid layer and inner phospholipid layer. Composition of this membrane is responsible for decreased drug penetration and transport. Transport of any drug molecule is mediated by: diffusion through porins in membrane, diffusion through bilayer or by regulated uptake mechanisms. Thus changes in membrane composition, pore size and selectivity due to mutations in lipopolysaccharide layer up regulate the resistance ability in microorganisms.

a) By modification of target:

   This mechanism interferes the interaction between the target site and antibiotic itself, thus disrupting drug molecule to bind at target site efficiently. In some cases, the modification in target site needed to produce resistance requires other changes in the cell to compensate for the altered characteristics of the target. Example: Methicillin- resistant *S.aureus* (MRSA) acquires penicillin-binding protein 2a (PBP2a) transpeptidase and this PBP2a further requires changes in composition and structure of peptidoglycan for the functioning of number of genes [5].

   - Peptidoglycan Structure alteration:

     The peptidoglycan component of bacteria provides a selective target for the antibiotics. Various enzymes involves in its synthesis provide targets for selective inhibition, such as mutations in the penicillin-binding domain of penicillin-binding proteins (PBPs) results in decreased affinity to beta-lactam antibiotics. Similarly, resistance to methicillin and oxacillin by *S.aureus* is due to acquisition of mobile genetic element-SCCmec, which contains resistant genes [5].

   - Protein synthesis inhibition:

     Resistance to antibiotics that interfere with protein synthesis or transcription via RNA polymerase is achieved by modification of the specific target. Example: Macrolide group of antibiotics block protein synthesis in bacteria by binding to 50S ribosomal subunit and resistance to these antibiotics is acquired by mutation in 23S rRNA component of 50S ribosomal subunit in range of organisms [5].

   - DNA synthesis interference:

     Resistance is acquire by mutations in the specific regions of genes resulting in the alterations in the enzymes preventing the binding of the antibiotics [5].

b) Direct modification of antibiotics:

Direct modification is mediated by hydrolysis, group transfer and redox mechanisms:

1. Modification by hydrolysis: Several enzymes released by organisms break bonds in the antibiotic structure thus degrading antibiotic itself, before it reaches its target site. Beta lactamases is the most classical hydrolytic enzyme that cleaves the beta lactam ring of the penicillin and cephalosporin antibiotics. Many Gram negative and Gram positive bacteria produce such enzymes. This enzymes are either chromosomal or plasmid encoded enzymes. Many other hydrolytic enzymes include esterases and epoxidases [5].
2. Modification by group transfer: The most diverse family of resistant enzymes include transferases. This enzymes inhibit antibiotic activity by chemical substitution (phosphoryl, acetyl group, nucleotidyl and ribitoyl groups' addition to periphery of the antibiotic molecule) [6]. This modification in antibiotics interferes its binding to specific target molecule. Such strategies include O-ribosylation, O-acetylation, N-acetylation, O-phosphorylation using co-substrates for their activity. Some of the co-substrates include ATP, NAD+ and glutathione. All this process is carried out in cytoplasm. Example: Aminoglycosides antibiotics are modified by this mechanism with the help of three modifying enzymes- acetyltransferases, phosphotransferases and nucleotidyltransferases [5].
3. Modification by redox process: Pathogenic bacteria exploit antibiotics by carrying out its oxidation or reduction. Example: Oxidation of tetracycline by TetX enzyme [5].

c) Increased efflux: Many Gram negative bacteria acquire intrinsic resistance to antibiotics due to their efflux pumps that actively transport antibiotic out of the cell. Overexpression of this efflux pumps results in conferring increased resistance to antibiotics. Some of this pumps have narrow or wide substrate specificity. Multiple drug resistance (MDR) efflux pumps are the most common pumps having wide substrate specificity. Most of the genes encoding MDR efflux pumps are present on the bacterial chromosome however, some are also present on plasmid and are thus, transferred from one bacteria to other. Well-studied examples include the multidrug efflux pump AcrB in *E. coli* and still many more are being studied. Pumps such as , AcrB are homotrimers that are present in inner membrane and form tripartite complex with the periplasmic adaptor protein such as AcrA and outer membrane channels such as TolC. Still many studies are going on in understanding the structure and function of these efflux pumps. Also, it is very important to understand the mechanism of overexpression these pumps. Overexpression in many cases is due to mutation in transcription factor or intergenic site. It can also occur in response to any specific environmental signals such as acrAB genes in *E. coli* are induced by small molecules such as indole, as a result of infection [5].

Commonly used antibiotics and their resistance mechanisms:

1. Beta- lactams:
   - Enzymatic destruction by Beta-lactamases: Cephalosporinases, Penicillinases, metallo-beta-lactamases.
   - Alteration of target by low affinity of PBPs.
   - Decreased uptake of antibiotic by efflux pumps.
2. Glycopeptides:
   - Alteration of target by modification of precursor.
   - Enzymatic modification carried out by: Acetylation, Adenylation, Methylation, and Phosphorylation.
3. Aminoglycosides:
   - Alteration of target
   - Decreased uptake by efflux pumps
   - Methylation of rRNA by methylases
4. Macrolides, Lincosamides and Streptogramin (MLS):
   - Decreased uptake by efflux pumps
   - Hydrolytic enzyme cause antibiotic inactivation
5. Tetracyclines:
   - Modification of antibiotic by enzymatic alterations
   - Ribosome protection
6. Chloramphenicol:
   - Enzymatic inactivation of antibiotic by chloramphenicol acetyltransferase
7. Sulfonamides: By the means of alterative pathways
8. Trimethoprim:
   - Overproduction of the enzyme dihydrofolate reductase (DHFR) enzyme at the target site due to mutation in the structural gene encoding DHFR enzyme
   - Decreased uptake of antibiotic by efflux pumps
9. Fluoroquinolones:
   - Reduced permeability of membrane thus limiting the drug penetration
   - Alterations in drug target enzymes (inhibition of DNA replication and transcription by inhibition of DNA gyrase and topoisomerase IV activity)

Solutions and Challenges

In order to overcome this problem, it is essential to obtain certain strategies such as reducing the consumption of antibiotics, sustainable antibiotic usage policies, disease prevention strategies, improving sanitation facilities and infection control practices. Various control strategies used to minimize the development of antibiotic resistance are:

1. Hygiene and sanitation: Improvement in basic hygiene and sanitation will reduce the spread of resistant organisms.
2. Vaccination: Vaccination reduces severity of disease and provide protection against pathogens.
3. Alternative therapies: The urge of pharmaceutical companies to invest in research and development of novel antibiotics necessitate the exploration of alternative therapies such as bacteriophage, probiotics and quorum sensing inhibitors.
    - Probiotics: Also referred as fecal transplant therapy (FTT). It involves the use of fecal material from pathogen free healthy donors to repopulate the microbiota of a recipient. Probiotics are able to destroy pathogenic microorganisms by producing antimicrobial compounds such as bacteriocins and organic acids, improve gastrointestinal microbial environment by adhering to intestinal mucosa thereby preventing attachment of pathogens and improve the digestion and absorption of nutrients. The most commonly used probiotics include *Pediococcus, Lactobacillus, Yeast, Bacteroides, Enterococcus, Streptococcus and Bifidobacterium* [2].
    - Quorum sensing inhibitors: This inhibitors represents and important antimicrobial target that may prevent, suppress or treat infectious diseases. The details of quorum sensing are different between Gram-negative and Gram-positive bacteria. Gram-negative bacteria utilize N-acyl L-homoserine lactones (AHL) while Gram positive bacteria uses oligopeptides. In response to antibiotics which kill or inhibit the growth of microorganisms, quorum sensing inhibiters simply attenuate bacterial virulence. This therapy has been carried out in variety of pathogens like *Pseudomonas aeruginosa, Vibrio fischeri, Staphylococcus aureus and Escherichia coli.* These studies have successfully exploited the bacterial quorum sensing system as potential target for treatment of bacterial infection.
4. Education: Health care providers and patients' needs to be educated and awared regarding the use and misuse of antibiotics which may contribute to the development of resistance.
5. Infection prevention & control: proper hospital infection control is required to prevent the spread of nosocomial pathogens and resistance microbes that may have easily been disseminated to the community if these measures were not in place.

It is therefore essential to understand the underpinning resistance events in organisms by the means of advances in genomics and structural biology. Increase in the level of understanding of resistance mechanisms provides new targets for the discovery and development of new drugs (genes encoding MDR efflux pumps). Another potential solution is therefore, to identify and develop new reliable drug, which is very costly as well as complicating process. High cost is involved in various aspects of new drug development such as use of various modern and efficient technologies for its discovery and development and phase 3 clinical trials, making it more uneconomical and unattractive. Despite global spread of antibiotic resistance, regulatory approval of new antibiotics has declined to 90% during past 30 years in US. Reason behind this drawbacks in drug discovery and development are the issues and challenges that needs to addressed. The major issue is the cost and time involved in research and development which subsequently leads to increase in the cost of treatment, not affordable by low income families.

Clinical trials too seemed to be very challenging due to changes in standards for clinical trials design made by US Food and Drug administration [3]. Also, additional new regulatory approaches are needed. Regulatory approval is the greatest obstacle in the path of a new antibiotic discover due to following reasons [3]:

1. Absence of clarity
2. Differences in clinical trial requirements among countries
3. Changes in regulatory and licensing rules and ineffective channels of communication.

Not enough new antibiotics are being discovered due to above mentioned hindering factors, to combat the threat of deadly drug resistant infections. Hence, modifications are being done in existing antibiotics to overcome this problem to some extent. It is an essential task to find an appropriate solution to overcome this 'global health emergency'. According to the data mentioned by WHO, around 700,000 people die every year as a result of drug resistant infections including drug resistant tuberculosis (TB), HIV and malaria [4]. Therefore, WHO warned that not only new antibiotics will solely eliminate this threat but also various strategies will be needed to regulate antibiotic distribution and usage in various fields of agriculture, animal healthcare and medicine.

The Infectious Diseases Society of America (IDSA) has proposed a new, limited population antibiotic drug (LPAD) regulatory approval pathway that has positive feedbacks from FDA officials [3]. This model can thus might enable smaller, less expensive and faster clinical trials. Thus, new steps must be exploited to manage crisis. The CDC assessed antibiotic-resistant bacterial infections according to seven factors: clinical impact, economic impact, incidence, 10-year projection of incidence, transmissibility, availability of effective antibiotics, and barriers to prevention [3]. The threat level of each bacteria was then classified as "urgent," "serious," or "concerning" [3] .Many new approaches are being studied in order to combat antibiotic resistance effectively such as [3]:

1. Inhibitors of resistance enzymes; co-drugs are supplied having antibiotic molecule and inhibitor of resistance enzymes that blocks the resistance ability of an organism efficiently.
2. To overcome resistance it is necessary to improve delivery or enhance the accessibility of antibiotic to their target site.

Many DNA sequencing technologies have helped to reconstruct the likely origins of many of the resistance genes currently circulating and evolving in human pathogens. The establishment and maintenance of databases and bioinformatics tools is essential to locate events combating resistance to antibiotics, particularly as the accumulation of whole- genome and next generation sequencing data rapidly expands our knowledge of resistant determinants. There are number of databases available for antibiotic a determinant, each of which has its own advantages and disadvantages [7]:

1. ARDB- Antibiotic Resistance Gene Database: http:/ardb.cbcb.umd.edu/
2. CARD- Comprehensive Antibiotic Resistance Database: https://card.mcmaster.ca/
3. RAC- Repository Antibiotic Resistance cassettes: http://rac.aihi.mq.edu.au/rac/
4. ResFinder - Resistance Gene Finder: https://cge.cbs.dtu.dk/services/Resfinder/
5. Resfams – Antibiotic Resistance Function: http://www.dantaslab.org/resfams/
6. ARG-ANNOT- Antibiotic Resistance Gene Annotation: http://en.mediterranee-infection.com/article.php

Other resistance and virulence determinants:

1. MvirDB- Virulence Factors and Toxins: http://mvirdb.llnl.gov/
2. PATRIC- Pathosystems Resource Integration Centre: https://www.patricbrc.org/portal/portal/patric/home#
3. BacMet- Biocide and Metal Resistance Genes: http://bacmet.biomedicine.gu.se/
4. Efflux pumps review: http://cmr.asm.org/content/28/2/337.short

Vectors and mobile elements:

1. INTEGRALL: The Integron Database: http://integrall.bio.ua.pt/
2. Integron Finder: https://github.com/gem-pasteur/Integron_Finder
3. ACLAME- phages, plasmids and transposons: http://aclame.ulb.ac.be/
4. IS Finder- Insertion Element Finder: https://www-is-biotoul.fr/
5. ICEBerg- Integrative Conjugative Element Analysis: http://db-mml.sjtu.edu.cn/ICEberg/
6. IslandViewer- Genomic island prediction: http://www.pathogenomics.sfu.ca/islandviewer/
7. PAIDB- Pathogenicity island database: http://www.paidb.re.kr/about_paidb.php
8. PlasmidFinder-In silico plasmid detection: https://cge.cbs.dtu.dk/services/PlasmidFinder/

There are three ways through genomics and sequence databases that focuses on antibiotic resistance that might help to inform about the future of resistance management [7]. The first is in identifying and understanding the interplay between the various agents involved in resistance: the resistome, the mobilome, the bacterial hosts, and their environmental compartments. The second way is rapid identification and tracking of both genes and species of interest. The third way is of examining the development of resistance in real time, using experimental evolution. Thus, genomics and metagenomics offer various opportunities for understanding the mechanism of gene transfer between bacteria, animal hosts, and environmental compartments. Investigation of resistome enables the detection of highly mobile resistance determinants and identifies hotspots for local transfer of resistance genes, such as wastewater treatment plants.

Several government regulatory agencies have engaged in national plans to combat this threat. Measures needed to be taken to expand the research and development of new antibiotics are: communication among companies working on antibiotic resistance, sharing compound libraries and providing financial incentives for early development on new antibiotics through clinical trials by governments. To highlight the area of antibiotic research and development, WHO has recently published a list of 'priority' pathogens as follows:

1. Priority 1 : CRITICAL

   Acinetobacter baumannii – carbapenem resistant

   Pseudomonas aeruginosa – carbapenem resistant

2. Priority 2: HIGH

   Staphylococcus aureus – methicillin resistant, vancomycin resistant

   Helicobacter pylori – clarithromycin resistant

   Neisseria gonorrhoea – 3rd generation cephalosporin resistant, fluoroquinolone resistant

3. Priority 3: MEDIUM

   Haemophilus influenza – ampicillin resistant

   Shigella spp. – fluoroquinolone resistant

Gram negative drug resistant bacteria are a major clinical problem nowerdays. These pathogens are transmitted to healthcare workers during nursing home care during different types of care (such as Toilet assistance, Hygiene, Diaper changing, device care or use etc.). Hence, emphasize is given on the importance of personalized protective equipment in all aspects of health care [8].

Modification of existing regulations is essential that has brought us to the current state of antibiotic resistance. There are various federal government bodies that aim to combat antibiotic resistance through implementation of strict federal regulations [9]:

1. FDA:

   - Checks the work of drug developers, demanding extensive information regarding safety and efficacy.

- Engages regularly in public education campaigns to minimize the spread of antibiotic resistance.
- It rationalizes antibiotic use by strict norms on distribution.
- It regulates antibiotic usage in food products in coordination with the Department of Agriculture.

2. National Institutes of Health:
   - Primary federal agency supporting biomedical research.
   - Consists of 27 Institutes and centres, the most relevant to antibiotic resistance is the National Institute of Allergy and Infectious Diseases (NIAID).
   - NIAID funds various grants to study antimicrobial resistance and also research against bioterrorism.
3. Centers for Disease Control (CDC):
   - It coordinates regional infection control as well as treatment practices.
   - Expands Public awareness programs
   - Maintains strategic drug stockpiles
4. Agency for Healthcare Research and Quality (AHRQ):
   - Funds for research related to aspects of antibiotic usage and treatment of drug resistant infections and control practices.
   - Generates surveillance reports on antibiotic resistant infections.
5. Public Health Service (PHS):
   - PHS officers serve in different settings to access antibiotic resistance patterns and associated infection control and treatment.
6. Veterans Health administration (VA):
   - Implements strategies such as strict limits on antibiotic usage and universal MRSA screening of patients admitted to specified clinical units

White House has implemented National strategy to combat antibiotic resistant bacteria. This strategy points out five interrelated goals that guide collaborative action by the U.S government in partnership with foreign governments, individuals, and organizations aiming to strengthen healthcare, public health, veterinary medicine, agriculture, food safety, and research and manufacturing. Those goals include:

1. Slow the emergence of resistant bacteria and prevent the spread of resistant infections.
2. Strengthen National One- Health Surveillance efforts to combat resistance
3. Advance development and use of rapid and innovative diagnostic tests for identification and characterization of resistant bacteria.
4. Accelerate basic and applied research and development for new antibiotics, other therapeutics, and vaccines; and

5. Improve international collaboration and capacities for antibiotic - resistance prevention, surveillance, control, and antibiotic research and development.

This National Strategy for Combating Antibiotic- Resistant Bacteria will be implemented in accordance with National Action Plan in order to combat this deadly threat. Various improved diagnostics are developed for detection and characterization of this resistant organism. These tests will greatly advance detection; control, and prevention of threats such as Carbapenem-resistant *Enterobacteriaceae* (CRE), Ceftriaxone- resistant *N.gonorrhoeae*, Methicillin- resistant *Staphylococcus aureus* (MRSA), and other multidrug resistant organisms (MDROs). This will efficiently help to reduce the development of resistance.

Biomedical Advance Research and Development Authority (BARDA) along with other government agencies in collaboration aims to advance innovative research on antibiotic resistance. Two programs are sponsored by BARDA that will file FDA New Drug applications for a new antibiotic by the end of 2018.

Thus, many strategies are being developed to combat this global threat of antibiotic resistance which can otherwise lead to numerous deaths among populations due to common infections.

One of the major concerns however, is the evolution of microorganisms which is uncertain natural phenomenon and hence, the timeline for the development of resistance is unpredictable. Development of resistance among organisms occurs naturally via selection through random mutation in response to selection pressures for survival even in extreme conditions. Studies have found that ribosomal mutations promote the evolution of antibiotic resistance (mutations in the gene encoding ribosomal components). Example: *Mycobacterium smegmatis* in which such mutation is found that confers resistance to several structurally and mechanistically unrelated classes of antibiotics and enhances survival following heat shock and membrane stress. Such mutations affect whole ribosomal assembly and cause large scale transcriptomic and proteomic changes such as up regulation of transcription factor, WhiB7 involved in innate antibiotic resistance [10].

References

Sustaining global action on antimicrobial resistance, United Nations Foundation.

James A. Ayukekbong, Michel Ntemgwa and Andrew N. Atabe, 2017.The threat of antimicrobial resistance in developing countries: causes and control strategies, BioMed Central.

C. Lee Ventola, MS, 2015. The Antibiotic Resistance Crisis, Part 1: Causes and Threats.

Maria Angeles Argudin, Ariane Deplano et.al. 2017. Bacteria from animals as a pool of antimicrobial resistance genes, MDPI Journal, Antibiotics, 6, 12.

Senka D`idi, Jagoda [u {kovi} and Bla`enka Kos, 2007. Antibiotic Resistance Mechanisms in Bacteria: Biochemical and Genetic Aspects, Food Technology, Biotechnology, 46 (1) 11–21.

Jessica M. A. Blair, Mark A. Webber, Alison J. Baylay, David O. Ogbolu and Laura J. V. Piddock, 2015. Molecular mechanisms of antibiotic resistance, Nature reviews, Volume 13.

Michael R. Gillings, Ian T. Paulsen, Sasha G. Tetu, 2017. Genomics and the evolution of antibiotic resistance, The New York Academy of Sciences, Volume 1388.

Transmission of Resistant Gram-negative bacteria to health care worker gowns and gloves during care of nursing home residents in Veterans affairs community living centres, Antimicrobial agents and Chemotherapy, 2017.

William M. Sage and David A. Hyman. Combating Antimicrobial Resistance: Regulatory Strategies and Institutional Capacity.

James E Gomez, 2017. Ribosomal mutations promote the evolution of antibiotic resistance in a multidrug environment.

Andrea Sageman, 2015. Antibiotic Resistance Mechanisms, Problems, and Solutions, Honors Projects, Paper 416.

Glenn Tillotson, 2016. The Fight against Bacterial Resistance - New Initiatives but Much Still Needed, Journal of Infectious Diseases and Therapy, DOI: 10.4172/2332-0877.1000e109.

Julian Davies and Dorothy Davies, 2010. Origins and Evolution of Antibiotic Resistance, Microbiology and Molecular Biology Reviews, Volume 74.

Jun Lin, Kunihiko Nishino, Marilyn Roberts, M.Tolmasky, R.Aminov and L.Zhang, 2015. Mechanism of antibiotic Resistance, Frontiers in Microbiology.

Richard Ofori- Asenso, 2017. "When the bug cannot be killed"- The Rising Challenge of Antimicrobial Resistance, MDPI Journal, Medicines, 4, 40.

Stuart B Levy & Bonnie Marshall, 2004. Antibacterial resistance worldwide: causes, challenges and responses, Nature medicine supplement, Volume 10.

Chapter 17

Surrogacy: The Dawn of Sterile Citizenry and the Legal Lacunae

Aiman Farhat

Advocate , LLM (Ist SEM), Sardar Patel Subharti Institute of Law, Swami Vivekanada Subharti University, Meerut, Uttar Pradesh, India.

Email: farhat.aiman@gmail.com

Abstract

The term "mothers" being associated with the term surrogate is indeed an example of the paradox that is in the society as India, where the adherence to the antiquarian norms of treating the woman as sacred and the goddesses as the objects of obeisance meets the 21st century formula of exploiting them for materialistic gains within the framework that the surrogacy industry has produced – that which ensures economic lucrativeness at the expense of the surrogate, moreover, another human.

Since the Vedic period it is well-settled that the mode of marriage has assumed religious connotation. Through the institution of marriage, men and women are united in wedlock for the purpose of procreation of a child. But due to growing problem of infertility, the desire to naturally have a child has caused grief and dissatisfaction in couples. At this point, the science of surrogacy acts as a boon to live up dreams of couples to raise a child.

In India, the web of surrogacy seems to be expanding in last two decades. Today, surrogacy is an accepted societal practice propelled by economic necessity and fuelled by the Reproductive Tourism Industry wantonly flourishing in India. The woman carrying an embryo has been in a grey zone, with uncertain legal and compensatory protection.

The Union Cabinet has taken the first step towards surrogacy regulation by approving the Surrogacy (Regulation) Bill, 2016, but it has many problematic provisions. Through this paper an attempt is made to look into the issues and problems related to surrogacy. It seeks to usher the pros and cons of Surrogacy (Regulation) Bill, 2016. Through concrete case laws a humble effort is placed to unveil the scope of surrogacy in Indian context. A comparative study of surrogacy regulation is made at global context. At last, possible suggestions are advanced that may assist in eliminating the legal lacuna on surrogacy.

Introduction

Surrogacy is one of those changes, which has challenged both society and law, in terms of its recognition & regulation. For many people, having a child is the ultimate dream. Sharing their love and raising a family can truly make their lifetime picture complete. Surrogacy can be viewed as a technique as well as a form of transaction, which parties resort to in order to give rise to new relation towards each other. The good news is that by using the services of a surrogate mother, these couples and individuals can still have the children that they desire, oftentimes with gene characteristics from one or both parents.

Surrogacy is a 'necessity' for those who are economically vulnerable and are unable to maintain themselves with the help of available resources, and a 'desire' of those who are otherwise unable to procreate or conceive the child of their own.

The natural desire to have one's own child has paved the way for recognizing the new techniques which aim at fulfilling the desire to have a child. Surrogacy is one such technique which is used across the globe. Surrogacy is a well-known method of reproduction, whereby a woman agrees to give birth to a child who she will not raise, but hand over to a contracted party. She may be the child's genetic mother (the more traditional form of surrogacy) or she may be, as a gestational carrier, carry the pregnancy to deliver after having been implanted in embryo.[1] Let us now analyze some of the authoritative explanations or definitions, which may further throw a light on the concept.

American Law Reports[2]defines surrogacy as a contract in the following lines:

> *"..a contractual undertaking whereby the natural or surrogate mother, for a fee, agrees to conceive a child through artificial insemination with sperm of the natural father, to bear and deliver the child to the natural father, and to terminate all of her parental rights subsequent to the child's birth."*[3]

Looking at the Indian scenario, the Indian Council for Medical Research[4] defines 'Assistive Reproductive Technology (ART)' as:

> "For the purpose of these guidelines, *ART would be taken to encompass all techniques that attempt to obtain a pregnancy by manipulating the sperm or/and oocyte outside the body, and transferring the gamete or embryo into the uterus."*

The Supreme Court of India[5] has defined surrogacy as:

> *"..a method of reproduction, whereby a woman agrees to become pregnant for the purpose of gestating and giving birth to a child she will not raise but hand over to a contracting party."*

---

1 J. Arijit Pasayat in *Baby Manji Yamada v. Union of India*,AIR 2009 SC 84 [hereafter *Baby Manji or Baby M*].

2 *In Re Baby M*, 1988 N.J.77 A.L.R.4th 1.

3 Smita Chandra, Surrogacy & India http://ssrn.com

4 Indian Council Med. Res. *National Guidelines for Accreditation, Supervision & Regulation of ART Clinics in India,* (Dec. 3, 2013).

5 *Baby Manji, supra* note 1.

Additionally, the Black's Law Dictionary[6] categorizes Surrogacy into two classes: traditional and gestational surrogacy. Altruistic surrogacy, wherein, the surrogate mother is only paid the medical expenses of the pregnancy and is also often a family relation of the commissioning couple, and, the other type being that of Commercial surrogacy, which involves payment to the surrogate mother for "renting" her body for the purpose of the procreation of the baby. Such a surrogate is a worker hired by the ART Clinics.

The Government of the country has been slow paced machinery when it comes to legal protection to the surrogate and the surfacing of various reports and news of the death of such surrogate mothers seems to become the beloved objects of their ignorance.

The Surrogacy (Regulation) Bill, 2016 has paved away the existence of commercial surrogacy in India. The said Bill is looked as a shield to protect the exploitation to the surrogate mother. It is pertinent to note here that, altruistic surrogacy has been allowed under the Bill on fulfilment of certain conditions and for specific purposes.

There are two types of Surrogacy: Traditional (straight) and Gestational (host).

Traditional surrogacy

Traditional or straight surrogacy is the simplest and least expensive form of surrogacy and is also known as artificial insemination. The surrogate uses an insemination kit to become pregnant using the intended father's semen. The baby will therefore be conceived using the surrogate's egg.

Some people prefer to use a clinic for inseminations, but it can also happen at home and can therefore seem a more natural and less 'medical' way of becoming pregnant than host surrogacy. It can, however, can be harder emotionally for both the surrogate and the intended Host (or gestational) surrogacy

Gestational Surrogacy

Gestational or host surrogacy is when IVF is used, either with the eggs of the intended mother, or with donor eggs. The surrogate therefore does not use her own eggs, and is genetically unrelated to the baby. It is physically more complicated and considerably more expensive than straight surrogacy and always takes place in a fertility clinic parents

Some Surrogates prefer this method as they may not be comfortable with using their own eggs in surrogacy. In essence, there are three stages to 'host' surrogacy:

1. Egg donation: the female IP, or the egg donor, undergo special procedures to extract a number of eggs.
2. Fertilisation: the egg is fertilised with semen in the laboratory.
3. Transfer: the fertilised egg is transferred into the womb of the surrogate mother.

6 Jyoti Bhakare, *Surrogacy- A Reality Eclipsed by Ethical, Social, Legal Issues-Indian Perspectives*, 2 Indian Journal of Law & Justice 80 (2011)

The fertilised egg can be transferred to the surrogate either 'fresh' or after having been de-frosted from egg storage. For a fresh egg transfer the monthly cycles of the surrogate and the egg donor must be synchronised, and this is done using hormone medications. In cases where embryos have been frozen already and the de-frosted embryos are being transferred some IVF clinics will insist on the surrogate taking hormone medications to 'ready' her womb lining.

What we commonly refer to as "surrogacy" in America is often called "commercial surrogacy" abroad. Commercial surrogacy is not an option in many other countries. Some countries only permit altruistic surrogacy agreements.

Altruistic Surrogacy

Altruistic surrogacy refers to those surrogacy agreements where the surrogate does not receive monetary compensation. In most altruistic surrogacy agreements, the surrogate is a close relation to the intended parents (family member/close friend).

Within the last two years, a story from Australia reached headlines about a positive altruistic surrogacy arrangement between strangers. The gestational surrogate decided she wanted to give back to someone faced with reproductive challenges. She connected with a family struggling to have a second child and agreed to be their gestational surrogate. This was a rare scenario.

Entering into an altruistic surrogacy with a known surrogate (i.e. family member, close friend) is a celebrated experience. However, even when the surrogate in an altruistic agreement is a close relation, complications or unforeseen expenses may arise.

Commercial Surrogacy

A commercial gestational surrogacy agreement includes a pre-determined monetary compensation to the surrogate, in addition to covering medical costs, etc. Some praise altruistic surrogacies and criticize commercial surrogacy agreements but some accuses commercial surrogacy of using women's wombs for profit, demoralizing the surrogates and sending "motherless" babies into the world.

Victimizing the Surrogates

The Social Stigma and the Ethical Dilemma

Mythology reveals the existence of surrogate mothers in India. Though Devika and Vasudeva were the biological parents to Krishna but were brought up by Devi Yashodha. However, in the modern scenario, surrogacy in India has been a matter of moral and ethical concern and was debated since ever. The main opposition to the practice of viable surrogacy is that it commoditises a woman's body, almost the same way as prostitution do, the most probable reason why this practice is also sometimes called as "womb prostitution". Moreover, this practice converts women essentially as breeders, putting their wombs up for hire to the premier bidders.[7]

Typically speaking, as far as the women, their status is concerned, then as per some intellects, this takes away from women's principal status as human

7 Anil Malhotra and Ranjit Malhotra, '*Surrogacy in India*', 2nd Ed., Universal Law Publishing, Lucknow (2015)

beings to a commodity only, providing an indispensable service; thereby treating women not as ends in themselves, but as a means to an end. Nonetheless, since time and again, the practice had finds it under regular assail from feminists, who vehemently condemn it.

Another issue that crops up is the exploitation of women. Surrogacy leads to the repression and subjection of poor women, who have almost no real say in the renting out of their wombs. Then there arise the issue of broker and commercial agencies that often keep most of the profit for them, with only a portion of the amount given as compensation reaching the actual beneficiary, i.e. the surrogate mother. Surrogacy, by the virtue of the long entrenched norms and principles embedded in the Indian culture, has come to be equated with prostitution and this reason has caused most to condemn the practice on a moral basis[8]. For example, it is found that in Asia, similar techniques similar to those employed under surrogacy arrangement are used to recruit women from the rural areas for prostitution and surrogacy, with the promise of a respectable job and ultimately subjecting them to sexual offences.[9]

Many human activists have regarded the recruiting process to be similar to those used by the human traffickers to lure women to sex work and wherein, they may sign contracts and are kept in a confined place till they execute the obligations listed under such a contract. This phenomenon is similar to the condition of the surrogate mothers that are confined to the surrogate hostels in isolation and subjected to strict and consistent surveillance by the clinic authorities - a breach of their right to privacy.

Commercial surrogacy, basically, ends up treating not only women, but even children as products, to be bought and sold altogether. Children are then seen as bits and pieces of contracts, subjected to sex- assortment and even abandonment in case of disability or a simple change of mind and mood. Also, then there arises a concern that commercial surrogacy is nothing more than the trafficking of children.

Similarly, as the decoy of the big bread earned by this practice, has also end up to the trafficking of women, who are forced into surrogacy against their will. Another important issue crops up relating to the psychological effect that the practice might have on the child, including the possibility of an identity crisis and the desire to meet his/ her gestational mother.

Surrogacy brokers are seeing the light of the day and it is forgeable at there may be a point of time where they become absolutely mainstream and even legal.[10] There are myriads of the very subtle social and class – based issues that make a surrogacy contract possible, and the never ending grievances of the poverty

8 *Indian Journal of Public Health,* Issue - 2 ,Volume - 57, 65-70 (2013) *Access at : https://nlsllmejournal.files.wordpress.com/2013/08/author_instructions.pdf*

9 *Surrogate Motherhood: A Violation of Human Rights,* International Centre for Law, Life, Faith and Family *http://icolf.org/surrogate-motherhood-a-violation-of-human-rights*

10 *Access at : http://www.iaac.ca/en/commercial-surrogacy-in-india-exploitation-or-mutual-assistance-4*

stricken surrogate mothers a reality. Surrogacy is a product of the capitalist patriarchal society.[11]

Trafficking of the children is also consequence of the largely unregulated commercial surrogacy in India is but illusory. A safeguard against such actions is the need of the hour. Although, it is true that there is a dire need for the nation to introduce strict and efficient legal protection for securing the surrogate mothers from the shackles of exploitation, it also stand true that commercial surrogacy cannot be overlooked by a third world nation as India, that is striving to attain the recognition so as to equate its development in all spheres with that of the superpowers.

The Reality of the Surrogacy Contract

It largely perceived that in most cases, the surrogate mother and her husband are barely educated and hence it poses as a difficulty for them to understand the details of the procedures in the surrogacy process or the complex medical jargons, that hold the information on the potential side effects and other medical conditions that may not be in the interest of the surrogate and disrupt her medical wellbeing.

Hence, by the reason of their this inability, the surrogate is apprised of the contents of the procedures in such terms and language that suits the interest of the Clinic authorities and which the surrogate cannot verify by any means. At present between the parties and ART Clinics, the surrogacy contract framed under the ICMR guidelines are the guiding force. Many times, the clinics also refrain from dispatching a copy of the contract to the surrogate, who is a signing party to the agreement, thus causing her to not have any written evidence concerning her pregnancy or the surrogacy arrangement.[12]

Sometimes, the clinics may refrain from signing such agreements under the surrogacy arrangement so as to eliminate any chances of them being held accountable in future.Most often the surrogates are also unaware of their legal rights and by the virtue of their degraded financial situation, they fail to avail the services of legal attorneys.[13]

Further, in most cases, there is the existence of the agent who undertakes the mediation between the surrogate mother and the commissioning couple, who is not mentioned as a party to the surrogacy contract under the ICMR guidelines. Such an agent, being concerned only with the monetary benefits that he may derive out of the process, may not relay the essential details of the medical complexities to the surrogate, thus displaying the act to be an instance of churning undue advantage out of the status of illiteracy and poverty of the surrogate.

11 *Surrogate Motherhood- Ethical or Commercial,* Centre for Social Research. *Access at : http://www.womenleadership.in/Csr/SurrogacyReport.pdf*

12 *Surrogate Motherhood- Ethical or Commercial,* Centre for Social Research, *Access at : http://www.womenleadership.in/Csr/SurrogacyReport.pdf*

13 The Surrogacy Motherhood ethical or commercial - ART

Physical & Psychological Exploitation of the Surrogates

An Analysis

The desperation of the commissioning couple to have a baby renders them to impart a blind faith on the clinics and the arrangements that they have in hand. Further, the doctors and the clinics are least concerned, in most cases, with the health of the surrogate mother but rather they lay emphasis on the health of the baby born as they need to fulfil the promises made to the commissioning couple. The well -being of the surrogate mothers, sadly, attract the attention of the doctors and the clinics only in relation to the health of the foetus.

In the Mother Jones case, an Indian surrogate died after giving birth. Upon delivery, she started haemorrhaging, and the clinic couldn't control her bleeding and subsequently, her husband was asked to call for medical help. As she died en route to the hospital, the clinic refused to take any responsibility for her demise.[14]

In the US, the surrogates are given not more than two embryos to secure their safety, contrary to that in India, where, the surrogates are implanted with up to 5 embryos to increase the chances of pregnancy, thus wreaking havoc on their health.[15]

Besides the health of the surrogates, during and before the pregnancy, there are possibilities of many post pregnancy problems as well as postpartum infections, breast engorgement which may even lead to breast infection, urinary and faecal incontinence etc. which she often might have to suffer. Side effects and medical risk occur across all methods of assisted reproductive treatment. Surrogacy is not a simple alternative to having a child. The process and surrounding issues are complex.

These are the complication that all surrogate mother will have to face once they decide to have that treatment. Post-Partum Depression is one of the side effect surrogate mother has to face. It is the sadness and depression after delivering the child or children. Besides, there is also rick associated with the pregnancy such as exhaustion, nausea, varicose veins, pre-eclampsia, placenta previa, gestational diabetes, constipation, indigestion, higher blood pressure, hormonal mood changes, abdominal and vaginal weakness, stretch mark because the skin expand as the baby grow and worse, death. Some of them will also facing with the reaction to fertility medication.

Different person will suffer different kinds of side effects and risk. It is all depends on the stamina and also the age of the surrogate as these risks are increased with the age of the surrogate. Furthermore, there is also the rare risk of transfer of HIV and/or hepatitis. To eliminate this risk, mandatory screening of everyone involved in surrogacy is required.

---

14 Scott Carney, *Inside India's Rent-a-Womb Business*, March – April (2010)

15 *Indian Journal of Public Health*, Issue - 2 ,Volume - 57, 65-70 (2013) *Access at : http://www.ijph.in/article.asp?issn=0019-557X;year=2013;volume=57;issue=2;spage=65;epage=70;aulast=Anu*

Clearly, the exploitation of the surrogates by the clinics and the agents employed as mediators is an easy process undertaken for several reasons one, with the lack of legal restriction and legal protection and two, due to the fact that they are mostly uneducated and hence lack the requisite knowledge and awareness before indulging in the surrogacy process.

In a country like India, where there is an alarmingly high maternal death rate, commercial surrogacy has caused the exploitation and the renting of the surrogate's body by the westerner, causing the industry to be termed as the wealth pronating tool for the capitalists and an epitome of capitalism. According to the ART Bill, a woman cannot give more than five live births including her own children, and that a surrogate mother shall not go for an embryo transfer more than three times for the same couple.

Further, whatever maybe the conditions of surrogacy, pregnancy is a somatopsychic event par excellence ,which is characterized as a time where the mother undergoes profound psychological and physiological changes. Separation from such an offspring nourished in her womb becomes the source of all emotional and psychological predicaments for the mother that fosters feelings for the child even with the firmly established realization of a non - genetic link up with the child, in most cases, and the realization of the inhuman duty to relinquish the new born.

In the US, the surrogacy agencies provide psychological support and discussion groups for the pregnant surrogate mothers so as to enable them to cope up with the separation from the offspring in an effective manner upon conception. However, no such provision has been incorporated in India either under the ICMR guidelines that are devoid of a legal backing or the proposed ART Bill that still strives to see the light of the day, as the surrogate mother also stands helpless in the face of the lack of basic medical amenities being made available to her in the crucial period of pregnancy and the post - pregnancy separation from the offspring.

The surrogacy arrangement also involves the separation of the surrogate mothers from their own families during the term of the pregnancy, when they are kept in the surrogate hostels in isolation, for reasons such as the possibilities of poor obstetrician care and social stigma imposed on her in her rural residence, difficulties concerning communication of the Clinic with the surrogate mother etc.

Moreover, these reasons are directed at the protection of the infant and the commissioning couple and no sound reason is projected on as to why the surrogate must be kept separated from her own children for a period of 9 months.

The central figures of the entire surrogacy process become the objects of apathy upon implementing the terms of the surrogacy contract,thus rendering another sound instance of the palpable commodification of women in this realm. The exploitation of the poor and uneducated is further aggravated with the addition status of being a woman, where the requirement of an informed consent is not justified in it's true meaning and the medical protection for the surrogates is only illusory.

Surrogacy Law in Foreign Jurisdiction

As far as the legality of the concept is concerned, reference of the Universal Declaration of Human Rights (UDHR), 1948 can be given, which ensures that *"men and women of full age without any limitation due to race, nationality or religion have right to marry and find a family."*[16]Under a wide interpretation of this provision, a surrogacy arrangement will be regarded as the opportunity for the infertile couple to have their own baby, which they were otherwise incapable of conceiving. States are under an obligation to respect this right under the head of right to reproduction ensured under this provision.

There are a few countries that have decided to incorporate surrogacy with a government imparted regulation, but these have also proved that the non-commercial nature of surrogacy is a difficult task to achieve. For example, in England, only a reasonable compensation is allowed, but in reality, is it so high that it qualifies as a payment.[17]It displays the downfalls of non-effective govt. control over the surrogacy transactions. However, there is also a belief among those in power that unpaid surrogacy will never meet the escalating demand since there won't be enough number of women volunteering for this occupation and then also, most of them may not qualify under the stringent rules and regulations governing the surrogacy arrangement.

In Germany[18], as the law stands today, surrogacy agreements are not recognized. Further, donation of eggs is prohibited and procedures such as artificial insemination or embryo donation are considered to be criminal offences but a recent ruling by highest court of Germany has paved a way towards the legalization of children born abroad via surrogacy by confirming status of Legal Parents.[19] The case was concerning two gay men whose child was born via surrogate in California. The baby, born in 2010, was registered in the United States as the child of the two men. Upon returning home, the couple had been unable to persuade the German authorities to recognize the child as theirs, though the baby has been living with the fathers in Berlin for the last three-and-a-half years. The issue was brought up before the German supreme court, which ruled that the decisions of foreign authorities in such matters must be respected as "part of a child's welfare to be able to rely on the parents to have continuous responsibility for its well-being," but maintained that surrogacy on German soil remains forbidden.[20] The situation is similar in Sweden, Norway, and Italy where the above-mentioned procedures may culminate into criminal prosecution[21]. But,

16 Universal Declaration of Human Rights, Art 16, G.A. Res. 217 (III) A, U.N. Doc. A/RES/217(III).

17 *Access at : http://www.nomaternitytraffic.eu/wordpress/wp-content/uploads/2015/09/2015-Contribution-HCCH-No-Maternity-Traffic EN.pdf*

18 Section 1(1) No. 7 German Embryo Protection Act and § 14b Adoption Placement Act

19 Richard Vaughn, Children Born Abroad via Surrogacy Entitled to Legal Parents, German Court Rules (December 23rd, 2014).

20 Deutsche Welle (DW-International Broadcaster), *Limited win for surrogacy, gay parenthood in Germany* (December 19, 2014).

21 Ukrainian Family Law Group, *The ABC's of Ukranaian Family Law*(2012).

some countries like Belgium, Netherlands and England are a little more liberal. In England, surrogacy arrangements are legal and the Surrogacy Arrangement Act, 1985 prohibits advertising and other commercial aspects of surrogacy[22]. The Act declares initiation and involvement in commercial surrogacy agreements to be a criminal offence.[23]

In United States of America, many states prohibit commercial surrogacy. The Uniform Parentage Act, 1987 of the USA Federal statute neither expressly precludes nor approves the use of techniques with the help of which it can be carried out. Article 7 of the Uniform Parentage Act, 2000 version, discusses the parental status of the donor to state that the donor is not a parent of the child conceived by means of assisted reproduction.[24] The Federal Supreme Court of USA in Eisenstad v. Baird[25]has recognized the 'right to privacy' as a fundamental right which includes the right to marriage, family, abortion, child rearing, procreation and education. The right to procreate, either as a married couple or as a single individual, was broadened or was given constitutional protection. Also, the Californian Supreme Court in Johnson v. Calvert[26]extended the constitutional protection to surrogacy contracts and held them to be valid on the grounds of public policy as the surrogacy contracts involve free, informed and rational choice by a woman to use her body.

In Australia, surrogate mother is regarded as the legal mother of the child that creates legal obligations between them and hence, any surrogacy agreement giving custody to others is void and not enforceable. This discourages surrogacy agreements by making it a criminal offence in cases involving transfer of custody after surrogacy transactions. The only legal arrangement to take custody is to take the surrogate child through adoption process which validates this transaction. Moreover, commercial surrogacy is illegal and recognition is given only to altruistic surrogacy.[27]

In Canada, the Assisted Human Reproduction Act, 2004 prohibits commercial surrogacy wherein a surrogacy arrangement involves an agreement with consideration. In France, surrogacy is completely prohibited irrespective of its nature as commercial or altruistic surrogacy. Thus, any surrogacy arrangement which involves transfer of custody of surrogate child is of no legal consequence.

Commercial surrogacy is legal in India, Ukraine, and California while it is illegal in England, many states of United States, and in Australia, which recognize only altruistic surrogacy. In contrast, countries like Germany, Sweden, Norway, and Italy do not recognize any surrogacy agreements. India has become a favorite

22 Legislation.gov.uk http://www.legislation.gov.uk/ukpga/1985/49 (last updated on May 27, 2015)

23 Margaret Ryznar, *International Commercial Surrogacy and its parties*, THE JOHN MARSHAL LAW REVIEW.

24 National Conference of Commissioners on Uniform State Laws, Uniform Parentage Act, (Feb. 10, 2003)

25 Eisenstad v. Baird, 40 5 U.S. 438, 453-54 (1979).

26 Johnson v. Calvert, 5 Cal. 484 (May 20, 1993).

27 *The Law Handbook*, http://www.lawhandbook.org.au/fact_sheets/ch38.php .

destination of fertility tourism. Each year, couples from abroad are attracted to India by so-called surrogacy agencies because cost of the whole procedure in India is as less as one third of what it is in United States and United Kingdom (10-20 lakhs).

The A.R.T. Bill and the Legal Lacunae

A Critical Analysis

Over the years, ***Assisted Reproductive Technology (ART)*** has turned out to be the boon for those deprived of progeny. ART has grown exponentially in the last few years and is now more and more available to the infertile couples in both developed and developing countries. India is poised to be the leader in the world of ART with rapid growths in ARTs.

The ***In Vitro Fertilization (IVF)*** is the most common form of ART. IVF is artificial technique of bestowing parenthood to those failing to conceive naturally. It involves fertilization by combining an egg and sperm in a laboratory dish manually and then transferring the embryo to the uterus. With infertility on the rise due to erratic life style and late marriages more and more couples are opting ART or adopted babies. The expansion and proliferation ARTs has been facilitated by economic globalization wherein reproductive tissues like sperm, ova and uterus are traded like any other commodity.

In 2008, the *India Council of Medical Research (ICMR)* Developed a draft for *ART Regulation Bill* and sent to the Ministry of Health & Family Welfare, which was the been revised by the *Ministry of Law & Justice* as **ART (Regulation) Bill, 2013**. The ART Regulation Bill came before the cabinet in 2016 for consideration. It was proposed to establish National, State Boards and National Registry of ART in India for accreditation and supervision of ART clinics and ART Banks, ensuring that services provided by these are ethical and that the medical, social and legal rights of all the concerned are protected with maximum benefit to all the stakeholders with ethical and good medical practices. This resulted into ***SURROGACY (Regulation) Bill, 2016*** by the *Health Ministry* that proposed to legalize altruistic, domestic surrogacy.

The bill although seeks to control exploitation of surrogate child and mother for unethical purposes. Despite this the bill in opinion of many ART experts failed. The major issue being lack of screening guidelines of couples based on their social economic background, criminal records in past, their heath , age and family information check. In absence of such screening guidelines the surrogate child's interest suffers risks and child's security. Further the bill is unclear if such a surrogate child is allowed to be abandoned or rejected or left in adoption home or orphanage.

Among the biggest misses of the bill is based on sex selective surrogacy or family balancing surrogacy to have child of pre-determined sex, in which the ART Bill prohibited and penalized the same by adding *PRE-NATAL DIAGNOSIS TECHNIQUES*. Further the bill does not talk about the trafficking or sale, abduction of surrogate child. On August 24, 2016 Union Cabinet approved the *Surrogacy Regulation Bill 2016.*

The bill acknowledges surrogacy agreements and their legal enforceability. The surrogacy agreements are treated at par with other contracts under the Indian Contract Act 1872 and other laws applicable to these kinds of agreements. Both the couple/single parent and surrogate mother need to enter into a surrogacy agreement covering all issues, which would be legally enforceable. Some of the features of proposed bill are that an authority at national and state level should be constituted to register and regulate the I.V.F. clinics and A.R.T centre and a forum should be created to file complaints for grievances against clinics and ART centre. The age of the surrogate mother should be 21-35 years, and she should not have delivered more than 5 times including her own children. Surrogate mother would not be allowed to undergo embryo transfer more than 3 times for the same couple. If the surrogate is a married woman, the consent of her spouse would be required before she may act as surrogate to prevent any legal or marital dispute. The surrogacy arrangement should also provide for financial support for the surrogate child in case the commissioning couple dies before delivery of the child, or divorce between the intended parents and subsequent willingness of none to take delivery of the child so as to avoid injustice to the child.

Commercial surrogacy was made legal in India with the landmark Supreme Court judgment in the Baby Manjhi case and later with the creation of the Indian Council of Medical Research (ICMR) Guidelines, 2005, which prescribed the use of ART procedures and treatment by the Assisted Reproduction Techniques Clinic (the ART Clinic). The Assisted Reproductive Technology (Regulation) Bill was passed in, and is formulated primarily to regulate the contractual relationship between the commissioning parents and the ART Clinic and legalizes commercial surrogacy by prescribing monetary compensation to the surrogate mother by the commissioning couple.

The Artificial Reproductive Technology (Regulation) Bill defines surrogacy as follows:

> "An arrangement in which a woman agrees to a pregnancy, achieved through assisted reproductive technology, in which neither of the gametes belong to her or her husband, with the intention of carrying it to term and handing over the child to the person or persons for whom she is acting as surrogate".

The ART clinics are also required to ensure utmost confidentiality of all the information that they obtain under the surrogacy arrangement. This implies that they are not to provide the information concerning the surrogate mother or potential surrogate mothers to any Centre for Social Research (CSR).

Under Clause 34 of S. 10,it is stated that that the birth certificate shall bear the name of the genetic parents of the baby.[28] Hence, the surrogate mother is to contract herself out of her parental duties prior to the commencement of pregnancy, agreeing to part from the child as soon as conception is terminated. The donor of the genetic material is also to relinquish the parental rights to the child.

28 Liz Bishop and Bebe Loff , The rights of the gestational mother and child in surrogacy: A Bill to regulate surrogacy in India , No. 3,Vol. 7, (2013)

The birth certificate of the child is issued in the name of the commissioning parents irrespective of the fact that the commissioning parents may not have contributed their genetic material to the pregnancy

The Bill does no impose a bar on the number of times a couple may employ surrogacy and there is no government body that has been instituted to discover the family background, the economic and social status etc. of the commissioning couple. This may lead to the further exploitation and corruption within the surrogacy framework as all the possible causes of any forcible problem within this framework are not being adequately assessed.

The Surrogacy (Regulation) Bill, 2016

A Glimpse

The Surrogacy (Regulation) Bill, 2016 proposes to regulate surrogacy in India by establishing National Surrogacy Board at Central level, State Surrogacy Boards and Appropriate Authorities in States and Union Territories. The proposed legislation ensures effective regulation of surrogacy, prohibit commercial surrogacy and allow ethical surrogacy to the needy infertile Indian couples.

The major objectives of the Bill are to regulate surrogacy services in the country, to provide altruistic ethical surrogacy to the needy infertile Indian couples, to prohibit commercial surrogacy including sale and purchase of human embryo and gametes, to prevent commercialization of surrogacy, to prohibit potential exploitation of surrogate mothers and protect the rights of children born through surrogacy.

The draft surrogacy Bill aims at regulating commissioning of surrogacy in the country in a proper manner.

- As per the 2009 Law Commission Report, the assisted reproduction treatment industry is 25,000 Crore industry.
- The Bill aims to prevent exploitation of women, especially those in rural and tribal areas.
- The Bill promises to ensure parentage of children born out of surrogacy is "legal and transparent."
- The new Bill proposes complete ban on commercial surrogacy. As per the Bill, only legally wedded Indian couples can have children through surrogacy, provided at least one of them have been proven to have fertility related issues.
- Foreigners, even Overseas Indians, are barred from commissioning surrogacy including NRI's. A woman will be allowed to become a surrogate mother only for altruistic purpose and under no circumstances money shall be paid to her, except for medical expenses.
- Unmarried couples, single parents, live-in-partners and homosexuals cannot choose for surrogacy as per the new bill.
- Surrogacy regulation board will be setup at Central and State level.

- To allow altruistic ethical surrogacy to intending infertile couple between the age of 23-50 years and 26-55 years for female and male respectively.
- The intending couples should be legally married for at least five years and should be Indian citizens.
- The intending couples have not had any surviving child biologically or through adoption or through surrogacy earlier except when they have a child and who is mentally or physically challenged or suffer from life threatening disorder with no permanent cure.
- The intending couples shall not abandon the child, born out of a surrogacy procedure under any condition.
- The child born through surrogacy will have the same rights as are available for the Biological child.
- The surrogate mother should be a close relative of the intending couple and should be between the age of 25-35 years. She can act as surrogate mother only once.
- The surrogate mother will carry a child which is genetically related to the Intending Couple. An order concerning the parentage and custody of the child to be born through surrogacy, is to be passed by a court of the Magistrate of the first class.
- An insurance coverage of reasonable and adequate amount shall be ensured in favour of the surrogate mother.
- National Surrogacy Board shall exercise the powers and shall perform functions conferred on the Board under this Act.
- The Board shall consist of the Minister in-charge of the Ministry of Health and Family Welfare, as the Chairperson, Secretary to the Government of India in- charge of the Department dealing with the surrogacy matter, as Vice-Chairperson and three women Members of Parliament, of whom two shall be elected by the House of the People and one by the Council of State as Members.
- The National Surrogacy board and State Surrogacy board shall be the Policy making bodies and Appropriate Authority will be the Implementation body for the Act.
- The appropriate authority shall comprise of an officer of or above the rank of the Joint Director of Health and Family Welfare Department, as Chairperson, an eminent woman representing women's organization, as member, an officer of Law Department of the State or the Union territory concerned not below the rank of a Deputy Secretary, as member and an eminent registered medical practitioner, as a member.
- The surrogacy clinics shall be registered under this Act after the Appropriate Authority is satisfied that such clinics are in a position to provide facilities and can maintain equipments and standards including specialised manpower, physical infrastructure and diagnostic facilities as may be prescribed in the rules and regulations.

- No person, organisation, surrogacy clinic, laboratory or clinical establishment of any kind shall undertake commercial surrogacy, abandon the child, exploit the surrogate mother, sell human embryo or import embryo for the purpose of surrogacy. Violation to the said provision shall be an offence punishable with imprisonment for a term which shall not be less than ten years and with fine which may extend to ten lakh rupees.
- The surrogacy clinics shall have to maintain all records for a period of 25 years Transitional provision-Subject to the provisions of this Act, there shall be provided a gestation period of ten months from the date of coming into force of this act to protect the wellbeing of already existing surrogate mothers

Surrogacy (Regulation) Bill, 2016

A Bane or Boon

There are certain advantages and disadvantages of Surrogacy bill,2016 which are as follows:

- Pros:
  1. The proposed Bill will help in preventing exploitation of women especially those from rural and tribal areas.
  2. By bringing in altruistic surrogacy and allowing a woman to be a surrogate only once in her lifetime, the government aims to ensure better health and life of the surrogate mother.
  3. It proposes that if any establishment undertakes commercial surrogacy, exploits the mother, abandons the child or tries to sell or import a human embryo, there would be punishment with imprisonment of not less than 10 years along with a fine up to Rs.10 lakhs.
  4. Adoption, an underutilized option for having a child can be taken into perspective where the orphan child and the couple's happiness will be ensured at the same time.
- Cons:
  1. The proposed provisions in the Bill might act as a ground that breeds underground illegal surrogacy. It is not necessary that all the medical clinics will adhere to law

     There will be corruption and unethical practices and exploitation of poor women.
  2. It has to be understood that a woman who enters into surrogacy is not out of will but because she is pushed towards it for a decent livelihood. Therefore, altruistic surrogacy will lead them to look for other means of living to sustain themselves.
  3. Given the nature of Indian society i.e. patriarchy, inheritance of property by the male child, a close relative might be forced by the family to become a surrogate mother for an infertile couple in the family without her will and there would be no place for her to complain.

4. If a couple gets married at the age of 38 years, then it would be very difficult for them to have a child through surrogacy at the age of 43 years as there are other health issues attached with increasing age.
5. The effectiveness of the proposed Bill will be questioned given the fact that there are laws in India which prohibit sex determination, female foeticide and organ donation with little achievement so far.

Bunch of Issues and Challenges

Surrogacy involves multi-factors & several issue that any legal system or law must keep in mind while formulating the regulations. Those factors range across emotional, natural, ethical, medical, financial and sociological aspects.

In India, there exists a peculiar situation where surrogacy is not being regulated efficiently.[29] However, the Union Cabinet has taken the first step towards regulation by approving the Surrogacy (Regulation) Bill, 2016, but it has many problematic provisions. These are questions that will remain even if the bill is passed.

- It is not clear if the ban and the allowance for altruistic surrogacy are meant to make an ideological point or to actually confront the ground situation.
- India's failure to administer the ban on organ donations and sex determination tests, it is anybody's guess how effective the ban on commercial surrogacy will be.
- How does it suddenly become acceptable if the surrogate mother is a relevant and uncompensated, besides probably being coerced, as women often are in intra- family decision making.
- An outright ban on surrogacy as it would be to push this industry underground, or shift it to another, increasing the vulnerability of women even more.
- The bill proposes that in the absence of close relatives, couples are 'free to adopt'. Why this selective imposition of the morality of adoption on only those who do not fit the hetero- normative ethics of the state?
- Is endorsing altruistic surrogacy over its commercialization is a formal declaration that women are obliged to be (reproductive) gift-givers, and need no compensation for loss of livelihood and the immense emotional and bodily labour of gestation involved in surrogacy.
- What if a close female relative, a sister or a sister-in-law does not want to be selfless? Will there be no shaming or penalty for that? Can we really convince ourselves that the coercion of a contract or the inducement of money is greater than the coercion of (patriarchal) family ties, especially in country like ours?
- Another related issue is the right of the child. Children born through surrogacy are entitled to know their personal history at an appropriate age.

29 *Jan Balaz vs. Anand Municipality*, AIR 2010 Guj 21 at ¶ 14. [hereinafter *Jan Balaz*]

- The proposed bill prohibits altruistic surrogacy benefits to homosexual's couples, live-in partners, single men and women. Does it not violate the fundamental right of equality?

Is Surrogacy Bill Violative of Right to Privacy ?

The view of the Government cannot be super imposed over the will of the people, say legal experts. Three months after the Union Cabinet passed the Surrogacy (Regulation) Bill, 2016, legal experts maintain that it will not stand the test of constitutional rights. In a panel discussion on the subject, Soli Sorabjee, former attorney general of India said that the bill imposes restrictions that are in *"violation of basic rights of privacy and fundamental rights of reproductive autonomy."*

The most controversial part, according to industry experts, is that overseas Indians, foreigners, unmarried couples, single parents, live-in partners and gay couples are barred from commissioning surrogacy. Only a close married blood relative who must have herself borne a child, and is not an NRI or a foreigner can be a surrogate mother once in a lifetime. Indian couples with biological or adopted children are prohibited to undertake surrogacy. Under the surrogacy contract, the commissioning parents will be allowed to only pay the medical expenses and not compensate the surrogate mother is any other way. Commercial surrogacy, amongst other offences, will entail a jail term of at least ten years and a fine of up to Rs. 10 lakhs.

"The right to life enshrines the right of reproductive autonomy, inclusive of the right to procreation and parenthood, which is not within the domain of the State, and does not warrant interference of a fundamental right. It is for the person and not the State to decide modes of parenthood. It is the prerogative of person(s) to have children born naturally or by surrogacy in which the State, constitutionally and legally cannot interfere or impose itself.

Surrogacy in India is relatively low cost and the legal environment is favorable. In 2008, the Supreme Court of India in the Manji's case (Japanese Baby) has held that commercial surrogacy is permitted in India with a direction to the Legislature to pass an appropriate Law governing Surrogacy in India. At present the Surrogacy Contract between the parties and the Assisted Reproductive Technique (ART) Clinics guidelines are the guiding force. Giving due regard to the apex court directions, the Legislature has enacted ART BILL, 2008 which is still pending and is expected to come in force somewhere in the next coming year. The law commission of India has specifically reviewed the Surrogacy Law keeping in mind that in India that India is an International Surrogacy destination.

International Surrogacy involves bilateral issues, where the laws of both the nations have to be at par/uniformity else the concerns and interests of parties involved will remain unresolved and thus, giving due regard to the concerns and in order to prevent the commercialization of the Human Reproductive system, exploitation of women and the commodification of Children, the law commission has submitted its report with the relevant suggestion:

> The Law Commission of India has submitted the 228th Report on "NEED FOR LEGISLATION TO REGULATE ASSISTED REPRODUCTIVE

TECHNOLOGY CLINICS AS WELL AS RIGHTS AND OBLIGATIONS OF PARTIES TO A SURROGACY." The following observations had been made by the Law Commission:

- Surrogacy arrangement will continue to be governed by contract amongst parties, which will contain all the terms requiring consent of surrogate mother to bear child, agreement of her husband and other family members for the same, medical procedures of artificial insemination, reimbursement of all reasonable expenses for carrying child to full term, willingness to hand over the child born to the commissioning parents. But such an arrangement should not be for commercial purposes.
- A surrogacy arrangement should provide for financial support for surrogate child in the event of death of the commissioning couple or individual before delivery of the child, or divorce between the intended parents and subsequent willingness of none to take delivery of the child.
- A surrogacy contract should necessarily take care of life insurance cover for surrogate mother.
- One of the intended parents should be a donor as well, because the bond of love and affection with a child primarily emanates from biological relationship. Also, the chances of various kinds of child-abuse, which have been noticed in cases of adoptions, will be reduced. In case the intended parent is single, he or she should be a donor to be able to have a surrogate child. Otherwise, adoption is the way to have a child which is resorted to if biological (natural) parents and adoptive parents are different.
- Legislation itself should recognize a surrogate child to be the legitimate child of the commissioning parent(s) without there being any need for adoption or even declaration of guardian.
- The birth certificate of the surrogate child should contain the name(s) of the commissioning parent(s) only.
- Right to privacy of donor as well as surrogate mother should be protected.
- Sex-selective surrogacy should be prohibited.
- Cases of abortions should be governed by the Medical Termination of Pregnancy Act 1971 only.

The Report has come largely in support of the Surrogacy in India, highlighting a proper way of operating surrogacy in Indian conditions. Exploitation of the women through surrogacy is another worrying factor, which the law has to address.

The recent Surrogacy (Regulations) Bill 2016 proposes for domestic altruistic surrogacy and prohibiting commercial, overseas or foreign surrogacy in India and permitting surrogacy only for such "Indian heterosexually married couples whose marriage has subsisted for five years or more wherein either couple are infertile". The recent cases of celeb single parent surrogacy has questioned the legality and raised debates on the permissibility of same.

While this Surrogacy bill awaits enactment, it is pertinent to refer and reiterate existing Supreme Court judicial pronouncement and the existing Law commission report and the Medical council guidelines on surrogacy, these seek to permit for single parent surrogacy. ICMR Medical Guidelines on regulating ART, Surrogacy 2005 contains no bar to surrogacy for single parent in India.

Supreme Court on Single parent surrogacy in India - In the landmark case of Baby Manji Vs. Union of India (2008)

The Supreme Court acknowledges the fact that "for certain individuals under typical medical situation "surrogacy is the only available option for parents who wish to have a child that is biologically related to them." In the course of judgement the apex court expressly states that the "intended parent may be a single individual" who may equally be allowed or permitted to commission surrogacy in India".[30] However the apex court directed the legislature to enact a regulatory statute on the same.

The Law Commission on Single Parent Surrogacy In India[31] recommendations on single parent surrogacy in India - "In case the intended parent is single, he or she should be a donor to be able to have a surrogate child".

On the other side, the single parenting through adoption is not only permitted but also made more flexible under the legal instruments, judicial developments. The Ministry of Women and Child Development Central Adoption Resource Agency (CARA) Guidelines governing adoption of children, 2015 permits single female to adopt a child of any gender, whereas single male person is allowed to adopt only male child and not adopt a girl child.

Secondly the age limit for single parent adoption has been lowered from 30 to 25 at present. The Delhi High Court in Shalu Nigam & Anr vs The Regional Passport Officer & others, 2016 held that "a single woman can be a natural guardian and also a parent" and "mother's name alone is sufficient in certain cases where she is a single parent in passport".

The Delhi HC held that "the single parent families are on the rise for various reasons by enumerating expressly single parent families as children born through IVF (in vitro fertilisation) technology" "surrogate mother". Therefore such inconsistent and varied approach for single parent surrogacy and single parenting through adoption or otherwise is questionable and arbitrary.

Another strongly favourable ground permitting single parent surrogacy finds its basis in constitutional right and international human rights under conventions. The single parent surrogacy falls within the ambit of right to health, right to access medical technology, right to family formation, right to privacy which are core constituents of right to life, personal liberty guaranteed under article 21 of Indian

30 (WP(C) No. 369 of 2008. (2008) 13 SCC 518., Para 11.)

31 -Law Commission report no 228 of the year 2009

constitution to every individual. A series of judicial precedents Kharak Singh v. State of Bihar (1963) Govind v. State of M.P, (1975), B. K. Parthasarthi v. Government of Andhra Pradesh (2000) have held "the right of reproductive autonomy, right to privacy, personal liberty, health, family formation of individual as facet of right to life under article 21 of Indian constitution".

These right are also guaranteed under series of international human right conventions as Universal Declaration of Human Rights 1948, International Covenant on Economic, Social and Cultural Rights 1966, (ICCPR) International Covenant on Economic, Social and Cultural Rights 1996 (ICESCR).Continuing on the right to privacy, reproductive freedom, it may be rightful to mention that any means of procreation or attainment of parenthood including adoption, fosterage or surrogacy, IVF or means of conception is essentially a subject matter of right to individual privacy, personal liberty.

Adoption is a socially benevolent choice and adoption is open for all including fertile and infertile couples, individuals under the Indian laws. Compelling the infertile alone who are already reeling under the stress of failed attempts of conceptions, medical treatments ailing couples to adopt is discriminatory and differential treatment of such couples or individuals on the ground of their medical incapacity. A same couple may adopt their first child and the same couple may have their second child through adoption, therefore putting adoption against surrogacy is neither desirable not pragmatic.

Ethical value of Surrogacy

Surrogacy is a boon given by the science to help the childless couple. Many couples, young women's don't think of the second child but if there is someone in family or in friend circle who is childless then definitely renting of womb is an option. The ethics of surrogacy include its brighter as well as its darker side:

The 'Con' voice against Surrogacy include some major ethical issues-

- Surrogacy is Like Prostitution- A typical objection to surrogacy particularly that of commercial surrogacy is comparing the physical aspects of surrogacy to a form of prostitution. In both cases it can be viewed that the women is selling physical, intimate, bodily services. Selling their bodies and their function for money.
- Surrogacy is a Form of Alienated Labour[32]- Many people work and are not emotionally attached to the 'product' of their work or the work process for that matter. This is physical alienated labor. Reproduction is something that many people believe belong in the private sphere and should be surrounded with respect and emotional attachment. According to people against surrogacy, women's reproductive capacities should not be used as physical labor and the status of a child, should not be relegated to that of a commodity.
- Surrogacy Turn Babies into Commodities- During a pregnancy a woman is supposed to bond with her unborn baby. Surrogacy prevents the

32 HEGEL's Philosophy of alienated labor.

mother from forming a natural bond to her baby and therefore forces her to emotionally detach herself from her pregnancy. Normally the child is the end goal in a pregnancy. For the surrogate mother the child becomes the means (as distinct from the goal), for something else, namely money. When the child becomes a means, the child is commoditized, speakers against surrogacy claim.

- Adoption Is Better for the World- The world is 'overpopulated' and that there are many orphans whose parents have died from decease or because of war. There are also many children who are living in children's homes because their parents couldn't afford to keep them. People have a moral duty to care for the already existing children in need of a loving caring family rather than proceed to make new babies into an already too crowded world.
- Surrogacy is for the Wealthy Only- Needless to say that surrogacy can be a very expensive affair and it is therefore not an option for those of few financial means. However, contrary to myth, many commissioning couples are not rich in the traditional sense but middle class / upper middle class. The surrogate mothers are typically, but not always, in the lower income range therefore the rich are exploiting the poor.
- Exploiting Third World Women as Baby Machines- Contrary to many Westerns countries, commercial surrogacy is legal in India and many Indian women have chosen to become surrogate mothers for Western couples. The typical reason for couples choosing Indian surrogate mothers over Western surrogate mothers is that they are cheaper.

The 'Pro' voice against Surrogacy include some major ethical issues-

- Fulfilling the deep seated wish for a family-Today upto 20% of women of every country have difficulties in getting pregnant. For couples who dream of their own children , infertility is frustrating and stressful. Having children and fulfilling the wish for a family with the help of surrogate mothers is therefore a possibility of living out that dream.
- Adoption is not that Easy process –Contrary to sensible logic (there are many children in need of a home - so adoption should be easy), being allowed to adopt a child is difficult and takes a long time.The whole paperwork process along with psychological evaluations and waiting list etc. may take many years
- Surrogate mothers are conscious of their choice- Under normal circumstances surrogate mothers are very conscious of their decision to carry someone else's child. They are well informed and well paid.

Most of these women have a positive experience and feel satisfied in what they perceive as an altruistic gesture (even though they are getting paid). While there are many religious organizations that frown upon the process of surrogacy, this concept is oftentimes the only option for some individuals to start a family. It is for this reason that some highly controversial and key ethical issues be addressed.

The Ethical Issues that are Pertinent in the Surrogacy Process

- Attachment with the Gestational Mother – In a surrogate situation, the gestational mother is the woman who carries the baby to term. This can be a very taxing process both physically and emotionally – and unique in that after the surrogate mother physically carries the baby throughout the pregnancy, she needs to physically and emotionally detach herself from the child once it is born.

Involvement with the Gestational Mother – Because the gestational mother will not likely be the child's primary caretaker, there could be legal questions that arise in terms of what – if any – involvement she will have with the child once born.

Identity of the Child – There are also ethical considerations that are brought to mind in terms of informing the child of his or her surrogate mother, as doing so may have an effect on the child's self-identity.

In addition to the above issues, there is also the factor of surrogate mother compensation. It is typically expected that the intended parents of the child will reimburse the surrogate mother for her medical and other related expenses. This can include a dollar amount for her hospitalization as well as incidentals such as her maternity clothing, meals, and other similar costs that she may be out during her time of pregnancy. With this in mind, it is thought by some that surrogacy could be thought of as being a luxury that is only available to the wealthy and in some cases it could even be thought of as pregnancy-for-hire.

The ever-rising prevalence of infertility world over has lead to advancement of assisted reproductive techniques (ART). Herein, surrogacy comes as an alternative when the infertile woman or couple is not able to reproduce. Surrogacy may be commercial or altruistic, depending upon whether the surrogate receives financial reward for her pregnancy.

Economic Marginalization of the Surrogates

Under the Surrogacy Framework

Although there are various opinions that have been put forth concerning the employment of a woman to conceive and the reception of a remuneration by her for the same, the fact stands that such women come from an impoverished background and hence the only way of ensuring justice to them, at least one level when they are employed within the surrogacy arrangement, is that they shall be duly paid the amount that they deserve and not be caught in the reins of economic and financial exploitation and dragged to the shadows of misery.

However, in reality, the amount of compensation paid to the surrogate mother is less than what is due, out of numerous factors which may include misappropriation of the fee by the clinic authorities or the agents employed etc. These are the examples of how the illiteracy of the surrogate mothers maybe taken inappropriate advantage of, primarily, because of the lack of legal protection to the surrogates and the deficiency in the measures to regulate the ART clinics by the Government.

Hence, it is of no surprise that in the West, about 50% of the total amount derived from the surrogacy arrangement is paid to the surrogate, whereas, in India most of the amount only stands misappropriated and becomes an object of the Clinic's arbitrary decision.[33] There is no provision concerning the fee that needs to be paid to her in case she is unexpectedly pregnant with twins or when the payment maybe delayed for months after relinquishing[34]or whether they shall have a say in such matters of payment etc.

The After Effects: Children as the Objects of Subjugation

A very significant problem that may take place concerning the child conceived as part of the surrogacy process is with regards to citizenship of such a child.

In the Baby Manjhi case[35],a Japanese couple had contracted with an Indian surrogate and a donor for the purpose of conceiving their child under the surrogacy arrangement. However, the couple divorced with the contracting mother being no longer interested to assume the parental rights over the child. The genetic father, further couldn't secure a Japanese passport for the infant as the policy in Japan is that the passport records the name of only the mother that gave birth to the baby, and in this case, the surrogate mother was to be recognized. The Indian law doesn't allow single men to adopt babies and it required the Japanese father to adopt the baby since a passport could not be issued to the child. Eventually, an identity certificate was issued to the child with the Japanese father being given a temporary visa. The baby's Japanese grandmother had to eventually adopt the baby.

In another case, Jan Balaz vs UOI case, [36] family used a surrogate and a oocyte donor for the surrogacy process and had twins in 2008.The twins had birth certificates issued to them by the Indian Govt. with the names of the intended parents mentioned on them. However, with the German Govt. not issuing a passport to the children due to the non-recognition of surrogacy there, the Indian Govt. had to do so, but, it eventually asked the family to return the passports and left the twins stateless. Later on, travel documents were issued to the twins so that proceedings of adoption could be instituted in Germany. The twins were then granted the German visas for them to be adopted by the German parent under the proceedings in Germany.

Another issue pertaining to the children born out of the surrogacy arrangement is concerning the risk of trafficking that they may become a victim of, A PIL was filed in the Delhi High Court, wherein advocate Nanita Roy apprised the court of the possibility of the children conceived as part of the surrogacy arrangement being subjected to unethical genetic engineering, prostitution and other serious crimes,

33 *Access at : http://www.iaac.ca/en/commercial-surrogacy-in-india-exploitation-or-mutual-assistance-4 Access at : http://www.communityhealth.in/~commun26/wiki/images/e/e8/Sama_Birthing_A_Market.pdf*

34 *Access at : http://www.communityhealth.in/~commun26/wiki/images/e/e8/Sama_Birthing_A_Market.pdf*

35 Baby Manji Yamada v. Union Of India & ANR. *[2008] INSC 1656 (29 September 2008)*

36 Jan Balaz Vs. Anand Municipality and 6 others.

on the ground, that there is neither the scrutiny of the commissioning couple nor an emotional tie between the child and the commissioning couple. The problem was raised that with the lack of scrutiny over the acts of the commissioning couple and a non-collection of any records concerning the development of the child under the parenthood of the commissioning parents, there are immense risks pertaining to the well-being of the child.

Infant malnutrition is yet another problem. Surrogates are required to breastfeed the child during the first few hours following birth. Induced lactation of the surrogate mother is undertaken due to which they don't produce the same quantity of milk as a new mother shall immediately after child birth. This may create problems in relation to infant nutrition.

Can single Parents Pursue Surrogacy?

As non-traditional families have become increasingly common, more and more individuals have become single parents by choice. Every year, thousands of single men and women add to their families, many of them through surrogacy. Single intended parents generally experience the same process, enjoy the same benefits and face the same challenges as couples pursuing surrogacy, with some exceptions.

Single Parent Surrogacy Process- In general, the surrogacy process is the same for single parents as for any other intended parents. In vitro fertilization (IVF) is used to create an embryo that is then carried to term by a surrogate mother.

In traditional surrogacy, a single man could hire a surrogate mother, whose eggs would be used to create the embryo. However, most intended parents pursue gestational surrogacy, in which the surrogate also called a gestational carrier is not genetically related to the baby. While many couples are able to use the intended mother's egg and intended father's sperm, every single intended parent will need to use an egg or sperm donor in gestational surrogacy. This is the main difference between single-parent surrogacy and surrogacy for couples.

Many surrogacy agencies will help you find a donor and surrogate concurrently, or they may be able to refer you to sperm banks and egg donors within their networks. Single intended parents may also choose to work with a known donor, such as a close friend. Once you have identified your donor, the surrogacy process will continue as it would for any other intended parent.

Single Parent Surrogacy Laws- In the United States, surrogacy laws are generally the same for single parents as they are for couples. However, the legal surrogacy process is far from simple. Regulations vary from state to state, and because surrogacy is a relatively new method of family-building, many of these laws are vague and can vary in application.

Pros and Cons of Surrogacy for Single Parents- Hopeful parents have many options when it comes to starting a family, and single intended parents should consider all of the benefits and challenges of surrogacy before committing to the process.

Here are some of the advantages and disadvantages of single-parent surrogacy:

- **PROS**

Surrogacy allows individuals to fulfill the dream of parenthood, even without a partner.

Intended parents have an opportunity to maintain biological ties with their child.

Surrogacy can create meaningful, long-term relationships between families and surrogates.

In some cases, single-parent surrogacy may be easier than adoption because many birth mothers choose two-parent homes.

- **CONS**

  Surrogacy is expensive, and single parents may face additional challenges budgeting with one income. Because of the high costs of U.S. surrogacy, many intended parents choose to work with surrogates overseas; however, international surrogacy laws may prevent single parents from working with surrogates in some countries.

  Single parents may face a stigma throughout the surrogacy process and following the birth of their baby, and managing time and resources as a single parent can be challenging.

Single-Parent Surrogacy vs. Single-Parent Adoption

For many individuals hoping to expand their families, the choice comes down to two main options i.e. surrogacy and adoption. Both can be fulfilling means of achieving parenthood, but there are some differences to consider when deciding which method is right. Surrogacy and adoption are each complex issues involving their own laws, processes and variations. In general, prospective parents can expect adoption and surrogacy to differ in the following ways:

- *Genetics:* Surrogacy allows the intended parent to be related to his or her child, whereas adoption involves the transfer of legal rights from the child's biological parents to the adoptive parent. This creates significant differences in the legal process. In adoption, for example, birth parents' rights must be terminated before the child can be adopted into a new family. In gestational surrogacy, the intended parent is legally recognized as the child's parent before birth, and the surrogate does not have parental rights that need to be terminated.
- *Cost:* Domestic infant adoption and surrogacy both involve a variety of expenses, including agency fees, advertising and matching services, legal costs and more. In addition, surrogates receive compensation throughout their pregnancy, which can make surrogacy significantly more expensive than adoption. Also, there are fewer grants, loans and tax credits available for intended parents than there are for adoptive families.
- *Wait:* Adoptive parents may wait months or even years to find a pregnant woman considering adoption. However, there are many surrogates waiting to find intended parents, often making the matching process much shorter.

- *Control:* Hopeful parents generally have more control over the surrogacy process than the adoption process. In surrogacy, the intended parent chooses a surrogate and donor, whereas the birth mother has the choice of adoptive family in adoption. Because the intended parent has legal custody of his or her child before birth and surrogacy contracts are signed ahead of the pregnancy, the intended parent does not have to worry about disruption and can ensure the surrogate is receiving proper prenatal care throughout her pregnancy.

Sushma Swaraj hits out at Celebrity Couples

Minister for External Affairs **Sushma Swaraj** has condemned the misuse of altruistic surrogacy. She hits out at star actors and celebrities saying that there are celebrity couples who have two kids and are going for surrogacy which is reprehensible. "Big celebrities who not only have one but two children, a son and a daughter, even then they went ahead with surrogacy. Just because their wife doesn't want to suffer pain you can't go for this," she said.

Cabinet has given approval to a bill to ban commercial surrogacy. It is an important bill and it will be revolutionary in improving the condition of females. In the last few years, a new business of renting a womb has come, where a poor woman's womb is used to produce a child and then the woman to left to her misery. According to reports, more than 2000 surrogate clinics are currently working in India. There is a complete ban on commercial surrogacy.

There was also an angle that there are couples who are not able to produce kids but their relatives are willing to help then why should the government come in between. This is what is called altruistic surrogacy. National surrogacy board constituted under the chairmanship of health minister. Three female MPs are member of the board and two MPs of Lok Sabha.

Only married couples are allowed to opt of surrogacy. Gay, single, live-in couples are not allowed. The marriage should be minimum of five years and the age of the woman should be from 23-50 and for the man 26-55. If the clinic violates any rule then they will face 10 years of imprisonment.

Commercial surrogacy has been legal in India since 2002, a practice that has been fully taken advantage of by many stars in the Hindi film industry. Recently producer and actor Karan Johar became the father of twins, a boy and a girl through a surrogate mother. While the name of the mother remains undisclosed in records, Johar is listed as the father.

India has been a favourite country for those wanting a surrogate child. The cheap availability of the service enables an overuse of the practice with commissioning parents arriving from various other countries as well. In 2002, the Indian Council of Medical Research (ICMR) laid out guidelines for surrogacy, which made the practice legal, but did not give it legislative backing. A study conducted in July 2012, backed by the UN, put the surrogacy business at more than $400 million with more than 3000 fertility clinics all over the country.

Surrogacy- A boon for Single Parents

UK law has never prohibited single dads or mums having children through surrogacy, but the legal issues are complicated to navigate. That is because parental orders which give parenthood to the intended parents after the birth and extinguish the status of the surrogate are only currently available to couples, making the issues around parentage and nationality difficult for single parents to resolve.

In 2008 (when parental orders were opened to same-sex and unmarried couples) an amendment to the law covering single parents were made. This was debated in Parliament, but unfortunately blocked by the government which said that government policy was to allow surrogacy only for couples. Ultimately the President of the High Court Family Division made a formal declaration that U.K surrogacy law was incompatible with the Human Rights Act as it discriminated against single parents and their children. In December 2016, the government told Parliament that, in response to that court ruling, it would be changing the law to enable single parents to apply for parental orders. The remedial order changed the law and introduced to Parliament in September 2017, which could see the new law in force by mid 2018. Being retrospective in nature, previously excluded single parents applied even if their children were more than six months old.

Surrogacy – The Islamic Jurisprudence

Surrogacy involves a woman agreeing to bear a child, and subsequently to surrender that child to be brought up by a person or persons other than herself. Surrogacy may be useful where a woman is unable to bear a child, due to severe pelvic disease or she has had a hysterectomy or because she has medical problems (e.g. heart or kidney disease) and pregnancy seriously threatens her life or health.

The first possible situation arises where a woman agrees to be a surrogate is because of the reasonable compensation, secondly she may receive payment beside the reasonable compensation, lastly the money is not necessarily that important part but the principle reason i.e. for instance, a sister may bear a child for her infertile sister, and the whole transaction may involve no payment of money or other rewards.

The above mentioned techniques no doubt allows an infertile couple to have a child who would have the genetic compliment of the husband, if the husband's sperm is used to fertilize the ovum of the surrogate woman but the problem arises when fertilizing the ovum of a woman by the sperm of a man other than her husband can be regarded as an adulterous union. Thus it would be illegal under Islamic Law. Here, it may be pointed out that Islam does permit Muslims to have their children breast fed by other women. If that is done, then the child would be like the child of the wet nurse. This means that if the wet nurse has her own biological children then the child she breast fed would not legally be permitted to marry any of her own biological children. But, it must be emphasised that this privilege can in no way serve as justification for the surrogate mother. No parallel can be drawn between the wet nurse and the surrogate mother. The wet nurse provides the basic nourishment to the already born child, while the surrogate mother carries the unformed child to term and literally gives birth to it.[37]

The Islamic Verdict- Scholars of Islam have pronounced the following fatwa (Islamic verdict) regarding surrogacy- *"It is illegal and immoral to introduce into a woman the sperm of any man other than her husband. The formation of the embryo outside the human body will only be permissible subject to certain strict conditions. It will be Haram (forbidden) to form the embryo by the fusion of a woman's ovum with the sperm of a man other than her husband. It is also not lawful to implant into a woman an embryo developed in a haram way."*[38]

Consequently, it will be quite obvious that it is Haram to introduce sperm or embryo into an unmarried woman. If, in violation of Allah's Law, either the sperm of a man other than the husband's has been introduced into an unmarried woman or a Haram formed embryo has been introduced into a woman, the rulings will be as follows:

> *"If the woman is married, the resultant child will legally be that of her husband even if it is confirmed that the sperm used was not that of her husband."*

The same ruling will apply if the child results from a haram embryo. Even if the embryo was formed by the fusion of the woman's ovum with the sperm of another man, the child will legally be that of her husband. The 'donor' of the sperm has no right whatsoever over the child even if prior agreement or contract was entered into to give him the right over the child. If the woman is unmarried, the resultant child will be illegitimate and would be regarded to be that of the surrogate mother.

Surrogate motherhood is definitely not allowed in Islam due to the fact that many evils may arise from this procedure, which can be listed as follows:

- Unmarried women could be tempted into *'leasing'* their wombs for monetary benefits, which would, in turn, undermine the very institution of marriage and family life. In order to relieve themselves of the agony of childbirth, married women could be tempted to resort to this technique. Islam abhors such action.
- Since pregnancy cannot be regarded as a burden, but in fact it is a blessing, a woman who passes away whilst in the process of delivering, is given the status of a martyr.
- Finally, surrogate motherhood violates the systematic planning of Allah in the normal process of procreation.

Status of Surrogate Mother in Islamic Prospective- Status of surrogacy in Islam is Haram that is, forbidden. The verdict pronounced is that it is illegal and immoral to introduce into a woman, the sperm of any man other than her husband. It is also not lawful to implant into a woman an embryo developed in a haram way. Therefore, it will be quite obvious that it is also Haram (forbidden) to introduce sperm or embryo into an unmarried woman.

---

37 www.alarbiya.net/art2011/01/AFP

38 Islamic Principles on Family Planning, Qasmi Publication (pp.150-153)

Allah the Almighty says, *"And those who guard their chastity (private parts from illegal sexual acts) except from their spouses.........."*[39] Only a husband has exclusive right to the womb of the woman he is married to. This is because fertilizing the ovum of a woman by the sperm of a man other than her husband can be regarded as an adulterous union. Allah the Almighty also has mentioned that, *"And do not approach unlawful sexual intercourse. Indeed, it is ever an immorality and is evil as a way."*[40] Thus, surrogacy would be illegal under Islamic jurisprudence.

A man may wish to have a child, but he has no partner or a gay couple that wish to have a child using their own sperm. The womb is known as *'Rahim'*. This word is also used to describe one of the attributes of Allah that is him being the most compassionate. Perhaps the reason behind it is that the manifestation of Allah's compassion to human kind begins while human are still in the dark recesses of our mother's womb.

Islam does allow man to married to four wives but in condition that he can afford to be fair among his entire wife. The woman can ask her husband to marry another woman so that they can have a child that has the father's genetic link so that the child can continue his father's generation. This option is rarely viewed as an acceptable option by woman themselves as they do not like to share her husband with another woman. Besides, they can also legally adopt an orphan child if they really want one. An orphan child need parents for him or her to feel loved and the infertile couple need a child to give their loved to. Indeed, they suit each other.

Surrogacy practise in Muslim & other Foreign Jurisdictions having some Muslim Domination- Surrogacy has been banned in France where in 1991 its highest court ruled that *'the human body is not lent out, is not rented out and is not sold'*. It has also been rejected by voters in Sweden, Spain, France, and Germany. In all of the Muslim countries surveyed including the Middle Eastern countries of Egypt, Iran, Kuwait, Jordan, Lebanon, Morocco, Qatar, and Turkey, as well as a number of non-Middle Eastern Muslim countries including Indonesia, Malaysia, and Pakistan sperm donation in IVF and all other forms of gamete donation were strictly prohibited.

There are also certain countries that allow people to do it including South Africa, United Kingdom and Argentina but an independent ethics committees are employed to evaluate surrogacy requests on a case-by-case basis.

In the United Kingdom and some states in the United States of America, commercial surrogacy has been declared illegal but such arrangement are subjected to certain rules and regulations. It literally means that surrogacy is still allowed to help alleviate the sufferings of childlessness for some couples, not for commercial purpose. India is also allowing this surrogacy since 2002 until very recently, there has been no law concerning surrogacy in India.

The issues involved in surrogacy arrangement are the ethical and moral issues. Surrogacy requires exposing and looking at the private parts of the surrogate

39 Reproductive Revolution (Singer, P., and Wells, D. Oxford: Oxford University Press 1984).

40 Islamic Principles on Family Planning, Qasmi Publication (pp.155-158)

mother in order to implant the fertilization between the sperm from the husband and the eggs from his wife. This procedure may need to repeat multiple times and just imagine how many times the surrogate mother has to open her private part. This is one of the reasons why Islam abhors the surrogacy. In conclusion, surrogacy is not only prohibited under Islamic family law, it is also not allowed under Islamic law of contract. Al-Quran and Sunnah is guidance for those who seek the correct path.

If the infertile couple really desires to have a child, they can do it with the right way. Intention doesn't make things halal (legal) or haram (forbidden). Allah has created every being in its own fitrah and he has appointed that no change should there be in that fitrah. Although Islam allows its believers to try their best to find cures for disease, there must be a limit to every act because act which tend to prejudice the rights of others are strictly prohibited in Islam.

Conclusion & Suggestion(S)

The Government of India has sent a clear message through this Bill that there are certain cultural and ethical values attached to India which it cannot fail to notice. However, it fails to address certain important issues that are required to be perceived upon keeping in view the modern trend emerging in the society such as issues concerning unmarried couple,live in partners etc. also, it does not guarantee the safeguard against exploitation of a lady delivering child out of altruistic surrogacy nor it concerns her will. Unfortunately, it seems, that this step may result in enhancement of corruption in this regard as now people will go for this method secretly and furtively, making situations bad to worse. Followed by, the infringement of the rights of single parents, as they have been kept out from this perspective. Hence, the question that whether the Surrogacy (Regulation) Bill, 2016 is able to address the concerns of all stakeholders involved or not is a matter that remains still and debatable.

Although the bill was made and passed with the intention of preventing this exploitation, some of the clauses had both the medical community and the general public outraged. For once the necessity of only a relative being a surrogate mother. This limits the possibility of surrogacy to a very large extent, especially since most times, surrogacy becomes the very last option a couple chooses. Even though adoption is always another choice, the adoption process is long and tedious. One also needs to keep in mind, the stigma attached to adoption and the desire of 'true' heir in Indian societies. Even if the state wanted to curb surrogacy in order to facilitate adoption, in order to stop the privileging of biological children; there needs to be a streamlining of adoption procedures. The idea of "altruistic surrogacy" expressed in the Bill, as has been reported, greatly limits both potential surrogate mothers as well as couples wanting children since women can become surrogates only once, and since couples who cannot find willing relatives have only one way out i.e. adoption.

It seems ironical that people are engaging in the practice of surrogacy when nearly 12 million Indian children are orphans. Adoption of a child in India is a complicated and a lengthy procedure for those childless couples who want to give a home to these children. Even 60 years of Independence have not given a comprehensive adoption law applicable to all its citizens, irrespective of the religion or the country they live in as Non-Resident Indians (NRIs), Persons of Indian Origin (PIOs) or Overseas Citizens of India (OCIs). As a result, they resort to the options of IVF or surrogacy.

The Guardian and Wards Act, 1890 permits Guardianship and not adoption. The Hindu Adoption and Maintenance Act, 1956 does not permit non-Hindus to adopt a Hindu child, and requirements of immigration after adoption have further hurdles. There is a strong need to modify and make the adoption procedure simple for all. This will bring down the rates of surrogacy. Altruistic and not commercial surrogacy should be promoted. Laws should be framed and implemented to cover the grey areas and to protect the rights of women and children.

If the problem of surrogate mothers are looked upon, things are even worse and unethical. The poor, illiterate women of rural background are often persuaded in such deals by their spouse or middlemen for earning easy money. These women have no right on decision regarding their own body and life. In India, there is no provision of psychological screening or legal counseling, which is mandatory in USA.

Additionally, limiting a woman's surrogacy choice to only one time is in a large way limiting the income of those who survive on this business. Again, it comes down to the issue of consent. If a woman willingly consents to being a surrogate mother, is assured of a safe delivery; and the baby is assured of a safe home, why should she be limited to only one surrogacy. After the surrogacy industry boomed, a lot of women were dependent on the same. The issue here seems to be that the woman is exploited for her body. And this too, is a legitimate issue. Just as in the case of sex work, when a woman is coerced into the business because she has no choice, and because she desperately needs the financial resources, it does not mean that she has fully consented to the job. It means that she has not been provided, or is not able to find, alternate employment to sustain herself. However, if she is consenting and is being paid the proper amount, then this should not be an issue at all. In certain European countries, sex work is fully regulated and sex workers have full constitutional rights, unlike in India. This is very different from agreeing to go into sex work for lack of any other options. Similarly, surrogacy laws should be set out in such a way that there is full consent of the woman in question. Here, instead of regulating the ways and policies in which a woman's exploitation is prevented, what the bill has done is eliminate the idea entirely.

Additionally, egg donations are also banned, perhaps in order to curb child trafficking and illegal surrogacy racket. However, again a blanket ban will not help in this situation. Policies need to be structured and laws need to be implemented in such a way that the issue is resolved without censoring the entire industry itself.

One of the most contentious points of the bill is its blatant ban on surrogacy rights of homosexual couples. This is the first time that the government's transparent homophobia has come out in the open. Sushma Swaraj very clearly stated that surrogacy for homosexuals is against "Indian ethos", although homosexuality has been constantly mentioned in various Indian texts. Now, even though this ban could be construed as a mere following of the law (Section 377 against "unnatural" intercourse), this would only make sense if heterosexual couples also violating the section were denied surrogacy rights. Since there is no way to conclusively find out, this is obviously a huge denial of justice to the queer community.

Furthermore, since according to marriage laws only heterosexual couples are allowed to get married; the explicit stating of the ban of surrogacy to homosexual couples means two very saddening things: one, since this is the first time there has been an explicit stating of "homosexuality", this only reveals that the government is not even open to the idea; and two, the government is almost stating that the community might as well cease to exist in the former's eyes, since the latter have almost no rights with regard to their sexuality. It is also pertinent to note here that, the Bill prohibits surrogacy benefits to live-in-relationship couples. However, these kinds of relationships are considered to be in nature of marriage under Section 2(f) of the Domestic Violence Act, 2005.

Therefore, there remains an ambiguity that why these couples are prohibited to enjoy the option of surrogacy to have a child. Moreover, inequality and contradiction also exist in regard to single parent who might want a surrogate child. It is relevant to note here that, under Hindu Adoption and Maintenance Act, 1956, adoption is allowed to single adults but under the 2016 bill, single men and women are deprived of this right.

However, sometimes we are quick to criticize policies without understanding the true extent of the situation. The bill is extremely necessary in certain places in India; for example, Gujarat, where 'baby farms' exist, i.e. underprivileged women are rounded up in scores and given out as surrogates to potential parents. In this industry middlemen play a large role and take huge slices of the amounts paid by the parents, and only about 25% ends up with the actual surrogate mothers.

Finally with the Islamic perspective Islam does not support surrogacy due to the fact that many bad things may arise from this procedure. Unmarried women could be tempted into 'leasing' their wombs for monetary benefits, which would undermine the institution of marriage and family life. It would not only up heave the very notion of family relations, but married woman could be tempted to escape themselves from the agony of childbirth by hiring or using other woman. Islam abominates such action. Few of them who didn't want to suffer the agony of childbirth regard the pregnancy as a burden. In this situation, they are wrong.

Pregnancy is actually a blessing because Prophet Muhammad S.A.W said, "a woman who passes away whilst in the process of delivering is given the status a martyr." The worst case scenario is surrogate mother violates the systematic planning of Allah in the normal process of procreation. There is a consequences if the sperm of a man other than husband's has been implanted into an unmarried woman or a forbidden formed embryo has been introduce into a woman. There are, the 'donor' of the sperm has no right over the child even if prior agreement or contract state that he has the right over the baby. If the woman is still unmarried, the child will be illegitimate. Illegitimate child is a child whose parents were not married to each other at the time of his or her birth. If the woman is married and she is force to implant the zygote or she is willing to conceive the baby, the result is that the child will be the child of her husband even if it is confirmed that the sperm used was not her husband.

In conclusion, surrogacy is not only prohibited under Islamic family law, it is also not allowed under Islamic law of contract. Al-Quran and Sunnah is guidance for those who seek the correct path. If the infertile couple really desire to have a child, they can do it with the right way. Intention doesn't make things halal (legal) or haram (illegal). Although Islam allows its believers to try their best to find cures for disease, there must be a limit to every act because act which tend to prejudice the rights of others are strictly prohibited in Islam.

Chapter 18

DNA Forensics: Ethical & Legal Issues in Red Biotechnology

Amit K Kashyap

Asst. Prof of Law, Institute of law, Nirma University, Ahmedabad, Gujarat, India

Email: amitılaw@gmail.com

Abstract

In 1990 the human genome project coordinated by the U.S. Department of Energy and the National Institutes of Health. With an expected duration of 15 years, the goal was to read ('sequence' in the scientific jargon) the entire human genome, all 3.3 billion nucleotides of it. Red Biotechnology also referred as biopharmaceuticals has completely revolutionized medicine. It involves getting organisms to produce new drugs. From establishing paternity to use in Forensic, DNA typing has recently become a powerful tool for establishing biological truths to be used as evidence in court of law. DNA Gateway and G8/Interpol Search Request databases, Interpol is able to collate DNA profiles provided by member states and make these available to investigators globally where a match has been recognized.

As Processes DNA Forensics brings into collaboration the disciplines of science and law, the objective of this paper is to address the Legal & Ethical issues in DNA Forensics & also reflect a special reference to Indian scenario.

Introduction

In 1990 the human genome project coordinated by the U.S. Department of Energy and the National Institutes of Health. With an expected duration of 15 years, the goal was to read ('sequence' in the scientific jargon) the entire human genome, all 3.3 billion nucleotides of it.[1] Since the mid-1990s, forensic labs have been using this newfound knowledge to provide criminal investigators with DNA fingerprinting that allegedly allowed to identify individuals with laser-like accuracy.[2] DNA evidence collected from a crime scene can implicate or eliminate a suspect. In countries like US, EU & the EU government regulates National DNA Index System which contains DNA profiles of individuals convicted of violent crimes or felony

1 Forensic Genomics and the Science of Solving Crimes | Raddington Report. (2017). Raddington Report. Retrieved 10 October 2017, from https://raddingtonreport.com/forensic-genomics-science-solving-crimes/

2 Ibid

sex offenses, depending on each state's law. Government databases of previous offenders are growing, allowing more crimes to be solved through DNA evidence in these states. As a result, a host of questions, many framed as elements of a broader privacy debate, emerged. The U.S. government has also recognized the need for a greater use of DNA forensics in the courtroom.[3] Each of DNA testing technique raises serious legal, social ethical & policy issues. As Processes DNA Forensics brings into collaboration the disciplines of science and law, the objective of this paper is to address the Legal & Ethical issues in DNA Forensics & also reflect a special reference to Indian scenario.

Red-Biotechnology & DNA Forensics

Red Biotechnology also referred as biopharmaceuticals has completely revolutionized medicine. It involves getting organisms to produce new drugs, or using stem cells to regenerate damaged human tissues and perhaps re-grow entire organs. The same process of DNA technology and sequencing allows us to perform DNA tests to determine paternity, to calculate the probability of developing a genetic disorder, and even to identify a missing person or murderer. DNA Forensics is the application of DNA technology and the knowledge of DNA genetics to the practice of forensic medicine and to the power of legal medicine.[4] Sources of DNA include blood, hair, semen, saliva, bone and tissue.

From establishing paternity to use in Forensic, DNA typing has recently become a powerful tool for establishing biological truths to be used as evidence in court of law. Another major use of legal DNA tests is for immigration applications which are most often taken in order to prove genetic relation between two people. This can be performed through one or more of many different techniques like;

- Polymerase Chain Reaction (PCR) Analysis
- Restriction Fragment Length Polymorphism (RFLP)
- Short Tandem Repeat (STR) Analysis
- Mitochondrial DNA Analysis
- Y-Chromosome Analysis

Out of these the most common form of DNA analysis is called polymerase chain reaction (PCR) & Restriction Fragment Length Polymorphism (RFLP). The Process works by taking very small amounts of DNA from biological evidence and making millions of copies of it. This process, often referred to as PCR amplification, creates enough DNA to allow a laboratory analyst to generate a DNA profile.[5] Restriction Fragment Length Polymorphism (RFLP) is used for the analysis of unique patterns in DNA fragments in order to genetically differentiate

3 Lyle, A., & Harris, M. (2017). DNA Forensics. BioWorld. Retrieved 15 June 2017, from http://www.bioworld.com/content/dna-forensics

4 Medical Definition of DNA forensics. (2017). MedicineNet. Retrieved 12 July 2017, from https://www.medicinenet.com/script/main/art.asp?articlekey=23307

5 Understanding DNA Evidence: A Guide for Victim Service Providers. (2001). Ojp.gov. Retrieved 14 September 2017, from https://ojp.gov/ovc/publications/bulletins/dna_4_2001/dna7_4_01.html

between organisms which is used in DNA Finger printing & Paternity tests.[6] With this minimal amount of contact required to yield a suspect profile comes tremendous crime solving potential, and a number of considerations for prudent application, and the maximization of evidentiary value.[7] Forensic DNA analysis is key to the conviction or exoneration of suspects and the identification of victims of crimes, accidents and disasters, driving the development of innovative methods in molecular genetics, statistics and the use of massive intelligence databases.[8]

The DNA Forensics is used in following ways:

- to determine whether two individuals have a biological parent (Father/Mother)-child relationship.
- Preservation facilities for biological samples like vaginal swabs, blood, bones, nails, skin cells and other evidences collected at the crime scene.
- To generate DNA Identity card for identifications
- In identifying victims of war, terrorism, airline crashes, crime, civil conflicts, and natural disasters.
- screening evidence and DNA analysis from both violent and nonviolent crime cases
- Resolving biological relationships for immigration, organ transplantation and property cases
- DNA identification from buried samples/remains

DNA Application to Criminal Law & Forensics

Forensic DNA has emerged as the world's greatest crime fighting technology. Many countries are effectively using forensic labs and protocols to collect, test and compare DNA at crime scenes.[9] DNA databases are used to identify, track, catalogue, apprehend, and prosecute the perpetrators of crimes. Today, national and international law enforcement agencies exchange DNA profiles found at crime scenes to identify serial perpetrators and to help solve crimes around the globe.[10] Forensic DNA analysis has played a crucial role in the investigation

6 Phillips, T. (2017). Learn About RFLP and How DNA Analysis Decodes Crime Scene Evidence. The Balance. Retrieved 17 December 2017, from https://www.thebalance.com/rflp-definition-and-dna-analysis-applications-375574

7 Wickenheiser, R. A. (2002). Trace DNA: a review, discussion of theory, and application of the transfer of trace quantities of DNA through skin contact. Journal of Forensic Science, 47(3), 442-450.

8 Jobling, M. A., & Gill, P. (2004). Encoded evidence: DNA in forensic analysis. Nature Reviews Genetics, 5(10), 739.

9 Time for India to adopt DNA forensics to solve crime. (2017). Governance Now. Retrieved 12 February 2017, from http://www.governancenow.com/news/regular-story/time-for-india-to-adopt-dna-forensics-to-solve-crime

10 DNA Forensics. (2017). Dnaforensics.com. Retrieved 11 September 2017, from http://www.dnaforensics.com/

and resolution of thousands of crimes since the late 1980s.[11] It first made its way into the courts in 1986[12], when police in England asked molecular biologist Alec Jeffrey's, who had begun investigating the use of DNA for forensics, to use DNA to verify the confession of a 17 year-old boy in two rape-murders in the English Midlands.[13] In 1987[14], forensic DNA analysis made its first appearance in a US courtroom.[15] DNA evidence has an overriding role in the detection, investigation and nabbing perpetrators besides exonerating innocent suspects.[16] In 1987, Florida rapist Tommie Lee Andrews became the first person in the U.S. to be convicted as a result of DNA evidence; he was sentenced to 22 years behind bars.[17] During the mid-1980s, the potential application of DNA typing or profiling was initiated by laboratories in the United Kingdom (UK), the United States (US), and Canada.[18] In 2010 DNA profiling helped to identify and convict an Afghan national of committing a number of violent sex attacks in California between 2002 and 2004 and of a rape in Austria in 2009.[19]

A highly notable example of governance through techno-science is the use of DNA profiling in government-sponsored forensic science, just one of the ways people are being exposed to new modes of biotechnological identification schemes. The United States maintains the largest DNA database, with the Combined DNA Index System (CODIS) holding over 9 million records as of 2011.[20] The United Kingdom maintains the National DNA Database (NDNAD), which is of similar size, despite the UK's smaller population.[21] Index System (CODIS), maintains DNA profiles obtained under the federal, state, and local systems in a set of databases that are available to law enforcement agencies across the country for law enforcement purposes. CODIS can compare crime scene evidence to a database of

---

11 Forensic DNA | National Institute of Justice. (2017). National Institute of Justice. Retrieved 17 October 2017, from https://www.nij.gov/topics/forensics/evidence/dna/pages/welcome.aspx

12 R v Pitchfork (Case No: 2008/04629/A1, EWCA Crim 963 (14 May 2009).)

13 Calandro, L., Reeder, D., & Cormier, K. (2005). Evolution of DNA Evidence for Crime Solving - A Judicial and Legislative History. Forensic Magazine. Retrieved 15 August 2017, from https://www.forensicmag.com/article/2005/01/evolution-dna-evidence-crime-solving-judicial-and-legislative-history

14 People v Wesley 198 3d 519 (Cal App, 1988) (Joseph Harris J)

15 Can DNA Demand a Verdict?. (2017). Learn.genetics.utah.edu. Retrieved 17 August 2017, from http://learn.genetics.utah.edu/content/science/forensics/

16 Thierry, M. B. (2016). Improving Rwandan Criminal Justice through Forensic DNA Evidence: An Appraisal. Beijing L. Rev., 7, 400.

17 James, R. (2009). Breaking News, Analysis, Politics, Blogs, News Photos, Video, Tech Reviews - TIME.com. TIME.com. Retrieved 12 October 2017, from http://content.time.com/time/nation/article/0,8599,1905706,00.html

18 Committee on DNA Technology in Forensic Science et al, DNA Technology in Forensic Science (National Academy Press, 1992) 28.

19 Muñoz, H. S., & Fiodorova, A. (2014). DNA and law enforcement in the European Union: tools and human rights protection. Utrecht L. Rev., 10, 149.

20 Kumar, S., Verma, A. K., Singh, P., & Singh, R. (2016). Current scenario of forensic DNA databases in or outside India and their relative risk. *Egyptian Journal of Forensic Sciences*, *6*(1), 1-5.

21 Ibid

DNA profiles obtained from convicted offenders.[22]

The EU has gone much beyond has adopted a Resolution on the exchange of DNA analysis results and invited EU Member States to establish compatible national DNA databases in order to exchange data from the non-coding part of the DNA molecule, in 9 June 1997. [23]

Further, DNA Gateway and G8/Interpol Search Request databases, Interpol is able to collate DNA profiles provided by member states and make these available to investigators globally where a match has been recognized. Interpol has 184 member countries and currently forty-nine members are making use of the DNA Database to varying degrees.[24]

Legal & Ethical Issues in DNA Forensics

Modern DNA forensic methods are powerful and sensitive, but great care must be taken to prevent miscarriages of justice. Forensic scientists examine and analyse evidence from crime scenes and elsewhere to develop objective findings that can absolve an innocent person from suspicion or assist in the investigation and prosecution of perpetrators of crime.

There's also a risk that contamination might implicate an innocent person. In the case of R v Jama[25], DNA evidence was the sole basis of the rape case. Only after 16 months' imprisonment was it revealed that the sample taken by the doctor was probably contaminated.[26]

Issue of DNA Forensic Evidence Admissibility

Government-administered DNA databases, such as the Federal Bureau of Investigation's (FBI) - Combined DNA Index System (CODIS), do help speed the process, but they also bring to light complex ethical issues involving the rights of victims and suspects alike.[27] Increase in databanks for storing DNA information on individuals convicted of certain crimes raises important legal and ethical issues on the use, collection and storage of DNA evidence.[28]

DNA evidence technically doesn't pinpoint a single suspect, but rather narrows it down to just a few possibilities within the human population. However, it's

22 Advancing Justice Through DNA Technology: Using Dna To Solve Crimes | AG | Department of Justice. (2017). Justice.gov. Retrieved 5 November 2017, from https://www.justice.gov/archives/ag/advancing-justice-through-dna-technology-using-dna-solve-crimes

23 Supra 19

24 Gruber, J. (2012). Gene Watch Page. Councilforresponsiblegenetics.org. Retrieved 16 September 2017, from http://www.councilforresponsiblegenetics.org/genewatch/GeneWatchPage.aspx?pageId=367

25 [2004] All ER (D) 159 (Apr)

26 Smith, J. (2017). From the crime scene to the courtroom: the journey of a DNA sample. The Conversation. Retrieved 14 December 2017, from http://theconversation.com/from-the-crime-scene-to-the-courtroom-the-journey-of-a-dna-sample-82250

27 Norrgard, K. (2017). Forensics, DNA Fingerprinting, and CODIS | Learn Science at Scitable. Nature.com. Retrieved 16 October 2017, from https://www.nature.com/scitable/topicpage/forensics-dna-fingerprinting-and-codis-736

28 Reilly, P. (2001). Legal and public policy issues in DNA forensics. Nature Reviews Genetics, 2(4), 313.

extremely accurate and useful as long as it is handled and analysed properly.[29] The chances of one individuals DNA profile matching another persons are extremely small -- about one in a billion by some estimates.[30] Errors in the collection and/or handling of the biological samples used for the DNA analysis can result in the exclusion of DNA evidence at trial. Thus Legal Ethics by Defence Lawyers has to be followed to minutely scrutinise & challenge the admissibility.

In order to evaluate DNA evidence properly, the jury must have sufficient understanding of DNA analysis and the statistical calculations used to determine its probative value.

In the United States, there are two main tests for admissibility of scientific information from experts.

The Frye Test

In Frye v. United States[31] the US Supreme court held that the scientific evidence is admissible if the method is sufficiently established to have gained general acceptance in the particular field in which it belongs.[32] Thus, admissibility of the evidence depends on the quality of the science underlying, as determined by scientists themselves.

"Helpfulness" standard

Helpfulness standard is suggested by the Federal Rules of Evidence. In determining admissibility according to the helpfulness standard under the Federal Rules of Evidence, without specifically repudiating the Frye rule, a court can adopt a more flexible approach.[33]

Admissibility Issue Analysis

In *State v. Woodall*, the West Virginia Supreme Court ruled on the admissibility of DNA evidence. The court upheld the defendant's conviction for rape, kidnaping, and robbery of two women. Subsequent DNA testing determined that Woodall was innocent, and he was released from prison[34]

In Spencer v. Commonwealth[35], The Virginia Supreme Court upheld the murder and rape convictions of Spencer, who had been convicted on the basis of DNA testing that matched his DNA with that of semen found in several victims.

---

29 How DNA Evidence Works - FindLaw. (2017). Findlaw. Retrieved 15 November 2017, from http://criminal.findlaw.com/criminal-procedure/how-dna-evidence-works.html

30 Ibid

31 293 F. 1013 (D.C. Cir. 1923)

32 Borenstein, J., & Henderson, C. (2015). Reflections on Daubert: A Look Back at the Supreme Court's Decision. The Journal of Philosophy, Science & Law, 15(1), 1-4.

33 Golanski, A. (2016). Legal Considerations of Forensic Applications of Epidemiology in the United States. In Forensic Epidemiology (pp. 3-24).

34 The Dna Revolution - The Dna Wars Are Over | The Case For Innocence | FRONTLINE | PBS. (2016). Pbs.org. Retrieved 16 October 2017, from https://www.pbs.org/wgbh/pages/frontline/shows/case/revolution/wars.html

35 238 Va. 275, 384

DNA Test Validity Challenge

Matching DNA from a crime scene to DNA taken from a suspect is not an absolute guarantee of the suspect's guilt. In US recently, DNA analysis methods are under the microscope, with scientists questioning their validity.[36]

Fair Trial Compromise

There is a chance that investigators may come to rely only on the new technology rather than on traditional methods of policing. So they may fail to obtain corroborating evidence like eyewitness testimony and other forms of evidence. Thus results in over-reliance of science in general & undermining the criminal procedure at large. As, DNA evidence can only tell us that a person was at a crime scene, it cannot "prove" that the person committed that crime. Legal Aid Society and the Federal Defenders of New York wrote the inspector general last year that; the medical examiner's office "has engaged in negligent conduct that undermines the integrity of its forensic DNA testing and analysis". Thus the accuracy of DNA test is in question.

Human Rights & Privacy Issue

In some countries, databases that used to contain records only from people convicted of serious crimes are being expanded to include many innocent people who have been arrested but not convicted and people convicted or given police warnings or other sanctions for minor crimes. These people are treated as a 'risky population' who may commit future offences.[37] In many cases it has been observed that the police try to interfere in the personal life of family relatives of suspects & disturbs there personal liberty & also some times arrest. With the collection, analysis and processing of DNA profiles different fundamental rights could be violated, e.g. the right to physical and moral integrity, the right not to be subject to degrading treatment, the right not to incriminate oneself, the right to family privacy together with that of not incriminating descendants or relatives in general, the right of children to personal development and the right to informative self-determination.[38]

Moreover, The DNA related data is linked to pedigree, thus, such sensitive data has raised concerns for individual and familial privacy. Identification of a suspect can potentially bring police officers to the doors of his or her relatives to ask questions about their genetic relationship to the offender.[39]

---

36 Kirchner, L. (2017). Traces of Crime: How New York's DNA Techniques Became Tainted. Mobile.nytimes.com. Retrieved 12 January 2018, from https://mobile.nytimes.com/2017/09/04/nyregion/dna-analysis-evidence-new-york-disputed-techniques.html

37 Rights, D. (2014). DNA Databases and Human Rights. Forensic Genetics Policy Initiative. Retrieved 18 June 2017, from http://dnapolicyinitiative.org/resources/dna-databases-and-human-rights/

38 Muñoz, H. S., & Fiodorova, A. (2014). DNA and law enforcement in the European Union: tools and human rights protection. Utrecht L. Rev., 10, 149.

39 Khaleda Parven, (2012). Forensic use of DNA information: human rights, privacy and other challenges. University of Western Sydney Law Review. Vol 17:41.

'Forced or non-consensual' collection of DNA samples from individuals constitutes a possible threat to bodily integrity.[40] When the sample is given to the agency doesn't includes the consent for using it any way or even distribute it as the consent is given only for the purposes it was originally collected. The introduction of the DNA technology is being perceived to pose serious challenge to some legal and functional rights of an individual such as "Right to privacy", "Right against Self-incrimination" Concerns can arise, however, when tissue samples, genetic information and personal data are stored indefinitely on a DNA database. There are fears that the government and the police may be able to misuse this data and threaten our individual rights as well as that of our families.[41]

To elaborate this issue with an example; Kuwait was the only country to require nationwide compulsory DNA testing. In 2016 the United Nations Human Rights Committee, which monitors implementation of the International Covenant on Civil and Political Rights, found that the law imposed "unnecessary and disproportionate restrictions on the right to privacy. [42]Last year, The Constitutional Court's decision on October 5, 2017 to strike down Kuwait's overly broad DNA law is a positive step for the right to privacy in the country.

Data Protection

One of the fundamental rights guaranteed by the Charter of Fundamental Rights of the European Union and the European Convention on Human Rights, is the right to the protection of personal data.[43] The national Laws with respect to data protection in DNA profiling & storage is not sufficient as repeatedly a DNA profile is used to be sent from one state to another & lacks data protection sanctions. As genetic databases become increasingly common in other countries (over 60 countries are now operating one) the sharing of data between international police forces is likely to increase.[44]

Data Sharing

One more ethical issue is the sharing of DNA confidential data with private companies. There are some instances where subsequent access by a third party has been permitted, where the question of ethics appears to have been ignored. As this data is also being used for statistical, educational and medical research purposes. DNA samples are a potential source of human genetic information and can reveal sensitive health information & this could be of great use to health related MNC, s.

40 Ibid

41 Ramachandran, N. (2017). Is profiling in India's DNA?. http://www.livemint.com/. Retrieved 2 February 2018, from http://www.livemint.com/Opinion/6wGBEP2ThTvjzT4175jVOO/Is-profiling-in-Indias-DNA.html

42 wallace, h. (2017). Kuwait: Court Strikes Down Draconian DNA Law. Forensic Genetics Policy Initiative. Retrieved 12 January 2018, from http://dnapolicyinitiative.org/kuwait-court-strikes-down-draconian-dna-law/

43 Supra 37

44 Is it ethical to have a national DNA database?. (2017). Yourgenome.org. Retrieved 12 August 2017, from https://www.yourgenome.org/debates/is-it-ethical-to-have-a-national-dna-database

Genetic Minority

The selection of better DNA has raised societal as well as practical implications. As the people could select spouse on the basis of this data & even can go ahead with selection for any partner etc. It could also give rise to discrimination against and stigmatisation of an individual or groups. This will result in creation of class which is genetically inferior. a person's DNA includes information about everything from eye color to genetic defects. Some people fear that the widespread use of DNA databases could encourage governments to discriminate against people because of information encoded in their DNA.[45]

Dna Testing & Forensics: India Scenario

There is no Specific legislation or guidelines in India which could direct the investigating agencies regarding DNA forensics & gathering evidences. Moreover, Indian Evidence Act, 1872 and Code of Criminal Procedure, 1973 is also silent in addressing science, technology and forensic science issues.

Due to lack of having any such provision, investigating officers have to face trouble in collecting evidences which involves modern mechanism to prove the accused person guilty.[46] Section 53 of Code of Criminal Procedure1973 authorizes a police officer to get the assistance of a medical practitioner in good faith for the propose of the investigation. But, it doesn't enable a complainant to collect blood, semen etc. for bringing the criminal charges against the accused.[47] The were some provisions like; Section 53-A, providing that an accused of rape can be examined by a medical practitioner, which will include taking of bodily substances from the accused for DNA profile.

According to Senior Advocate Rupinder Singh Suri, President Bar Association Supreme Court of India; *"DNA evidence is key to justice delivery system! An invaluable tool, with 100% accuracy and reliability for exonerating individuals who have been wrongfully convicted. The conventional methods of investigation by the I.O/police are a passé being obsolete and unproductive. It is the scientific investigation only which kick starts the hunt for the criminal."*[48] Recently, In a draft Bill, titled the 'DNA-Based Technology (Use and Regulation) Bill, 2017', the Law Commission of India has proposed human DNA profiling, and proposed to set up Central as well as state-

45 Garden, H., Science, L., & Science, G. (2018). How DNA Evidence Works. HowStuffWorks. Retrieved 7 February 2018, from https://science.howstuffworks.com/life/genetic/dna-evidence6.htm

46 Bhan, A. (2017). DNA and Indian legal system. www.greaterkashmir.com. Retrieved 12 January 2018, from http://www.greaterkashmir.com/news/opinion/dna-and-indian-legal-system/265178.html

47 Ibid

48 Experts Demand Use of DNA Evidence to Solve Crime in India. (2017). Businesswireindia.com. Retrieved 4 November 2017, from https://businesswireindia.com/news/fulldetails/experts-demand-use-dna-evidence-solve-crime-india/55582

level statutory bodies for the same.[49] The draft DNA Based Technology (Use and Regulation) Bill, 2017 permits processing of DNA samples and puts in place safeguards against the misuse of data.[50] The bill is based on the recommendations of 271st Law Commission Report on DNA Profiling.

The Draft bill is result of a Public Interest Litigation filed by an NGO called Lokniti Foundation. The NGO raised an issue that thousands of unclaimed dead bodies that are reported annually in India but there is no national DNA database to maintain record of that. Thus, advocated that maintaining of the DNA profiles for this.

While addressing a Live Debate on where is the DNA, On November 1, 2017, Tim Schellberg, President, Gordon Thomas Honeywell Governmental Affairs (GTH-GA), said that; *"DNA is the world's greatest crime fighting tool. Consequently, DNA should be aggressively collected, tested and compared to the accused. DNA testing is happening in India, but not nearly enough,"*

Various legal & ethical issues as addressed in the paper are also a big problem for India. The was no legal infrastructure to safeguard the privacy and the safety of the DNA profiles against both thefts and contamination as well as the time period till availability to the stakeholders concerned, namely scientists, law enforcement and other agencies.[51] In India, the bill was first proposed in 2007 and its drafting began in 2012. Worldwide, this bill is already a standard law in more than 25 countries.

The bill has assumed relevance given the recent Supreme Court debates surrounding the right to privacy as a fundamental right.[52] In short, The bill introduce a set of legislative provisions that will allow licensed laboratories, police stations and courts around the country to collect DNA samples from certain groups of people, analyse them for unique information about the persons' identity, store them in a 'databank', use them as evidence during trials and to identify missing or unidentified persons.[53]

Conclusion

DNA Forensics has proved to be a worthy investigative tool for releasing the innocent citizens and bringing forth the person responsible for serious crimes but yet there is requirement of a robust legal infrastructure top address the legal & ethical issues like human rights, privacy etc. The DNA databases is rising very

49 Venkataraman, R. (2017). Another violation of 'right to privacy'? Law Commission proposes DNA profiling. CatchNews.com. Retrieved 4 February 2018, from http://www.catchnews.com/india-news/another-violation-of-right-to-privacy-law-commission-proposes-dna-profiling-74397.html

50 Supra 42

51 All you need to know about India's DNA profiling Bill. (2017). Moneycontrol. Retrieved 17 December 2017, from http://www.moneycontrol.com/news/trends/current-affairs-trends/all-you-need-to-know-about-indias-dna-profiling-bill-2327979.html

52 Ibid

53 Mukunth, V. (2017). The DNA Profiling Bill Is Back in a New Avatar – Here's the Lowdown - The Wire. The Wire. Retrieved 18 November 2018, from https://thewire.in/163958/dna-profiling-fingerprinting-bill-dbt-crime-scene/

firstly & also is traveling cross border, thus raises issues as to the efficiency, confidentiality, commensurability and infringement of privacy.

References

Gowrishankar, J., & Nandineni, M. R. (2016). Forensic science: Why India is rooting for its DNA identification Act. *logy*, 29.

Bhatti, S., Aslam Khan, M., Abbas, S., Attimonelli, M., Gonzalez, G. R., Aydin, H. H., & de Souza, E. M. S. (2017). Problems in Mitochondrial DNA forensics: while interpreting length heteroplasmy conundrum of various Sindhi and Baluchi ethnic groups of Pakistan. *Mitochondrial DNA Part A*, 1-10.

Schmitt, S., & Mazoori, D. (2017). Jurisdiction, Privacy, and Ownership: DNA Technology and Field Dynamics in Conflict-Related Mass Fatalities. *Genocide Studies and Prevention: An International Journal, 11*(1), 8.

Scudder, N., McNevin, D., Kelty, S. F., Walsh, S. J., & Robertson, J. (2017). Massively parallel sequencing and the emergence of forensic genomics: Defining the policy and legal issues for law enforcement. *Science & Justice*.

Bond, J. W., & Weart, J. R. (2017). The Effectiveness of Trace DNA Profiling—A Comparison Between a US and a UK Law Enforcement Jurisdiction. *Journal of forensic sciences, 62*(3), 753-760.

Jamieson, A., & Bader, S. (2016). *A Guide to Forensic DNA Profiling*. John Wiley & Sons.

Kayser, M. (2015). Forensic DNA phenotyping: predicting human appearance from crime scene material for investigative purposes. *Forensic Science International: Genetics, 18*, 33-48.

Butler, J. M. (2015). US initiatives to strengthen forensic science & international standards in forensic DNA. *Forensic Science International: Genetics, 18*, 4-20.

Chapter 19

Pre-natal Sex Selection and Infanticide: Advanced Technology *vs* Social Issues, Global Perspective

Viralkumar B. Mandaliya,

Assistant Professor (Research),
Gujarat National Law University, Attalika Avenue,
Knowledge Corridor, Koba, Gandhinagar - 382007 (Gujarat, INDIA)
E-mail: viral_mandaliya@yahoo.com

Abstract

Girl Child Campaign, Government of India with its prime line "A happy girl is the future of our country" which focused on burning issue of "Save the Girl Child". Since a long it's pertaining that mayhems against women in various forms has become an integral part of the civilization. Shamelessly, India has witnessed most barbaric acts against humanity that not only includes dowry deaths and sati, but also female infanticide and female foeticide. Technologies are invented for the betterment of society. Techniques such as amniotic fluid test and pre-natal diagnostic tools were introduced to identify any genetic abnormalities and to cure any potential birth defects and associated conditions. Mankind in his quest start to misuse of the scientific tools. PCPNDT [Pre-Conception and Pre-Natal Diagnostic Techniques (Prohibition of Sex Selection)] Act, 1994 aimed to control medical practitioners who try to influence the sex of child before conception by using techniques such as sperm sorting. The common medical practice of female fetuses' abortion after pre-natal sex determination has become most prominent issue even the legal regulations banning the same. Alternatively, people starts to move outside of India for sex determination. The misuse of techniques became a call of death for the tiny unborn female fetuses. It has been a most important topic as a social-legal awareness to the global perspective. There is need to create a transparency in legal form at global level to minimize misuse of medical practice and to save the girl child.

Introduction

The unborn child waiting for an aid, just because our fondness towards child especially boy child. Girl Child Campaign, Government of India with its prime line "A happy girl is the future of our country" which focused on burning issue of

"Save the Girl Child"[1]. Since a long it's pertaining that mayhems against women in various forms has become an integral part of the civilization[2]. Shamelessly, India has witnessed most barbaric acts against humanity that not only includes dowry deaths and sati, but also female infanticide and female foeticide[3] (Figure 1).

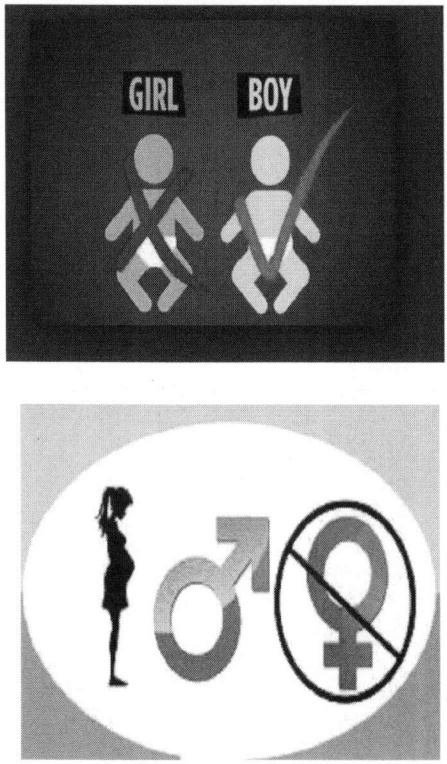

Figure 1. Child as boy selected against girl and became the reason of female infanticide and female foeticide.

Introduction of Medical Technologies

Technologies are invented for the betterment of society. Techniques such as amniotic fluid test and pre-natal diagnostic tools were introduced to identify any genetic abnormalities and to cure any potential birth defects and associated conditions[4]. Mankind in his quest start to misuse of the scientific tools. These

1 http://laadli.org, Laadli – A girl child campaign, Population First's campaign against sex selection and falling sex ratio, accessed on 20th March, 2017.

2 http://www.ndtv.com/topic/girl-child-campaign, NDTV, Section: Girl Child Campaign, accessed on 20th March, 2017.

3 http://ncw.nic.in/, National Commission for Women, The apex national level organization of India with the mandate of protecting and promoting the interests of women, accessed on 20th March, 2017.

4 Carlson LM, Vora NL (2017). Prenatal Diagnosis: Screening and Diagnostic Tools. Obstetrics and Gynecology Clinics of North America. 44(2): 245-256. doi: 10.1016/j.ogc.2017.02.004.

techniques just became a tool for sex determination (Figure 2).

There are number of invasive and non-invasive prenatal diagnosis techniques available for detecting genetic disorders/ abnormalities[5] summarized in Figure 3.

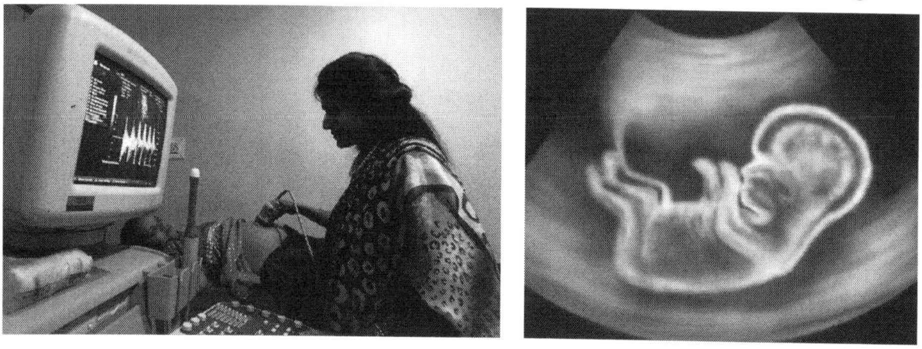

(a) (b)

Figure 2. Use of Ultra sound technology as a tool for sex determination. (a) The specialist is using the Ultra Sound Technology. (b) The developing fetus inside the womb observed under the Ultra Sound Technology.

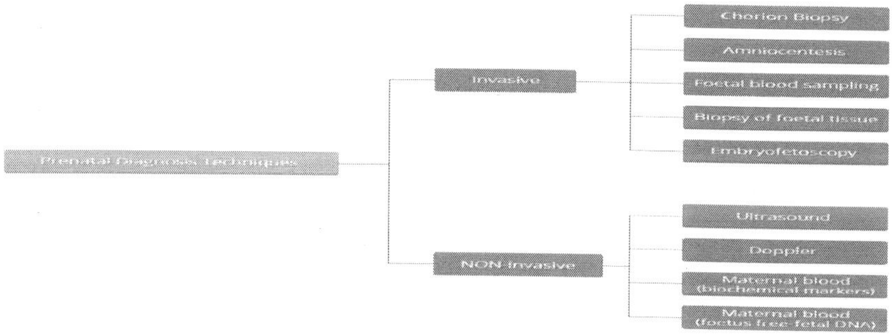

Figure 3. Invasive and non-invasive prenatal diagnosis techniques for detection of genetic disorders/ abnormalities.

Generally, various advanced prenatal diagnosis technologies used to sex determination[6] (Figure 4) and sampling for identification of fetus based on Y Chromosome staining[7] (Figure 5).

---

https://www.ncbi.nlm.nih.gov/pubmed/28499534.

5 http://lagenetica.info/en/prenatal-diagnosis/prenatal-diagnosis-techniques, Prenatal Diagnosis Techniques, accessed on 22th March, 2017.

6 Colah RB, Gorakshakar AC, Nadkarni AH (2011). Invasive & non-invasive approaches for prenatal diagnosis of haemoglobinopathies: Experiences from India. The Indian Journal of Medical Research. 2011;134(4):552-560. https://www.ncbi.nlm.nih.gov/pmc/articles/PMC3237256.

7 https://ghr.nlm.nih.gov/chromosome/Y, National Institute of Health, US, Y chromosome, accessed on 25th March, 2017.

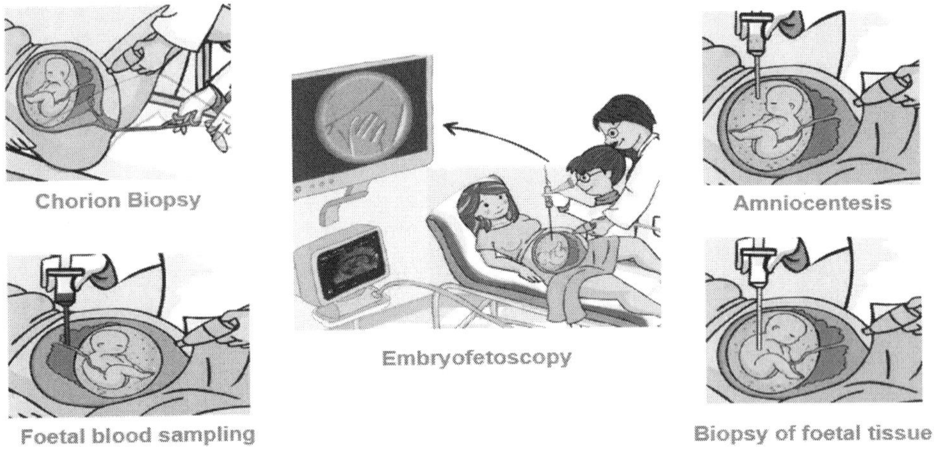

Figure 3. Various advanced prenatal diagnosis techniques for detection of genetic disorders/ abnormalities[8].

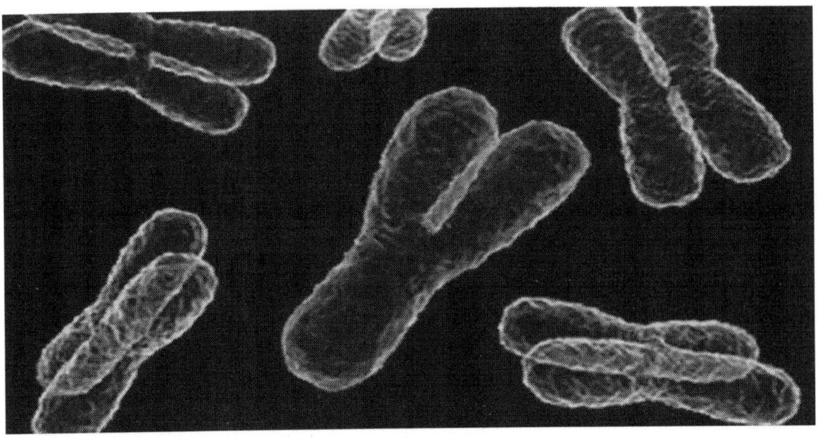

Figure 4. Identification of Y chromosome, leads to determination of Sex

The advent of advanced technologies for pre-natal diagnostic techniques leads to worldwide decrease in child ratio, especially the counties like India and China, where people more fond of boy as their child[9] (Figure 5). While Figure 6 summarizes the child ratio as number of girls for every 1000 boys since 1961-2011, prepared based on the Indian Census Reports of respective years[10].

8 http://lagenetica.info. Prenatal Diagnosis Techniques, accessed on 25th March, 2017.

9 https://soapboxie.com/social-issues/Female-Feticide-Causes-Effects-and-Solutions, Female Feticide: Causes & Effects of Sex-Selective Abortion, accessed on 26th March, 2017.

10 www.censusindia.gov.in, Census of India, accessed on 26th March, 2017.

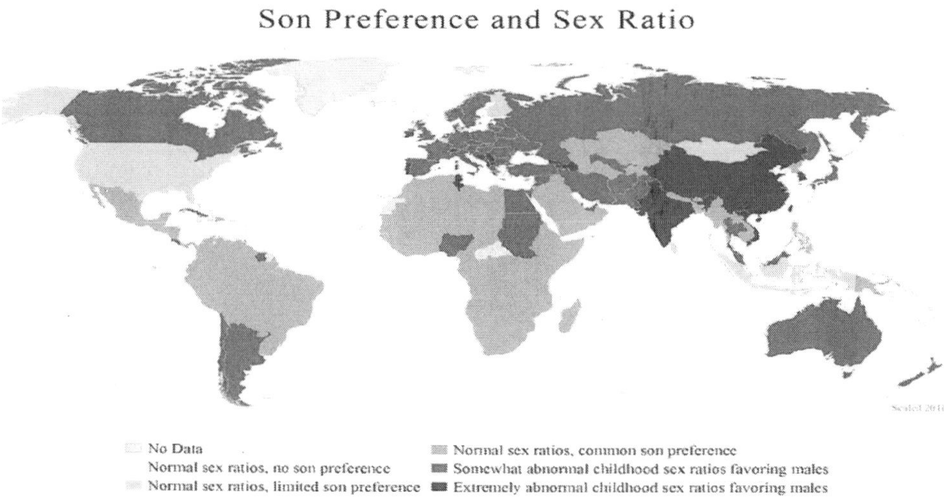

Figure 4. World scenario showing the son preference and status of sex ratio.

Figure 5. Indian scenario showing the child ratio as number of girls for every 1000 boys since 1961-2011.

An Evolution of PC-PNDT Act, 1994

Pre-Natal Diagnostic Techniques (Regulation and Prevention of Misuse) Act, 1994 was came into force in 1996[11] against the falling sex ratio and fears misuse of ultrasound technologies for determination sex of foetus. Then amended in 2003 as Pre-Conception and Pre-Natal Diagnostic Techniques (Prohibition of Sex Selection) Act, 1994[12].

The amendment was aimed to control medical practitioners who try to influence the sex of child before conception by using techniques such as sperm sorting. The common medical practice of female fetuses' abortion after pre-natal sex determination has become most prominent issue even the legal regulations banning the same. Alternatively, people starts to move outside of India for sex determination.

The 2011 Census conducted by Government of India, it is most alarming that a sharp decline in the Child Sex Ratio (CSR) highest in urban area rather to rural. It's directly suggestive that technology acquiring urban people misused well of it and resulted in decline of CSR[13]. Amongst the Southeast Asian countries, India

11 http://pndt.gov.in/writereaddata/mainlinkFile/File51.pdf, The Pre-Natal Diagnostic Techniques (Regulation And Prevention Of Misuse) Rules, 1996 and Pre-Conception And Pre Natal Diagnostic Techniques (Prohibition Of Sex Selection) Rules, 1996, accessed on 30th April, 2017.

12 http://pndt.gov.in/writereaddata/mainlinkFile/File50.pdf, The Pre-conception and Prenatal Diagnostic Techniques (Prohibition of Sex Selection) Act, 1994, accessed on 30th April, 2017.

13 www.censusindia.gov.in, Census of India, accessed on 25th May, 2017.

represents a one of most adverse CSR figures. It is reflecting a highly undesirable reversal of the norms of nature.

Awareness and Policy Development

A Socio-legal awareness among academicians, lawyers, doctors, researchers, and societal people towards Save the Girl Child based on conferences and workshops. This idea will cultivate inter alia connection and provide opportunities for exchange of views among them to discuss and find solution on scientific and ethical issues prevailing in the country.

Thus, there is need of actual ground of implementation and prospective of this guidelines and/or legislation for Pre-Natal Diagnostic Techniques. Global forum should be formed and such issues should be addressed to work out the Remedies for Female Infanticide and Female Foeticide.

Concluding Remarks

Girls are most important section of society and equally participate in life existence on the earth. The misuse of techniques became a call of death for the tiny unborn female fetuses. It has been a most important topic as a social-legal awareness in the global perspective. There is need to create a transparency in legal form at global level to minimize misuse of medical practice and to save the girl child.

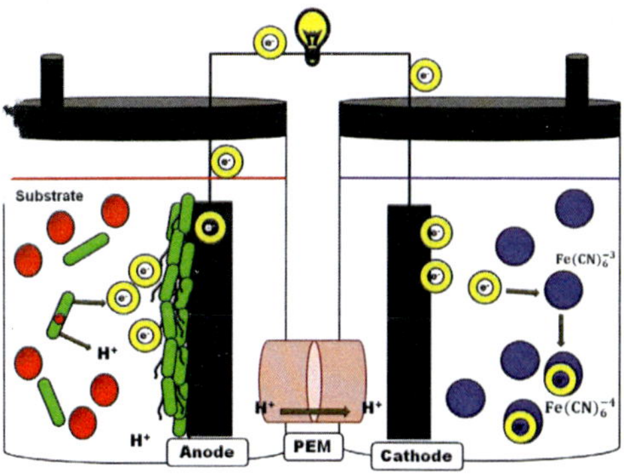

Basic H- type Microbial fuel cell design (p. 3)

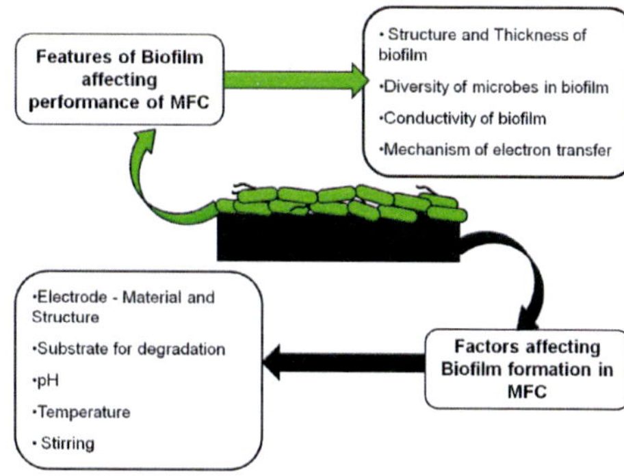

Conditions affecting biofilm formation in MFC and features of biofilm which can affect the performance of MFC. (p. 4)

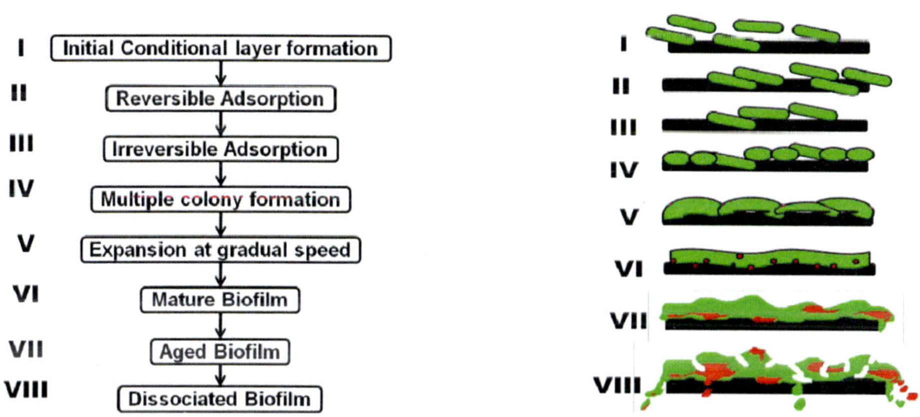

Flow chart 1: Flow chart depicting "The Process of Biofilm Formation" (p. 5)

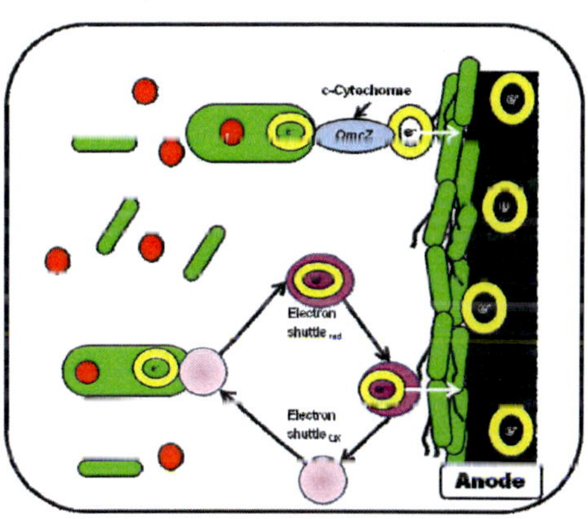

Cytochrome and electron shuttle mediated electron transfer from the microbial cell to the electrode (p. 11)

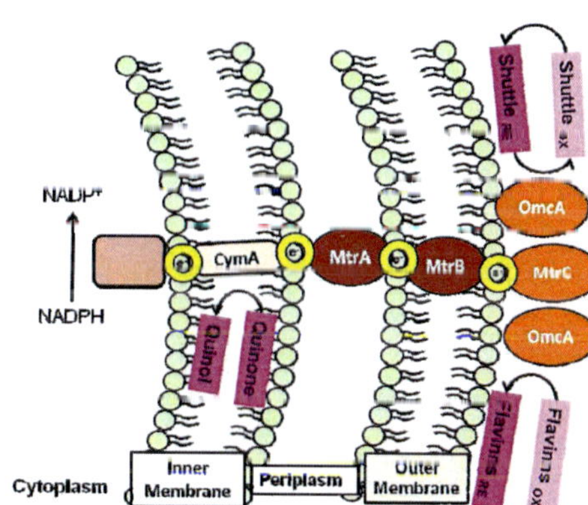

Extracellular electron transfer from the *Shewanella* cell to the electrode (p. 13)

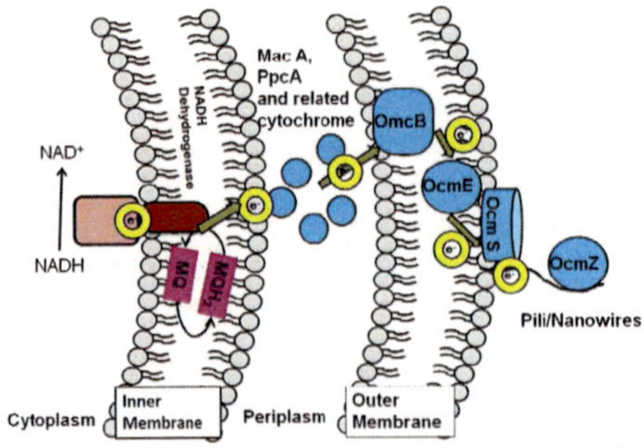

Long distance extracellular direct electron transfer via Pili/Nanowire from the *Geobacter* cell to the electrode; MQH2-menaquinol, MQ- menaquinone. (p. 14)

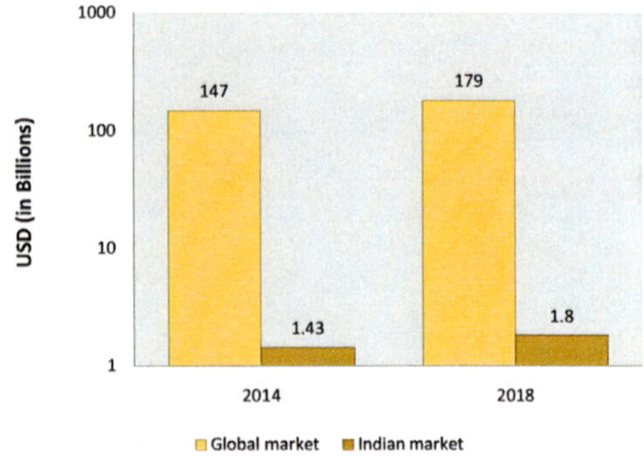

Market value of Technical textile (data from Indian Textile Journal, April 2017) (p. 50)

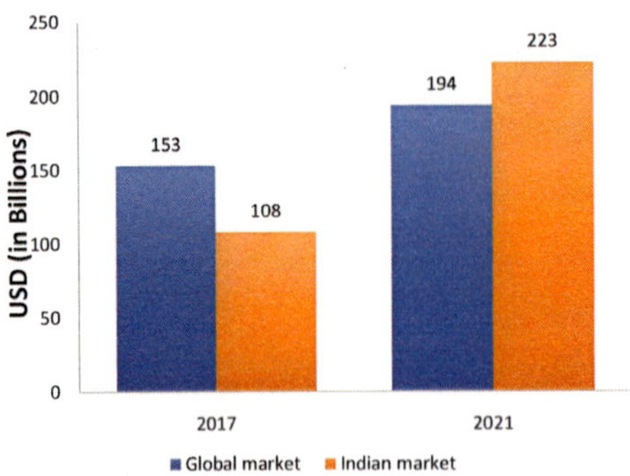

Market value of Technical textile (data from Indian Textile Journal, April 2017) (p. 51)

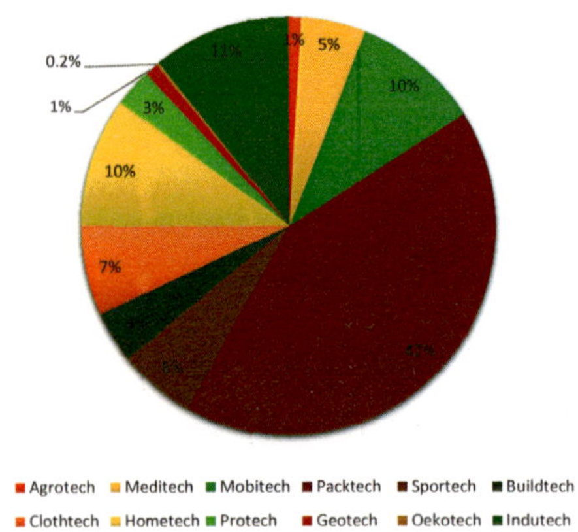

Segment Wise Sharen Technical Textiles Market 2017-1018(P) [Indian Textile Journal, April 2017] (p. 52)

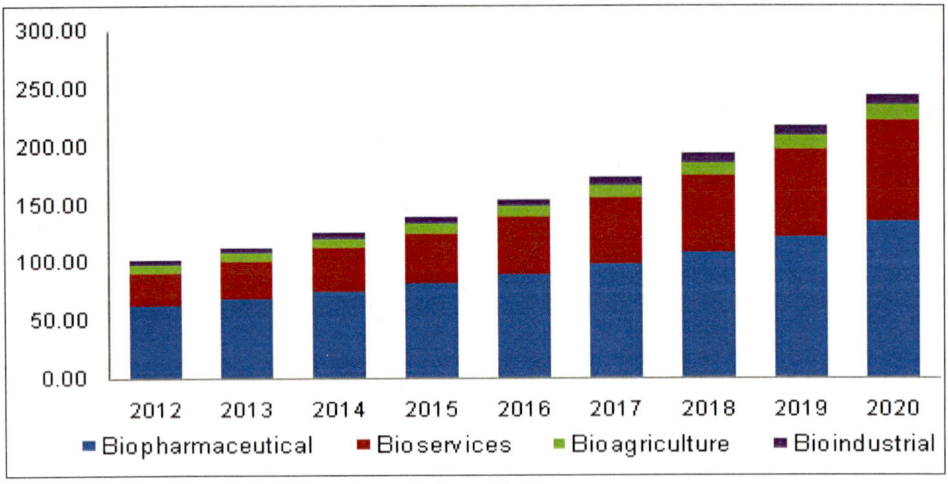

(p. 110)

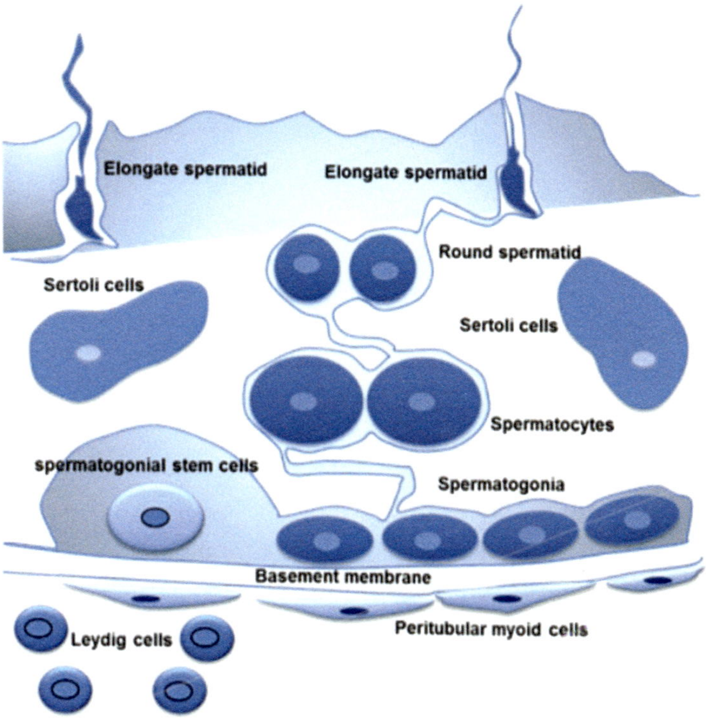

Spermatogenesis is the process in which rodents produce spermatozoa from spermatogonial stem cells by way of mitosis and meiosis. The initial cells in this process are diploid spermatogonia, producing primary spermatocytes by mitosis. The primary spermatocytes divide meiotically (meiosis I) into two secondary spermatocytes; each secondary spermatocyte divides into two spermatids by meiosis II, making a total of four haploid spermatids. These develop into mature spermatozoa. (p. 134)

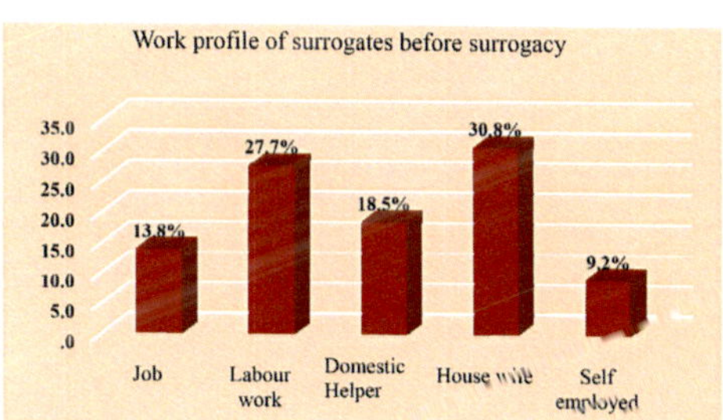

Work profile of Surrogate mothers before surrogacy (p. 162)

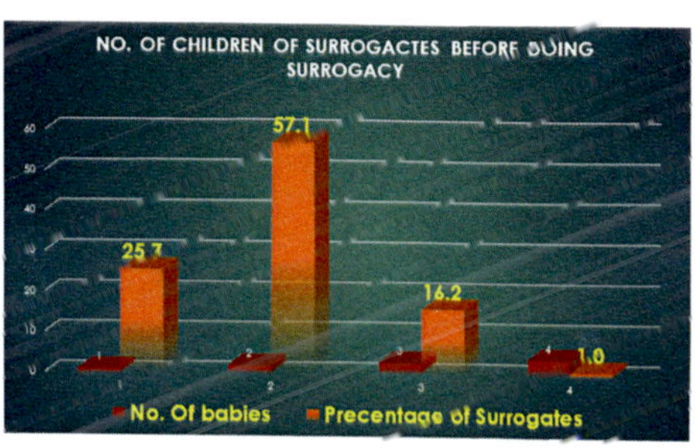

Motives of surrogate mothers behind practicing surrogacy (p. 163)

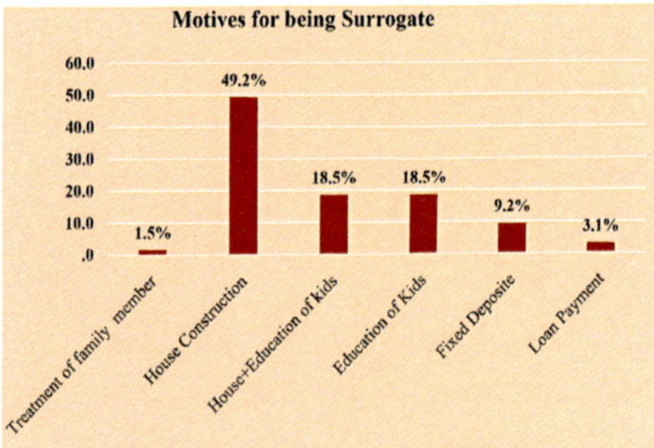

Motives of surrogate mothers behind practicing surrogacy (p. 163)

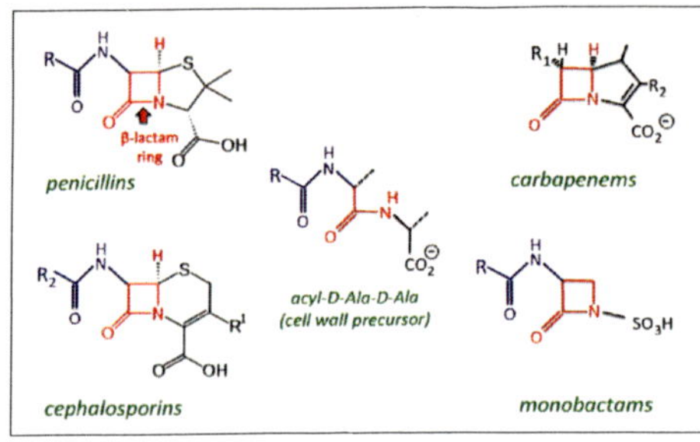

Structure of β-lactam antibiotics, similarity between β-lactam structure with cell wall precursor and site of inactivation by β-lactamase enzyme (Arrow). The 4-member β-lactam ring is shown in red. (p. 192)

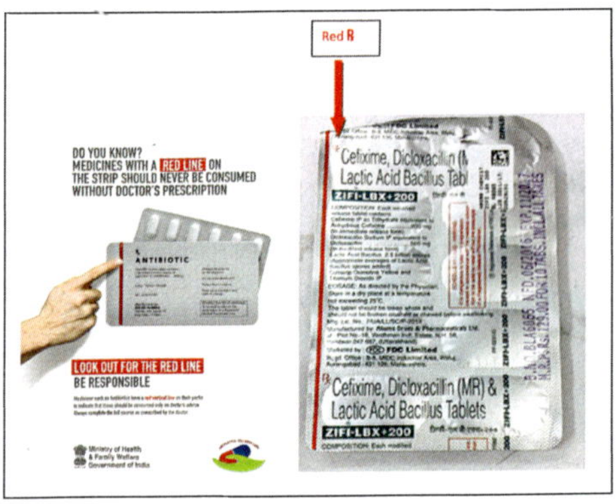

Increasing Public Awareness (p. 193)

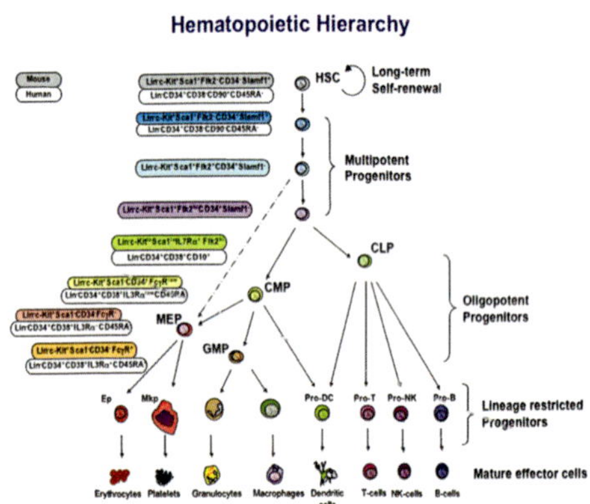

Differentiation scheme of haemopoietic stem cells (4) (p. 203)

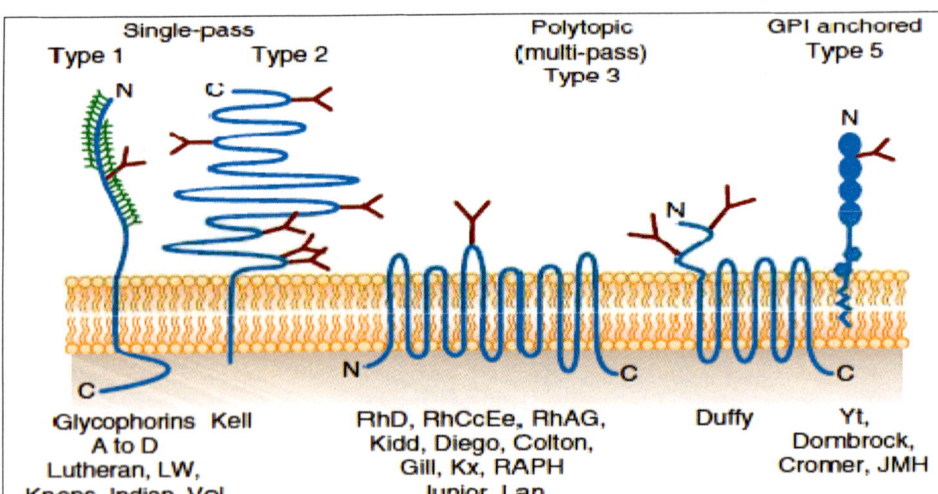

Diagram of different types of blood group active proteins and glycoproteins based on their integration into the red cell surface membrane. Listed are examples of blood group antigens for each type. (Type 4 proteins are cytoplasmic and not present in red cells.) (p. 218)

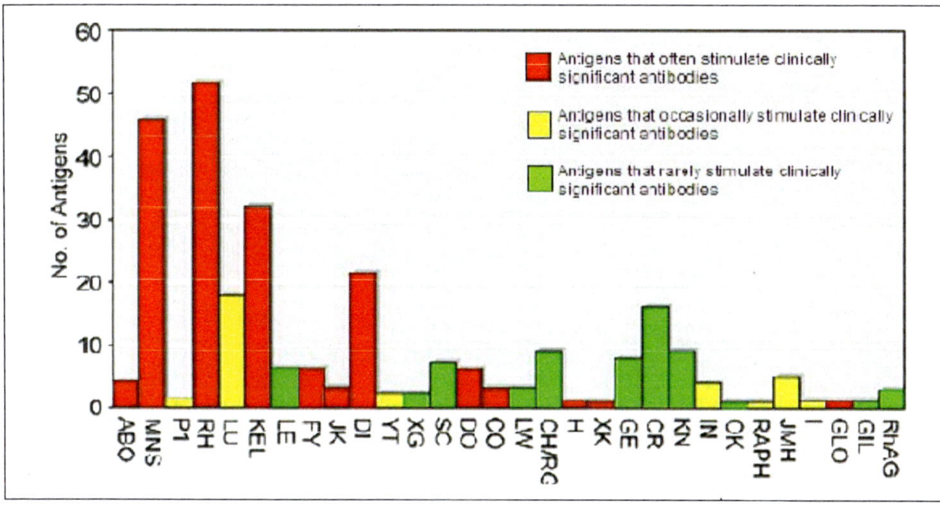

Clinical importance of different blood group specific antibodies [12] (p. 219)

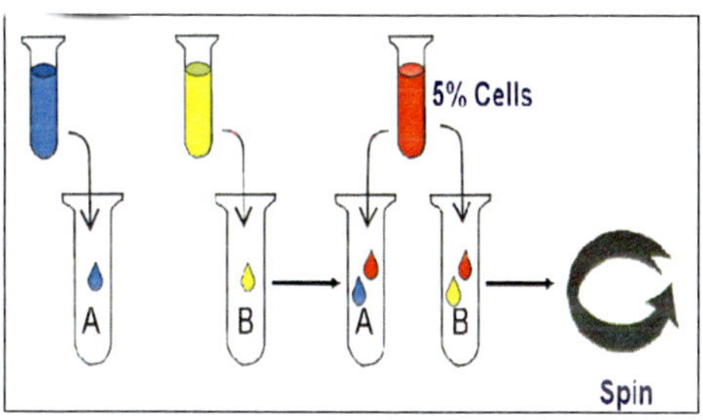

ABO forward grouping (p. 224)

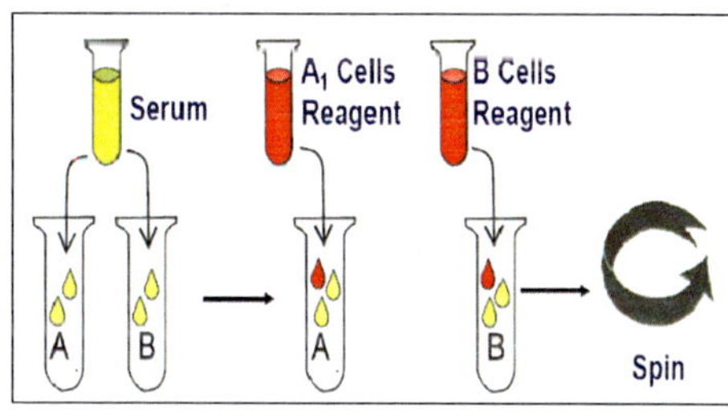

ABO reverse grouping (p. 225)

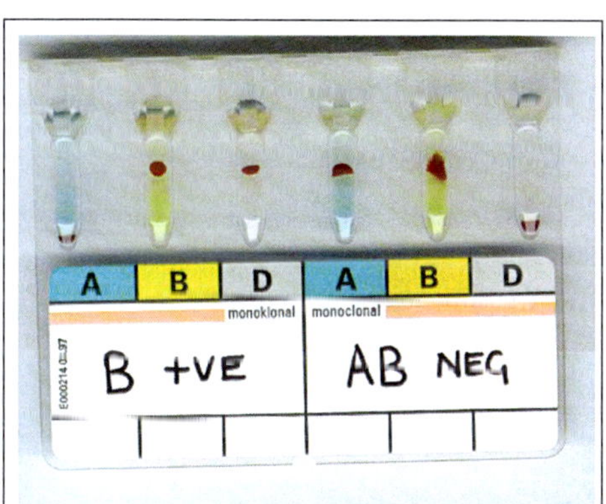

Gel cards showing blood grouping (p. 225)

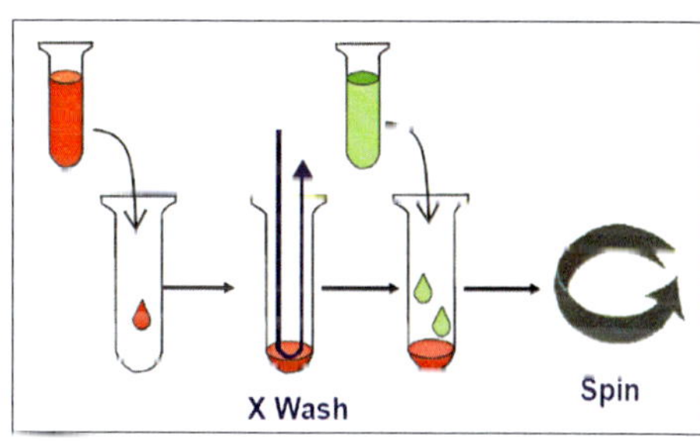

Direct Coomb's Test [DCT] (p. 226)

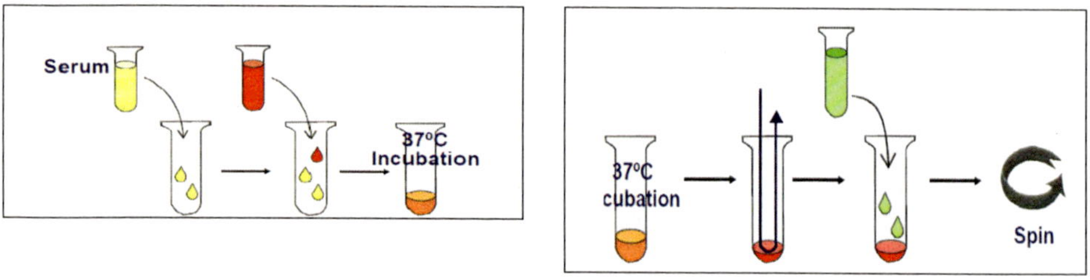

Indirect Coomb's test (ICT) (p. 227)

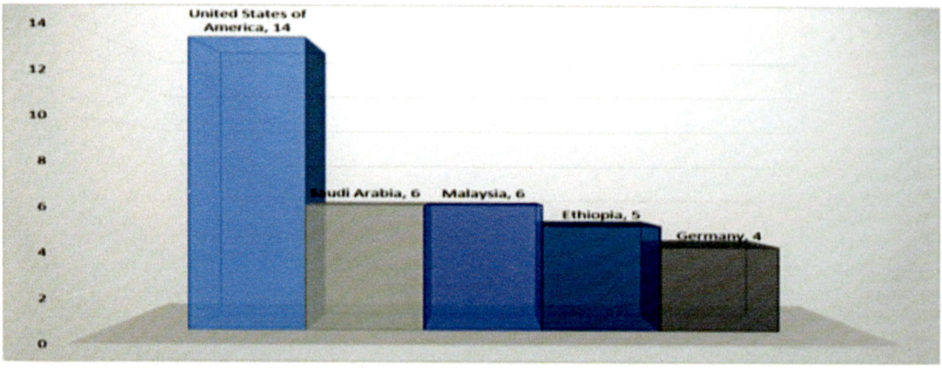

Top countries for their collaboration in the sector of "Medicinal Plants" (2004-17) (p. 254)

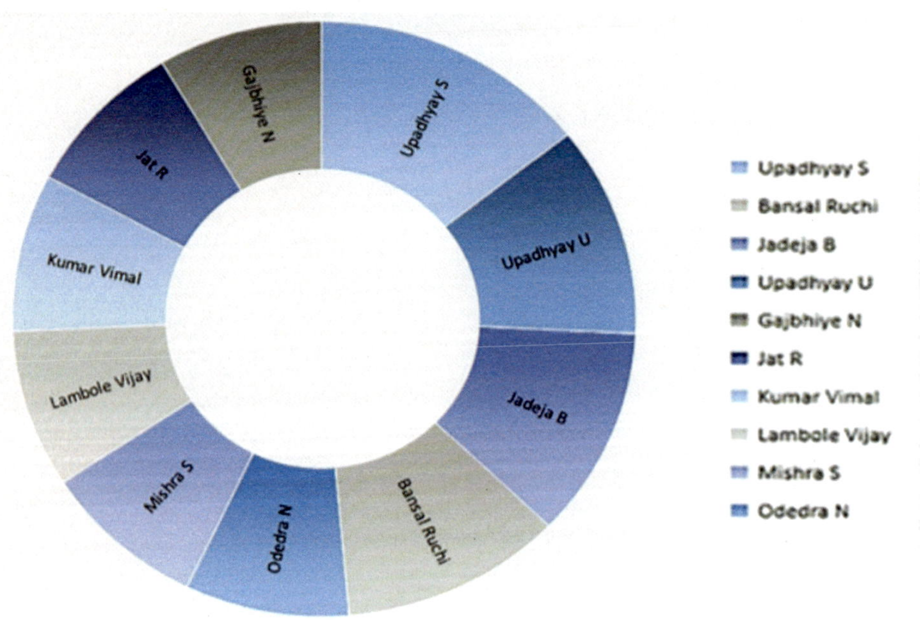

Top ten authors from Gujarat on the sector "medicinal plants" identified from Indian Citation Index (2004-17). (p. 255)

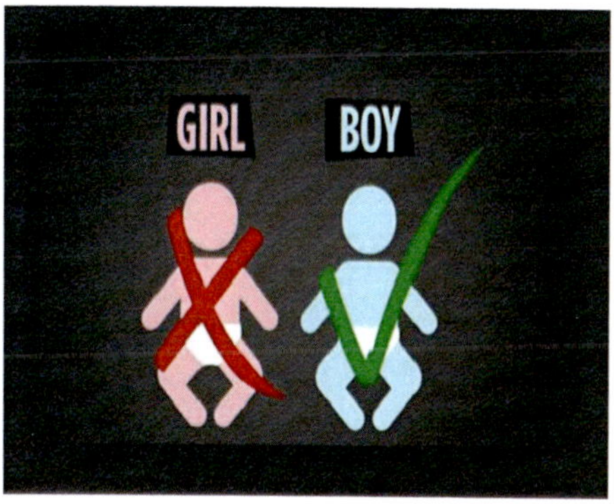

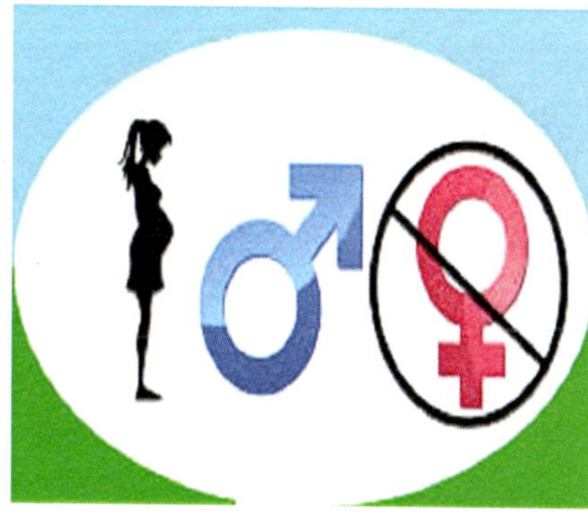

Child as boy selected against girl and became the reason of female infanticide and female foeticide. (p. 320)

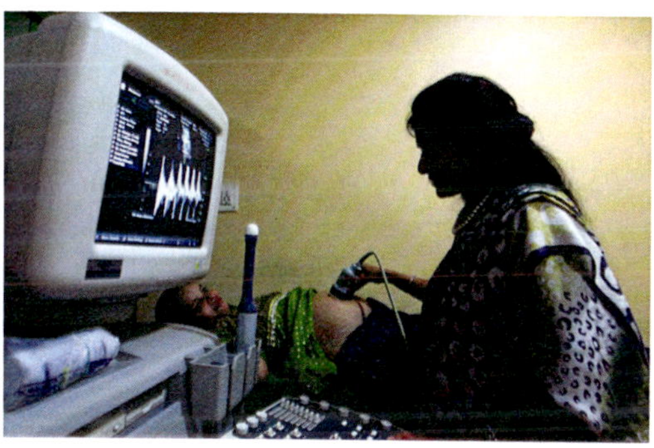

(p. 321)

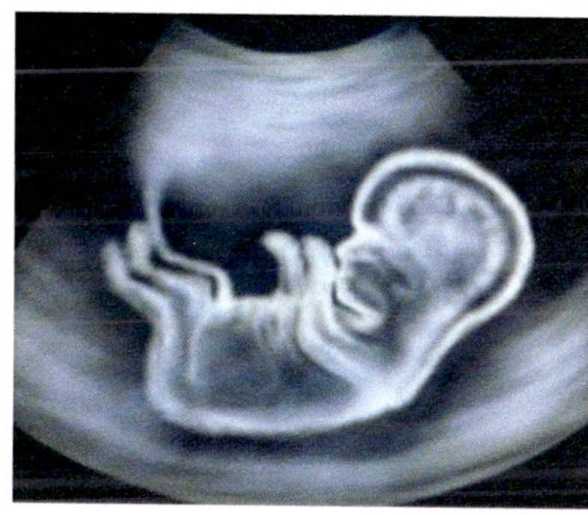

(p. 321)

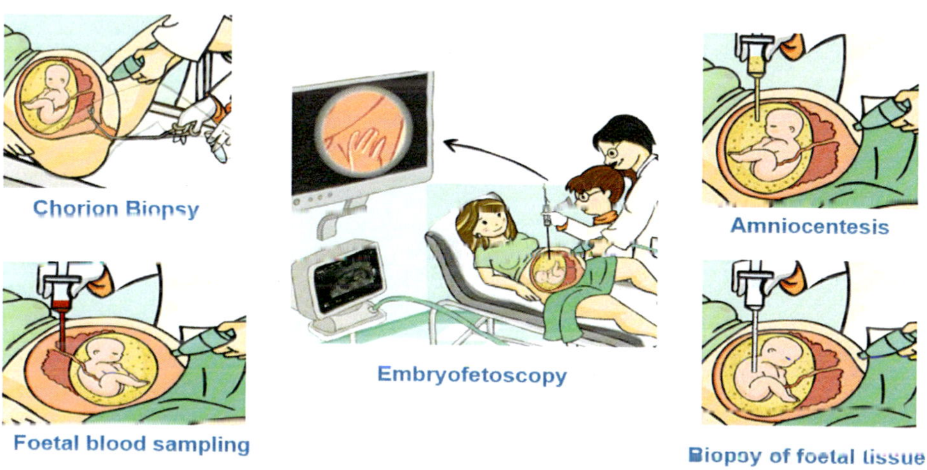

Various advanced prenatal diagnosis techniques for detection of genetic disorders/ abnormalities. (p. 322)

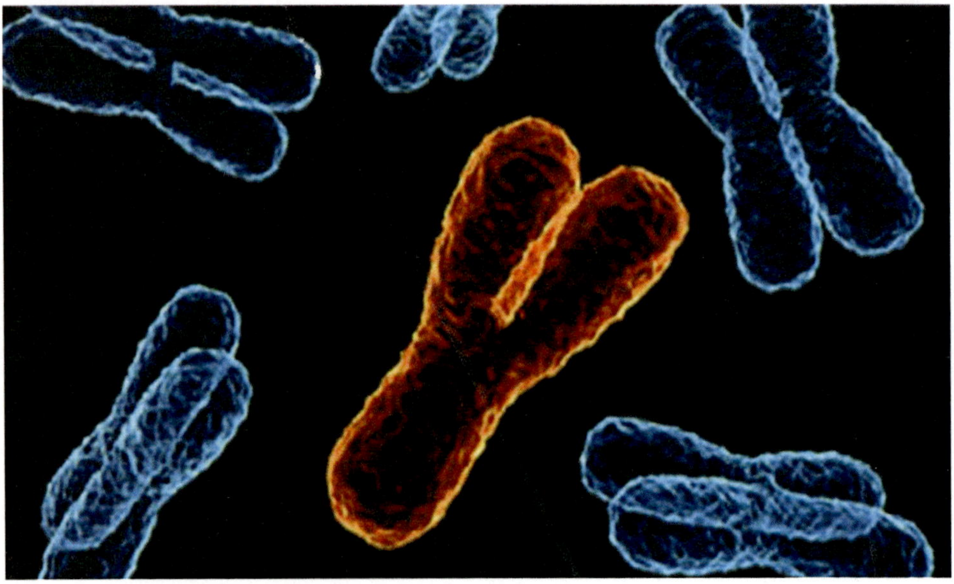

Identification of Y chromosome, leads to determination of Sex (p. 322)

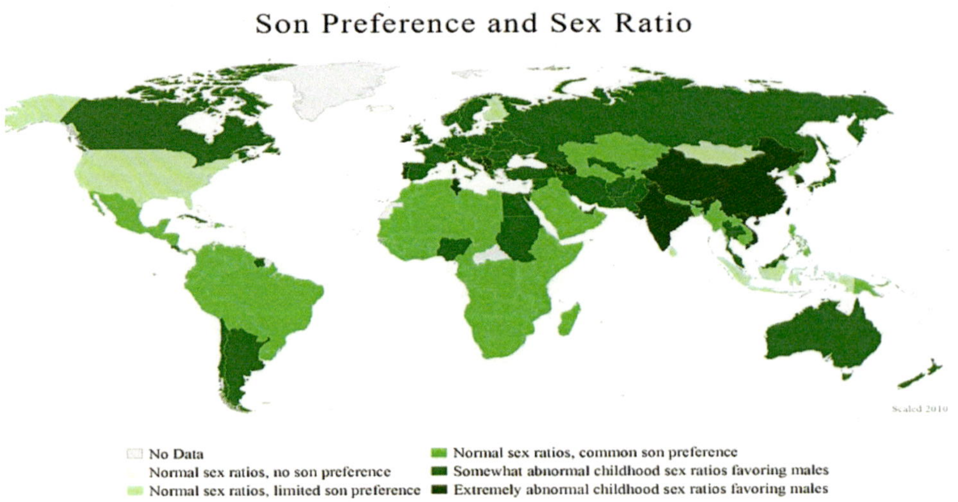

Figure 4. World scenario showing the son preference and status of sex ratio. (p. 323)